Introduction to Public Health in Pharmacy

Introduction to Public Health in Pharmacy

SECOND EDITION

EDITED BY

BRUCE LUBOTSKY LEVIN, DRPH, MPH

ARDIS HANSON, PHD

PETER D. HURD, PHD

OXFORD
UNIVERSITY PRESS

OXFORD
UNIVERSITY PRESS

Oxford University Press is a department of the University of Oxford. It furthers
the University's objective of excellence in research, scholarship, and education
by publishing worldwide. Oxford is a registered trade mark of Oxford University
Press in the UK and certain other countries.

Published in the United States of America by Oxford University Press
198 Madison Avenue, New York, NY 10016, United States of America.

© Oxford University Press 2018

First Edition published in 2007
Second Edition published in 2018

Library of Congress Cataloging-in-Publication Data
Names: Levin, Bruce Lubotsky, editor. | Hanson, Ardis, editor. | Hurd, Peter D., editor.
Title: Introduction to public health in pharmacy / edited by Bruce Lubotsky Levin,
Ardis Hanson, Peter D. Hurd.
Description: Second edition. | Oxford ; New York : Oxford University Press, [2018] |
Includes bibliographical references and index.
Identifiers: LCCN 2017035085 | ISBN 9780190238308 (pbk. : alk. paper)
Subjects: | MESH: Pharmaceutical Services | Public Health
Classification: LCC RA427 | NLM QV 737 | DDC 362.1—dc23
LC record available at https://lccn.loc.gov/2017035085

9 8 7 6 5 4 3 2 1

Printed by Sheridan Books, Inc., United States of America

Contents

Contributors

Barry A. Bleidt, PhD, PharmD, RPh, FAPhA, FNPhA
Professor, Sociobehavioral and Administrative Pharmacy
College of Pharmacy–Ft. Lauderdale Campus
Nova Southeastern University
Fort Lauderdale, FL

Patrick J. Bryant, PharmD
Clinical Professor in Division of Practice and Administration
Director, Drug Information Center
University of Missouri Kansas City School of Pharmacy
Kansas City, MO

Krystal Bullers, MA, AHIP
Research and Education Librarian; College of Pharmacy Liaison
Shimberg Health Sciences Library
University of South Florida
Tampa, FL

Melody Chavez, MPH, RDN, LD/N
Doctoral Student
Department of Community and Family Health
College of Public Health
University of South Florida
Tampa, FL

Carmita A. Coleman, PharmD, MAA
Associate Professor and Interim Dean
College of Pharmacy
Chicago State University
Chicago, IL

Daniel Forrister, PharmD
Assistant Professor
College of Pharmacy
University of South Florida
Tampa, FL

Angela S. Garcia, PharmD, MPH, CPh
Assistant Professor
Pharmacotherapeutics and Clinical Research
College of Pharmacy
Department of Pharmacy Practice
University of South Florida
Tampa, FL

Scott K. Griggs, PharmD, PhD
Assistant Professor
Department of Pharmaceutical and Administrative Sciences
St. Louis College of Pharmacy
St. Louis, MO

Justinne Guyton, PharmD
Assistant Professor of Pharmacy
    Practice
St. Louis College of Pharmacy
St. Louis, MO

Ardis Hanson, PhD
Assistant Director
Research and Education
Morsani College of Medicine
University of South Florida Health
    Shimberg Library

Peter D. Hurd, PhD
Professor of Pharmacy
    Administration & Chair,
    Department of Pharmaceutical
    and Administrative Sciences
St. Louis College of Pharmacy

**Bruce Lubotsky Levin,
DrPH, MPH**
Associate Professor & Head
Behavioral Health Concentration
Department of Community &
    Family Health
College of Public Health and
Associate Professor & Director
MS Degree in Child & Adolescent
    Behavioral Health Program
Department of Child & Family
    Health
College of Behavioral & Community
    Sciences
University of South Florida

Earle Buddy Lingle, PhD, RPh
Professor and Associate Dean
Student and Professional Affairs
School of Pharmacy
High Point University
High Point, NC

Stephanie Lukas, PharmD, MPH
Assistant Professor of Pharmacy
    Administration
Department of Pharmaceutical and
    Administrative Sciences and
Assistant Director Office of
    International Program
St. Louis College of Pharmacy
St. Louis, MO

Robert L. McCarthy, RPh, PhD
Professor of Pharmacy Practice
Dean Emeritus
School of Pharmacy
University of Connecticut
Storrs, CT

Aimon Miranda, PharmD, BCPS
Assistant Professor
Department of Pharmacy Practice
College of Pharmacy
University of South Florida
Tampa, FL

Carol A. Ott, PharmD, BCPP
Clinical Professor of Pharmacy
    Practice
Clinical Pharmacy Specialist,
    Psychiatry
Eskenazi Health/Midtown
    Community Mental Health
Purdue University College of
    Pharmacy
Indianapolis, IN

**Donna J. Petersen, ScD,
MHS, CPH**
Senior Associate Vice President
University of South Florida Health
Professor and Dean
College of Public Health
University of South Florida
Tampa, FL

Silvia E. Rabionet, MEd,
EdD, FAACP
Associate Professor of Public Health
Sociobehavioral and Administrative
    Pharmacy Department
College of Pharmacy–
    Ft. Lauderdale Campus
Nova Southeastern University
Fort Lauderdale, FL

Lauri Wright, PhD, RDN, LD/N
Assistant Professor and Director
Doctorate in Clinical Nutrition
    Program
Department of Nutrition and
    Dietetics
Brooks College of Health
University of North Florida
Jacksonville, FL

Samuel H. Zuvekas, PhD
Senior Economist
Agency for Healthcare Research and
    Quality
Rockville, MD

Foreword: A Public Health Perspective

DONNA J. PETERSEN

The publication of the first edition of this text marked a milestone in our understanding of the importance of integrative approaches to improving population health, linking public health directly to pharmacy practice in ways not considered previously. Since that time, substantive and, in some cases, disruptive changes in the health care environment have demonstrated the importance of collaborative approaches in addressing the complexities of disease surveillance, services delivery, and responses to emergent and persistent health problems. Public health has become ever more significant with increased globalization of the marketplace, changing disease transmission patterns, and continued human interference in the ecosystem creating environmental hazards and different patterns of natural disasters. These forces challenge us to think differently about how we promote healthy communities, leading us to further consider how health care professionals can contribute to solutions to increasingly complex health conditions.

Pharmacists are among the most visible and accessible group of health professionals, and, as such, they are uniquely positioned to educate the public on disease prevention and health promotion. They can facilitate the transmission of important health information, monitor the responses of providers and consumers to that information, and correct misinformation regarding treatment options, medications, and alternative therapies. Pharmacists are also integral components of interdisciplinary health care teams, providing additional perspectives on patient care and medication management. However, to keep pace with the fields of public health and pharmacy requires pharmacists to be aware of the literature examining integrative and global perspectives.

Featuring national scholars from the fields of both public health and pharmacy in the development of each chapter, this second edition illustrates the benefits of an integrative public health pharmacy approach. In addition, it provides a more global perspective, introducing and comparing pharmacy and public health practices and policies throughout the text. Each chapter closes with implications for pharmacy practice, a feature that assists the reader in summarizing the importance of the chapter to the larger public health pharmacy field.

This text elegantly provides the critical linkages to expanding this understanding, providing for pharmacists an introduction to public health and an in-depth discussion of the role of pharmacy professionals in promoting and protecting the public's health. Incorporating practice, research, and policy, this text examines critical issues for public health pharmacy within an increasingly globalized world. Clearly illustrating the critical partnership between pharmacy and public health to improve and sustain the population's health, this text should be on the required reading list for all pharmacy students and individuals in pharmacy practice. Public health professionals would do well to also explore in these pages further insights into the role of pharmacy professionals in achieving population health goals, goals we all share.

Foreword: A Pharmacy Perspective

ROBERT L. MCCARTHY

In writing the foreword for the first edition of *Introduction to Public Health in Pharmacy*, I noted that the public health community faces daunting challenges in the 21st century much like it did a century ago. All health care professionals, including pharmacists, have essential roles to play in ensuring the public at-large is educated about and protected against the myriad of threats ranging from environmental concerns to resistant microorganisms. Given these potential hazards, I noted that it is more important now than perhaps during any other time in our recent past for pharmacists to be grounded in the principles of public health, enabling them to bring to bear their significant expertise in medication therapy management to the care of populations, especially those at risk.

The first edition of *Introduction to Public Health in Pharmacy* provided a primer for pharmacy students and practicing pharmacists in the principles of public health. The book's publication received wide acclaim as the first text that uniquely addressed public health issues from the perspective of pharmacy and pharmacists.

Building upon the strengths of the first edition, *Introduction to Public Health in Pharmacy* (second edition) provides a greater global perspective by providing additional international examples, including health challenges and diseases. The references have been updated in order to share the most current thinking and public health approaches; additional examples have also been included. The content of the book has been revised to reflect instructor experiences using the text in the classroom.

This new edition also has been restructured to allow readers easier access to subjects of interest. American and global public health and pharmacy are presented in distinct chapters, enabling readers to compare public health in the United States and throughout the world. New chapters in nutrition and health literacy have been added. The chapter focused on financing public health services has been reworked

xiii

into a discussion on federal programs, financing, and insurance. The text concludes with a chapter focused on education and leadership.

Finally, this new edition adds to the useful, practical public health information for pharmacists found in the first edition of *Introduction to Public Health in Pharmacy*. For the pharmacy student, it provides an introduction to the public health field and the important contributions pharmacists can make to population-based health care. For the practicing pharmacist, it offers both a refresher and a litany of possibilities. All readers should come away with an enhanced understanding of public health and a deep appreciation of the essential role both pharmacy and public health plays in helping to ensure the health of society.

Preface

When the original edition of this book was conceptualized, it was heavily influenced by the CAPE 2004 Educational Outcomes from the American Association of Pharmacy and the discussions surrounding *Healthy People 2010*. Both of these documents created strong linkages between pharmacy and public health. Since that time, we have seen continued emphases on the global burden of disease and the effects of the social determinants of health at both the national and international levels.

This second edition continues to build upon the updated CAPE Educational Outcomes (2013) and *Healthy People 2020* in emphasizing the importance of evidence-based practice, health promotion and disease prevention, health literacy, cultural sensitivity, patient-centered care and advocacy, medication management, cultural sensitivity, and awareness and analysis of emerging theories, information, and technologies in public health and pharmacy. The text also focuses on global health concerns, such as monitoring global infectious diseases, measuring national and international capacity, and responding to emerging social issues and environmental conditions. Finally, the text weaves a global perspective of the challenges and benefits public health and pharmacy face in addressing the social determinants of health.

The pairing of public health and pharmacy is a logical combination since we believe these disciplines are inextricably woven together in so many ways and across so many areas. Combining population health, individual patient health, and community-based health perspectives provides a more complete understanding of the public health challenges facing community pharmacists and public health practitioners. However, we still have a ways to go in encouraging individuals with pharmacy degrees to engage more fully in public health. We believe that many pharmacists have opportunities to integrate public health in their practices that go unrecognized and unrealized; hence a more substantive grounding in public health may make these opportunities more apparent.

Features in This Volume

This second edition features collaboration by chapter contributors who collectively have strong backgrounds in public health and pharmacy. The combined expertise of chapter contributors from public health and pharmacy help substantiate the relevance and authenticity of the text for students and practitioners. A second feature of this edition is the "Implications for Public Health and Pharmacy Practice" section, which appears in each chapter of the text. Our chapter contributors describe the significance of their chapter to the larger fields of public health and pharmacy. The third feature is the global perspective, which is addressed in every chapter.

In this edition, all chapters are original contributions. While it is difficult to include a chapter representing all possible relevant topics to public health and pharmacy, the editors have tried to include a broad spectrum of chapter topics to both stimulate and increase engagement in public health and pharmacy issues.

New chapters include those on global health, nutrition, heath literacy, and evidence-based practice. Some chapters retained their original chapter contributors but have been substantially revised to address current challenges and concerns. Other chapters have new contributors who bring new perspectives and content to the topic. For increased consistency from chapter to chapter, the editors participated as chapter contributors.

We have stressed concepts and issues in public health that pharmacy students and pharmacists need to establish a working knowledge base in public health. First, we framed services and systems in the United States and globally. Then we examined traditional and emerging public health areas for pharmacy students and practitioners who are interested in a larger population health/community services perspective.

For practitioners who want to work at the population health level, disease prevention and health promotion activities have expanded beyond tobacco cessation programs to include counseling for nutritional and behavioral health problems. Programmatic and administrative perspectives are organized to address financing and insurance, pharmacoeconomics, evidence-based services, and informatics. Finally, how do we best educate and train practitioners to deal with continually evolving public health and health care environments, especially when natural and manmade disasters occur with increasing frequency?

We hope this book stimulates the interest of pharmacy practitioners and public health professionals to increase their participation across their respective fields and engage more fully in cross-professional activities.

1

Public Health and Pharmacy in the United States

BRUCE LUBOTSKY LEVIN, ARDIS HANSON, AND PETER D. HURD

The World Health Organization (1948, p. 1) defines health within a socioeconomic framework with the intent to allow individuals to live productive lives: addressing physical, mental, and social well-being, not just the absence of disease or infirmity. This definition, which has remained the same since 1948, is mirrored in the United States' *Healthy People* initiatives, most recently *Healthy People 2020*. *Healthy People 2020* also addresses the relationships among the social determinants of health (Public Health Emergency, 2017) and how they affect and influence population health outcomes. *Healthy People 2020* is noteworthy because it identifies the most significant public health issues in the United States and acts as a guide in improving the public's health at local, state, and national levels. It is a 10-year "temporal snapshot" of what the United States sees as the most important health issues to address. In this chapter, we provide an overview of the US public health systems and pharmacy practice, research, and education.

Although many definitions of public health focus on disease prevention and health promotion, the preferred definition is by Charles-Edward Amory Winslow, a pioneer in public health practice in America. Winslow saw public health as both an art and a science that had, as its goals, the development of a healthy standard of living to maintain or improve the health of society (Winslow, 1920, pp. 6–7). Although the phrase "public health" has been revisited many times since 1920, Winslow's definition guides all subsequent discussion on what is public health.

While health is multidisciplinary in its approach to patient care and services delivery, its focus is *the* patient using evidence-based practice. The field of public health also utilizes a multidisciplinary approach in its examination of health problems in at-risk populations. However, unlike health, public health has a population-based focus. It draws heavily from the areas of biostatistics and epidemiology, environmental and occupational health, health policy and management, community and family health, and global health. Its professionals include nurses, physicians, epidemiologists, statisticians, health educators, environmental health specialists, industrial hygienists, sanitarians, food and drug inspectors, toxicologists, laboratory technicians, environmental scientists, crisis and disaster professionals, veterinarians, economists, social scientists, attorneys, nutritionists, dentists, social workers, administrators, and managers, among many other professionals.

Although pharmacy includes many aspects of patient care (e.g., immunizations, adherence, and drug information) as well as more product-related responsibilities including the preparation, dispensing, and proper utilization of medications, we see pharmacy as a bridge between patient-centered health care and public health. Within community pharmacy, the individual patient *and* the community in which the patient resides are equally important in the practice of pharmacy. In 2014, CVS, a national pharmacy retail chain, ceased the sale of tobacco products to be better aligned with its new name of CVS Health, giving up roughly $2 billion in sales to reflect a health orientation to the retail customer (Ziobro, 2014). While tobacco-free pharmacies are not new in the United States, the public health impact of decreasing the locations where cigarettes can be purchased can help decrease the sale of tobacco products to individuals and potentially increase the health of the community.

While some people think of a pharmacy as a place where medicines, including prescription medicines, are sold, the practice of pharmacy continues to shift its focus from a product-orientation to a health care orientation. Community pharmacy and hospital pharmacy are important components of US health care systems, and clinical pharmacy, which can be practiced in the community, the hospital, the nursing home, or some other health care setting, focuses on efforts to optimize the use of medications for the patients using them. Pharmacy, as a source of information to maximize medicine benefits, is the key to its future.

History of Public Health and Pharmacy

Public health is not a new concept. Starting with the Greco-Roman conceptualization of population health, through the plagues of the Middle Ages and pandemics of the modern age, public health has addressed the biological and social determinants of disease. Hippocratic texts were among the first to relate environmental factors to disease. The Roman emphasis on sanitation and the establishment of public hospitals was the start of Western public health systems. Early theories of contagious disease and disease transmission by Girolamo Frascatoro in 1546 and the discovery of environmental and occupational diseases by Bernardino Ramazzini in 1713 contributed to the emerging field of public health (Rosen, 1958). Epidemiologic methods, the gathering of vital statistics, the use of regional and national health surveys, the association between poverty and disease, and the use of sanitary reforms to reduce the spread of infectious diseases were all central to the rise of national public health systems in Europe and the United States (Cassedy, 1969; Chadwick, 1843; Coleman, 1982; Rosenberg, 1962). These early years also saw the rise of the profession of pharmacy.

In the United States, pharmacy was already commonplace. Elizabeth Greenleaf was practicing pharmacy in Boston in 1727 (Griffenhagen, 2002). The first pharmacy in colonial America operated from 1729 to 1825 in Philadelphia (Ellis, 1903). In 1777, the Continental Congress created the position of Apothecary General (Worthen, 1928), a position that ended after the Revolutionary War. In 1798, the U.S. Congress established the U. S. Marine Hospital Service, the predecessor of the current U.S. Public Health Service. In 1871, the post of U.S. Surgeon General was formally established.

The Philadelphia College of Pharmacy, established in 1821, marked the beginning of the first pharmacy society as well as the first school of pharmacy in the United States (England & Kramer, 1922). The American Pharmaceutical Association was founded on October 6, 1852. Many of today's pharmacy associations trace their roots back to the American Pharmaceutical Association: the National Association of Retail Druggists (1898, now the National Community Pharmacy Association); the American Conference on Pharmaceutical Faculties (1900, now American Association of Colleges of Pharmacy); and the American Society of Hospital Pharmacists (1942, now American Society of Health-System Pharmacists). The American College of Clinical Pharmacy (AACP, 2008) defined clinical pharmacy as both the science and practice of rational medication use and as accountable for the optimum use of medication therapy in the prevention and treatment of disease. These discussion points from clinical pharmacy are appropriate in all health care settings. As an example, medication therapy management would include such pharmacy services as medication therapy reviews, immunizations, pharmacogenomics applications, and medication safety, as well as public health pharmacy (American Pharmacists Association, 2014). The links to public health (American Association of Colleges of Pharmacy, 2004) and population health (American Association of Colleges of Pharmacy, 2013) have become central components of the pharmacy curriculum through the recommendations of the Center for the Advancement of Pharmacy Education (American Association of Colleges of Pharmacy, 2004, 2013).

In 1872, the American Public Health Association (APHA) was founded (Ravenel, 1921), with public health courses offered at the University of Pennsylvania in 1909 (Fee, 1992), and additional programs offered at the Harvard School of Public Health in 1913 (the oldest continuously operating school of public health in the United States). Johns Hopkins School of Hygiene and Public Health was established in 1916 (Fee, 1992). Unlike public health education systems of Great Britain or Europe, public health education in the United States was independent of medical schools and state public health services (Ravenel, 1921). Welch and Rose (1915) argued the US public health educational system should represent "both the scientific and the practical aspects of hygiene and public health" and acknowledged the importance of the relationship between the modern social welfare and public health movements.

From those early years, the roles of public health and pharmacy have been refined and redefined through legislation, societal changes, technology, and health care delivery systems. In 1988, the Institute of Medicine's (IOM) Committee for the Study of the Future of Public Health (IOM Committee) closely examined public health programs and the coordination of services across US government agencies and within state and local health departments (LHDs). Its subsequent report, *The Future of Public Health* (IOM, 1988), defined both the *substance* and the *mission* of public health, which reified Winslow's community-based prevention and promotion foci with the larger societal goal of promoting healthy neighborhoods and lifestyles.

Working with the larger public health community, three core functions for public health were determined: (a) assessment, (b) policy development, and (c) assurance (of providing necessary public health services in the community), and identified which level of government (federal, state, and local) would be best suited to handle these core functions.

While pharmacists in the U.S. Public Health Service provided direct patient care support activities at the National Institutes of Health, the U.S. Food and Drug Administration, and the Indian Health Service (IHS; Church, 1987, 1989), the American pharmaceutical industry was undergoing significant changes with the advancement of biotechnology, new product research and development, and new pharmacy services to accommodate social and economic changes in patient care, drug delivery, and pharmacy management (Doluisio, 1989; Penna, 1987). Pharmaceutical education was also under revision, as the needs of community and hospital pharmacy were recognized (Oddis, 1988). What followed were a number of recommendations in pharmacy, including calls to address pharmaceutical science as an academic discipline (Lemberger, 1988), changes in residency training programs, and the emphasis on the doctor of pharmacy (PharmD) degree as the sole entry-level degree for pharmacy practitioners (Smith, 1988). The "reprofessionalization" of pharmacy suggested a return to its preindustrial origins in "valued, complex, specific, and committed public service" (Hepler, 1988, p. 1071), with an emphasis on quality assurance in patient care and pharmaceutical services (Oddis, 1988).

In 1993, work began on again redefining public health within the parameters of proposed national health care reforms, such as the Omnibus Budget Reconciliation Act of 1990 (OBRA-90; Pub.L. 101–508, 104 Stat. 1388) and the proposed American Health Security Act of 1993 (H.R. 1200, 103rd Congress). The proposed American Health Security Act emphasized extending access to health care, containing health care costs, assuring the quality of care, financing reform, and improving the health care infrastructure to maintain and improve health and well-being (Committee on Assessing Health Care Reform Proposals, 1993).

Legislative changes, such as the Medicaid rebate provisions of the Omnibus Budget Reconciliation Act of 1990, and the Medicare outpatient drug benefit in the proposed American Health Security Act would impact pharmacy practice. Although OBRA-90 was meant to ensure Medicaid patients received specific pharmaceutical care, the legislation required the same type of care be rendered to all patients, not just Medicaid patients. Pharmacists would now be required to provide pharmacist counseling, meet prospective drug utilization review requirements, and engage in new record-keeping mandates.

By 1994, the U.S. Public Health Service Core Public Health Functions Steering Committee developed "10 Essential Public Health Services" needed to carry out the basic public health core functions in any community. As seen in Figure 1-1, the essential services are iterative and can be easily grouped into the three focal functions: (a) assessment, (b) policy development, and (c) assurance.

By 2000, there were a number of changes in federal policy regarding public health. The Surgeon General had released his report on mental health, thereby making mental health a national priority. The "Decade of the Brain" project had ended, with considerable strides made in the neuroscience of physical and mental diseases. In addition, the *Healthy People 2000* initiative was ending, and the *Healthy People 2010* was just beginning. As the decade advanced, additional changes reflected the move to a managed health care financing model, the incorporation of evidence-based (decision-making) practices, the increase in intersectoral (public–private) health

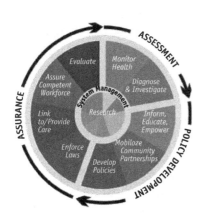

1. Monitor health status to identify community health problems;
2. Diagnose and investigate identified health problems and health hazards in the community;
3. Inform, educate, and empower people about health issues;
4. Mobilize community partnerships to identify and solve health problems;
5. Develop policies and plans that support individual and community health efforts;
6. Enforce laws and regulations that protect health and ensure safety;
7. Link people to needed personal health services and assure the provision of health care;
8. Assure a competent public health and personal health care workforce;
9. Assess effectiveness, accessibility, and quality of personal and population-based health; and
10. Research for new insights and innovative solutions to health problems.

Figure 1-1. Ten essential services of public health.

partnerships, calls for accountability in the public health systems, and enhanced communication within and among the broader public health systems. Public health was described as "complex, adaptive systems in which population health occurs" (Committee on Assuring the Health of the Public in the 21st Century, 2002, p. xiii). Policymakers and practitioners wanted evidence-based recommendations to improve public health practice and population health outcomes, such as specifications regarding under what conditions population health improves and what can be done to affect those conditions (Brownson, Fielding, & Maylahn, 2009; Victora, Habicht, & Bryce, 2004). Health communication and workforce development/ capacity were acknowledged as a crucial process in the effective delivery of health care services and the promotion of public health (Anderson et al., 2005; Hill, Alpi, & Auerbach, 2010).

The importance of public health re-emerged during 2011 to 2012. The IOM wrote a series of reports titled *For the Public's Health*. The first report focused on measurement of population health and related accountability across national, state, and local government. The IOM Committee on Public Health Strategies to Improve Health (2011b) stressed the role of measurement and the data that provides us with ways of understanding health status in different ways (determinant or underlying cause), with different types of evidence (national, local, or comparative) regarding the performance of the many stakeholders in the US public health system and if outcomes are successful based upon the investments made to the system. Although it is difficult to establish causality between actions of the health system and health outcomes, measurement is fundamental.

The second report described the laws that establish the structure, duties, and authorities of public health departments and reviewed how statutes and regulations prevent injury and disease and optimize health outcomes (Committee on Public Health Strategies to Improve Health, 2011a). It also addressed legal and regulatory authority, model public health legislation, and social and policy implications of public health laws and regulations.

The third report considered resources necessary to maintain and sustain a robust population-based national health system. There is a significant knowledge base about the distal (actual) and proximal (auxiliary) causes of death and disease, as well as existing social and economic conditions that impair health and increase health risks (Committee on Public Health Strategies to Improve Health, 2012, p. 2). However, new benchmarks are needed to see how the health of the nation is faring. Two new benchmarks are longevity and per capita health spending as national targets for health system performance. Administrative rule changes and procedural changes in existing funding streams (e.g., contracts, grants, and cooperative agreements) are also recommended to create a more flexible, adaptive, and efficient use of increasingly scarce resources. More importantly, the IOM urged the creation of a "*minimum package of public health services*, which includes the *foundational capabilities* and an array of *basic programs* that no health department can be without" (Committee on Public Health Strategies to Improve Health, 2012, p. 5), based on the three core public health functions and the 10 essential public health services.

With the passage of the Patient Protection and Affordable Care Act (Affordable Care Act [ACA], Pub. L. No. 111-148), a number of public health initiatives were created, including establishing the National Prevention, Health Promotion, and Public Health Council, creating a fund for prevention and public health and requiring nonprofit hospitals to redefine their roles in the community (Roundtable on Population Health Improvement, 2013). In addition, the ACA also permanently reauthorized the Indian Health Care Improvement Act legal authority for the provision of health care to Native Americans and Alaska Natives (Indian Health Care Improvement Act, 25 U.S. Code Chapter 18). These initiatives were in response to a broader understanding of population and health that is based on distribution of health outcomes across individuals living within geographical or geopolitical boundaries (Jacobson & Teutsch, 2012; Kindig & Stoddart, 2003).

Healthy People 2020, Public Health, and Pharmacy's Role in Public Health

There are 1,200 objectives that span 42 distinct public health topic areas identified in *Healthy People 2020*. The objectives and topics are clustered into 22 priority areas. Of the 22 priority areas, the first 21 areas pertain to health promotion, health protection, and preventive services; the 22nd area addresses the development of an infrastructure to track the objectives and to identify and evaluate emerging public health issues at the national, state, and local levels. Since the *raison d'etre* for the *Healthy People* initiative is to improve the public's health in the United States, roles for pharmacy and pharmacists can be found in a number of its objectives.

Within the objectives for *Healthy People 2020*'s Educational and Community-Based Programs (ECBP), objective ECBP-17 requires that core clinical prevention and public health content be included in PharmD-granting colleges and schools of pharmacy. Objectives 17.1 to 17.6 specifically address counseling for health promotion and disease prevention content, cultural diversity content, the evaluation of health sciences literature content, environmental health content, public health systems content, and global health content, respectively. Data is drawn from the American Association of Colleges of Pharmacy Survey of Professional and Graduate Degree Programs. In 2012, baseline data was at 99.2, with the target established at 100%.

Considering the six content areas added to graduate pharmacy education, we see a growth in the areas for pharmacists within public health to contribute to *Healthy People 2020* objectives. One area is "Access to Health Services" (AHS-6.4), which seeks to reduce the number of persons who are unable to obtain or have delays in obtaining necessary medical care, dental care, or prescription medicines.

A second area is "Disability and Health" (DH). The DH-1 objective seeks to increase the number of population-based data systems, such as pharmacy management systems that use a standardized core set of questions to identify people with disabilities. Also within this objective (DH-3) is a requirement for US master of public health programs to offer graduate-level courses in disability and health. For pharmacists who wish to practice in public health or community settings, courses such as these provide additional insights into the needs of persons with a range of disabilities.

A third area is in "Public Health Infrastructure" (PHI). The first three objectives (PHI-1–3) address the incorporation of "Core Competencies for Public Health Professionals" into job descriptions and performance evaluations, continuing education programs, and public health graduate school curricula. The "Core Competencies for Public Health Professionals" (Core Competencies), developed by the Council on Linkages Between Academia and Public Health Practice (2014), are defined by and linked to the "10 Essential Public Health Services" (see Figure 1-1). As such, the Core Competencies reflect "foundational skills that are essential for public health professionals who are researchers, practitioners, and/or educators." Organized into eight domains and three tiers, each domain addresses a skill area within public health, and each tier represents a career stage (entry level, supervisory, executive). The domains include analytic/assessment skills, policy development/program planning skills, communications skills, cultural competency skills, community dimensions of practice skills, basic public health sciences skills, financial planning and management skills, and leadership and systems thinking skills. With the emphasis on public health within schools of pharmacy and the Center for Excellence in Pharmacy Education (CAPE) Outcomes, these same core competencies may also be addressed in graduate programs in schools of pharmacy.

Data collection is another major area under PHI, whether it is increasing the number of tribal, state, and local public health agencies involved in data collection for *Healthy People 2020* objectives (e.g., epidemiology, surveillance), conducting system-wide assessments using national performance standards (PHI-14), implementing health improvement plans that are linked to state plans (PHI-15), conducting quality improvement processes (PHI-16), or increasing the number of accredited public health agencies (PHI-17). There are many opportunities for pharmacists to be involved at the practice and policy levels in PHI.

Other new objectives that are also of interest to public health or community pharmacists are preparedness, whose objectives are taken from the *National Health Security Strategy of the United States of America* (Public Health Emergency, 2017), a focus on specific populations: early and middle childhood; adolescent health; older adults; lesbian, gay, bisexual, and transgender health; and global health.

The US Public Health Structure: Federal, State, and Local

The US public health systems evolved as a separate health system following World War II. As mentioned earlier, the medical sector focused on individual patients, with an emphasis on the biological mechanisms of disease and the use of technologically sophisticated diagnosis and treatment. The public health sector concentrated on populations, with an emphasis on the social determinants of health, prevention, and safety-net primary care.

The U.S. Public Health Service is comprised of a Commissioned Corps, one of the seven uniformed services of the United States, who serve throughout 13 offices and agencies of the Department of Health and Human Services (DHHS), and 11 non-DHHS offices and agencies. The Commissioned Corps is overseen by the U.S. Surgeon General and is comprised of over 6,500 public health professionals, including physicians, nurses, pharmacists, dentists, behavioral health professionals, clinical and rehabilitation therapists, dietitians, engineers, environmental health scientists, health services professionals (clinical care providers, health information management, public health education, and public health administration), science and research health professionals, and veterinary medicine professionals (Table 1-1).

Public health systems in the United States are commonly defined as "all public, private, and voluntary entities that contribute to the delivery of essential public health services within a jurisdiction" (National Public Health Performance Standards Program, n.d., p. 3). Hence, a state or local public health system would work with numerous agencies and organizations across public health, environmental health, public safety, health care providers, tribal health, faith institutions, human services, charities and philanthropies, economic development, education, youth development, community centers, recreation centers, and the arts (see Figure 1-2).

However, to describe that infrastructure *in toto* is beyond the scope of this chapter. We focus on what most people understand as the public health system: the infrastructure established within the United States and its relationship with the Centers for Disease Control and Prevention (CDC).

CENTERS FOR DISEASE CONTROL AND PREVENTION

At the national level, the CDC is one of the 11 operating divisions within the Department of Health and Human Services, which is the principal agency for protecting the health of all Americans. Since its inception in 1946, the CDC has protected the health of the nation and promoted quality of life for Americans through the prevention and control of disease, injury, and disability. The CDC is seen as a liaison, a facilitator of training, a provider of administrative and program management

Table 1-1 **Agencies Where the US Public Health Service Commissioned Core Serve**

1. Agency for Healthcare Research and Quality	2. District of Columbia Commission on Mental Health Services
3. Agency for Toxic Substances and Disease Registry	4. Environmental Protection Agency
5. Centers for Disease Control and Prevention	6. Federal Bureau of Prisons
7. Food and Drug Administration	8. National Oceanic & Atmospheric Administration
9. Health Resources and Services Administration	10. National Park Service
11. Centers for Medicare and Medicaid Services	12. U.S. Department of Agriculture
13. Indian Health Service	14. U.S. Department of Defense
15. National Institutes of Health	16. U.S. Department of Homeland Security
17. Office of the Assistant Secretary of Health	18. Division of Immigration Health Services
19. Office of the Secretary	20. U.S. Coast Guard
21. Program Support Center	22. U.S. Marshals Service
23. Substance Abuse and Mental Health Services Administration	24. Office of the Assistant Secretary for Preparedness and Response

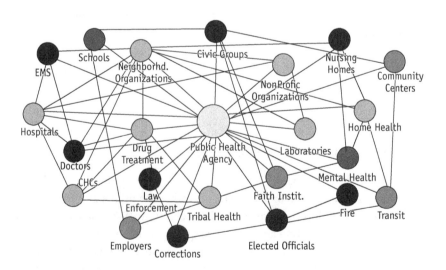

Figure 1-2. The *de facto* public health system.

support, and a sharer/disseminator of information to states (Fischer, Ellingson, McCormick, & Sinkowitz-Cochran, 2014). The CDC works closely with the state and territorial, tribal, and county/city public health offices with a variety of services, ranging from epidemiological studies, infectious disease assessment and identification, and technical assistance. In addition, the CDC, working with the Centers for Medicare and Medicaid Services and the Agency for Healthcare Research and Quality, has increased national awareness of health care–associated infections, developed public awareness campaigns, and provided an improved infrastructure and tools to diagnose and treat these infections (Srinivasan, Craig, & Cardo, 2012).

Organizationally speaking, the CDC is comprised of a number of centers, institutes, and offices (see Figure 1-3). It is one of the largest health care agencies in the world, with over 15,000 employees located in more than 50 countries worldwide, employing staff in over 168 occupational areas, including behavioral scientists,

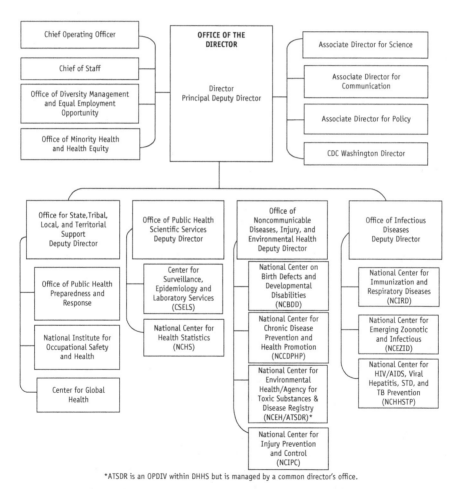

Figure 1-3. CDC organizational chart.

biologists, emergency-response specialists, epidemiologists, health education specialists, health informatics specialists, health scientists, medical officers, microbiologists, pharmacists, public health advisors, and public health analysts, to name just a few of the 168 staff categories.

The CDC plays a vital part in the network of public health organizations at the national level. The Office for State, Tribal, Local and Territorial Support (OSTLTS) was formed to advance national public health agency and system performance. OSTLTS initiatives and programs include the National Public Health Improvement Initiative, the National Public Health Performance Standards Program, the National Voluntary Accreditation for Public Health, the national Public Health Law Program, and the national Town Hall Teleconferences.

TYPES OF PUBLIC HEALTH DEPARTMENTS

There are state and territorial, tribal, and local health departments. Generally, each state or territory has a department of health, which oversees public health activities in the state, with a county health department located in each county. A county health department has a primary health office and may have a number of branch offices. Each county health department provides a number of programs, ranging from clinical and family health services, immunization programs, patient care and case management services, disease control and surveillance programs, social service programs, and environmental health services. In 2010, there were 2,790 LHDs and 261 regional or district health offices in the United States and Washington, D.C. (Association of State and Territorial Health Officials [ASTHO], 2011).

State and Territorial Health Departments

State and territorial health departments (SHAs) have full or shared fiscal and programmatic responsibility for federal initiatives, including Women, Infants, and Children (a program administered by the Food and Nutrition Service of the United States Department of Agriculture), the CDC Preventive Health and Health Services Block Grant, Title V Maternal and Infant Health Services, the National Cancer Prevention and Control Program Grant, HIV Pharmacies, and Health Professionals Shortage Area Designations (ASTHO, 2011). In cases where they do not have sole responsibility, state health agencies often share responsibility with another state agency; a local governmental agency, including local public health agencies; or nonprofit organizations. The state and territorial health agency workforce includes over 100,000 full-time employees, with different governance structures, including centralized, shared, decentralized, or a mixed governance structure. Fifty-five percent of state health agencies are free-standing, independent agencies; the remaining state health agencies are part of a super or umbrella agency (ASTHO, 2011).

State and territorial health agencies have three main roles: health protection, health promotion and disease prevention, and health treatment. Within those areas, they screen and treat for diseases and other health conditions, provide technical assistance and training, run state laboratory services, and collect epidemiologic data and surveillance. As such, they provide many population-based primary prevention services, helping to inform and educate people about health issues in states and territories. In 2010, for example, 88% of state health agencies offered tobacco prevention and control services, 84% had HIV prevention programs, and 80% operated injury prevention programs (AHTSO, 2011). Almost 60% of the care state health agencies provide is for infectious diseases, such as tuberculosis and sexually transmitted diseases, including HIV/AIDS (AHTSO, 2011). However, almost 80% of the agencies also provide services to children with special health care needs. In addition to providing population-based services, state health agencies also enforce laws and regulations that protect health and ensure safety.

Tribal Health Departments

In addition to state and territorial health agencies, the US public health system also includes tribal health departments. A tribal health department is a "health department corporation or organization operated under the jurisdiction of a federally recognized tribe, or association of federally recognized tribes, which is funded by the tribe(s) and/or contract service(s) from the Indian Health Service" (National Indian Health Board, 2011).

Established in 1955, the IHS, an agency within the Department of Health and Human Services, is authorized to provide health care to approximately 568 native American/Alaska Native tribes (approximately 5.4 million members; Bureau of Indian Affairs, 2012; U.S.Census Bureau, 2012) through the Indian Self-Determination and Educational Assistance Act of 1975 (Pub. L. 93-638). In 2011, 36 out of 51 states (70%) reported they worked with Native American/Alaska Native populations (ASTHO, 2011).

Since tribes are recognized as independent sovereign nations, they have a unique government-to-government relationship with the US federal government. Each tribe decides which programs and services are negotiated and contracted with the IHS. Each tribe also identifies, addresses, and prioritizes community health needs. In addition to tribal health departments, three other types of facilities also provide health care services: (a) IHS facilities, (b) an Area Indian Health Board or Inter-Tribal Councils, and (c) Urban Indian Health Centers (National Indian Health Board, 2011).

Local (County/City) Health Departments

A LHD is defined as "an administrative or service unit of local or state government, concerned with health, and carrying some responsibility for the health of a jurisdiction smaller than the state" (National Association of County and City Health Officials [NACCHO], 2011, p. 3). The first study in the United States of local public health infrastructure and practice, *Report of the Sanitary Commission of*

Massachusetts, was written in 1850 by Lemuel Shattuck (Turnock & Barnes, 2007). It presaged the beginning of LHDs. By 1911, county-based LHDs were appearing throughout the United States. By 1943, there were 178 LHDs in 31 states (Turnock & Barnes, 2007). In 2010, there were 2,565 LHDs, excluding Hawai'i and Rhode Island, since those states operate under the state health departments and have no subunits. Although a 1945 report suggested that local health systems could be most effectively organized to serve no fewer than 50,000 people, today LHDs serve populations from less than 25,000 (1,067 LHDs) to populations serving over 1 million or more (41 LHDs; NACCHO, 2011). LHDs provide a range of services, including adult and child immunizations, infectious/communicable disease surveillance, tuberculosis screening and treatment, environmental health surveillance, school/day care center inspections, population-based nutrition services, food service establishment inspections, and safety education.

Local Boards of Health

A LHD differs from a local board of health in that the latter is a legally designated governing body whose role is to provide oversight to the public health agency, focusing on community health assessments, assurance, and policy development. Approximately 75% of LHDs serve a jurisdiction that has a local board of health (NACCHO, 2011). Jurisdictionally, a local board of health may be a city, county, or district-level board. City boards of health are appointed by the city council and have jurisdiction over public health matters within the city. County boards of health are appointed by the county board of supervisors and have jurisdiction over public health matters within the county. District boards of health are appointed by county boards of supervisors from the counties represented by the district and have jurisdiction over district public health matters. The boards of health generally report to the State Department of (Public) Health.

In 2013, the CDC and the National Association of Local Boards of Health developed an update to the *National Public Health Performance Standards Local Public Health Governance Performance Assessment Instrument* (version 2.0). Version 2.0 allows local boards of health and the state public health system to assess the activities and capacities of their public health systems in providing the essential public health services in their jurisdictions.

PUBLIC HEALTH AGENCY ACCREDITATION

In 2011, the Public Health Accreditation Board (PHAB) established a voluntary national accreditation program for state, local, and tribal health agencies (Bender, Kronstadt, Wilcox, & Lee, 2014; Ingram, Bender, Wilcox, & Kronstadt, 2014; Marshall et al., 2014; Matthews, Markiewicz, & Beitsch, 2012; Thielen, Leff, et al., 2014). There are three quality improvement and planning prerequisites: (a) a state health assessment, (b) a state health improvement plan, and (c) an agency-wide strategic plan. In addition, the PHAB requires agencies to implement a performance management system with performance standards, performance measures, reporting of progress, and quality improvement.

Standards may include national, state/territory, or scientific guidelines such as *Healthy People*. Quality improvement approaches include nationally recognized programs, such as plan-do-study-act (or plan-do-check-act; Livingood et al., 2013), Balanced Scorecard (Weir, d'Entremont, Stalker, Kurji, & Robinson, 2009), Baldrige Performance Excellence Criteria (Gorenflo, Klater, Mason, Russo, & Rivera, 2014), and Six Sigma (Robbins, Garman, Song, & McAlearney, 2012). The PHAB also recognizes disease/clinical-specific approaches, such as the CDC's Winnable Battles (Blanck & Collins, 2013) or the Network for the Improvement of Addiction Treatment, which is used in behavioral health care settings (Quanbeck et al., 2012).

The actual number of PHAB accreditations is low. By 2012, only 6% of LHDs and 27% of SHAs had submitted an application or statement of intent to accredit (Shah et al., 2014). However, 26 states have a mandate that requires one or more of the PHAB prerequisites, with one state within the 26 requiring PHAB accreditation (Thielen, Dauer, Burkhardt, Lampe, & VanRaemdonck, 2014). There is significant national and global interest in moving toward public health accreditation. To do so will require a number of actions, such as governmental support (e. g., policy and funding), the enactment of legal mandates, and the growth of a health care market large enough to justify the cost and labor involved to achieve accreditation (Bender et al., 2014; Braithwaite et al., 2012; Thielen, Leff, et al., 2014). This is an opportunity for pharmacists to become involved in policy, practice, and education issues within a community framework.

Public Health Links to Pharmacy

The intersection of public health and pharmacy education is not new. As early as 1932, public health instruction was being taught in schools of pharmacy (Gibson, 1972a). This trend continued through the 1950s and 1960s (Blauch & Webster, 1952; Gibson, 1966). A series of surveys in the 1970s reiterated the importance of public health in pharmacy education and practice (Gibson, 1972a, 1972b, 1973). Bush and Johnson (1979, p. 249) argue "not nearly enough pharmacists are now engaged in public health activities" and "pharmacy education has failed to recognize the potential for pharmacists in public health." They emphasized the need for macro-level pharmacists, who could focus on the health status of a community and not the individual. These pharmacists would actively engage in services planning, delivery, assessment, and evaluation and also participate in policy development. Later, the APHA Pharmacy Services Committee would publish a position paper that addressed four activities for pharmacists in public health. These included

(a) community policy and planning of pharmacy services; (b) consumer outreach and access; (c) addiction programs; and (d) health care delivery, such as intra- and interagency drug delivery systems and coordination with private-sector drug systems (Milne & Johnson, 1979).

In 1980, the APHA adopted a position paper, "The Role of the Pharmacist in Public Health," which described what it saw as core pharmacist activities within public health. The paper mirrored many of the activities on Bush and Johnson's (1979) list and included counseling, educating, and screening patients; it also encouraged formal educational training in public health (APHA, 1980).

A decade and a half later, in 2006, the APHA released a new policy statement on "The Role of the Pharmacist in Public Health," superseding its earlier 1980 policy statement. The new policy stated there were "many functions of public health that can benefit from pharmacists' unique expertise that may include pharmacotherapy, access to care, and prevention services" (APHA, 2006, para. 1). Building on that statement and its historical support for the role of pharmacy in public health, the association formally began to clarify pharmacy as a profession within the public health workforce, public health education, disease prevention and health promotion, services within the core public health functions, public health preparedness, and policy development.

CENTER FOR EXCELLENCE IN PHARMACY EDUCATION OUTCOMES AND PUBLIC HEALTH PHARMACY EDUCATION

In 2004, the American Association of Colleges of Pharmacy recognized the important role pharmacists can play in public health by including population-based care in its CAPE educational outcomes. These outcomes, revised in 2013, emphasize the importance of population health, including public health, but also the important role the entire community plays (including industry, community leaders, health disparities, and the social components of health) that can help optimize the health of population.

CALLS FOR PUBLIC HEALTH IN PHARMACY

The APHA (2006) also recognized the importance of the pharmacist's role within the community, stating the pharmacist's "centralized placement in the community and clinical expertise are invaluable" in the execution of the public health mission (para. 1), offering "an accessibility that is rare among health care professionals" (para. 3). Hence, pharmacy plays an essential role in public health.

The American Association of Colleges of Pharmacy is part of the Association for Prevention Teaching and Research Healthy People Curriculum Task Force, whose mission is to implement the educational objectives of *Healthy People 2020* and to collect data for two of its objectives: ECBP-12-18 (to "increase the inclusion of core clinical prevention and population health content in health professions education") and ECBP-19 (to "increase the proportion of academic institutions with health professions education programs whose prevention curricula include interprofessional educational experiences"). To help achieve that mission, the task force released the "Clinical Prevention and Population Health Curriculum Framework," which consists of 23 domains under four major components: (a) 10 Foundations of Population Health, (b) Clinical Preventive Services and Health Promotion, (c) Clinical Practice and Population Health, and (d) Health Systems and Health Policy (Association for Prevention Teaching and Research, 2015 2011).

Implications for Public Health and Pharmacy Practice

Transdisciplinary professionalism can be defined as interprofessional collaboration, shared values, and shared accountability for improved patient health outcomes. Such an approach would involve interprofessional teamwork, synthesis and extension of discipline-specific expertise, new ways of engaging individual patients and providers, and improving health outcomes. With the passage of the Affordable Care Act, health care providers must work together to provide integrated, coordinated care. Hence, the need of an understanding or creation of a model of transdisciplinary professionalism is pertinent. The IOM (2013, pp. 1–2) identified seven key questions regarding transdisciplinary professionalism.

1. How can the "shared understanding" be integrated into education and practice to promote a transdisciplinary model of professionalism?
2. What are the ethical implications of a transdisciplinary professionalism?
3. How can health and wellness be integrated into transdisciplinary education and practice?
4. How is "leadership" taught and practiced within a model of transdisciplinary professionalism?
5. What are the barriers to transdisciplinary professionalism?
6. What measures are relevant to transdisciplinary professionalism?
7. What is the impact of an evolving professional context on patients, students, and others working within the various health care systems?

We also see these questions as central to any discussion on the integration of public health and pharmacy as a profession, as an academic discipline, and for policymaking. More importantly, we want to emphasize the synergistic and symbiotic roles the fields of public health and pharmacy have with each other. Although much of this chapter has addressed the importance of pharmacy students, educators, professionals, and researchers understanding public health principles and practice, it is equally important that public health students, educators, professionals, and researchers understand pharmacy principles and practice. We look forward to a continued dialogue and engagement among public health and pharmacy professionals.

References

American Association of Colleges of Pharmacy. (2004). *Center for Excellence in Pharmacy Education (CAPE) educational outcomes.* Alexandria, VA: Author.

American Association of Colleges of Pharmacy. (2013). *Educational outcomes.* Alexandria, VA: Author.

American College of Clinical Pharmacy. (2008). The definition of clinical pharmacy. *Pharmacotherapy, 28*(6), 816–817. doi:10.1592/phco.28.6.816

American Pharmacists Association. (2014). *What is medication therapy management?* Washington, DC: Author.

American Public Health Association. (1980). The role of the pharmacist in public health. Washington, DC: Author. Retrieved from https://www.apha.org/policies-and-advocacy/public-health-policy-statements/policy-database/2014/07/07/13/05/the-role-of-the-pharmacist-in-public-health

American Public Health Association. (2006, November 8). *The role of the pharmacist in public health* (Policy Number: 200614). Washington, DC: Author. Retrieved from https://www.apha.org/policies-and-advocacy/public-health-policy-statements/policy-database/2014/07/07/13/05/the-role-of-the-pharmacist-in-public-health

Anderson, L. M., Brownson, R. C., Fullilove, M. T., Teutsch, S. M., Novick, L. F., Fielding, J., & Land, G. H. (2005). Evidence-based public health policy and practice: Promises and limits. *American Journal of Preventive Medicine, 28*(5 Suppl.), 226–230. doi:10.1016/j.amepre.2005.02.014

Association for Prevention Teaching and Research. (2015). *Clinical prevention and population health curriculum framework, version 3.* Washington, DC: Author. Retrieved from http://www.aptrweb.org/resource/resmgr/HPCTF_Docs/Revised_CPPH_Framework_2.201.pdf

Association of State and Territorial Health Officials. (2011). *ASTHO profile of state public health* (Vol. 2). Arlington, VA: Author.

Bender, K., Kronstadt, J., Wilcox, R., & Lee, T. P. (2014). Overview of the public health accreditation board. *Journal of Public Health Management and Practice, 20*(1), 4–6. doi:10.1097/PHH.0b013e3182a778a0

Blanck, H. M., & Collins, J. (2013). CDC's winnable battles: Improved nutrition, physical activity, and decreased obesity. *Child Obesity, 9*(6), 469–471. doi:10.1089/chi.2013.9506

Blauch, L. E., & Webster, G. L. (1952). *The pharmaceutical curriculum.* Washington, DC: American Council on Education.

Braithwaite, J., Shaw, C. D., Moldovan, M., Greenfield, D., Hinchcliff, R., Mumford, V., ... Whittaker, S. (2012). Comparison of health service accreditation programs in low- and middle-income countries with those in higher income countries: A cross-sectional study. *International Journal for Quality in Health Care, 24*(6), 568–577. doi:10.1093/intqhc/mzs064

Brownson, R. C., Fielding, J. E., & Maylahn, C. M. (2009). Evidence-based public health: A fundamental concept for public health practice. *Annual Review of Public Health, 30*, 175–201. doi:10.1146/annurev.publhealth.031308.100134

Bureau of Indian Affairs. (2012). Indian entities recognized and eligible to receive services from the Bureau of Indian Affairs. *Federal Register, 77*(155), 47868–47873. Retrieved from http://www.loc.gov/catdir/cpso/biaind.pdf.

Bush, P. J., & Johnson, K. W. (1979). Where is the public-health pharmacist? *American Journal of Pharmaceutical Education, 43*(3), 249–252.

Cassedy, J. H. (1969). *Demography in early America: Beginnings of the statistical mind, 1600–1800.* Cambridge, MA: Harvard University Press.

Centers for Disease Control and Prevention. (n.d.). *National Public Health Performance Standards Program: Local public health governance performance assessment instrument, version 2.0.* Atlanta, GA: Author. Retrieved from http://www.cdc.gov/nphpsp/documents/governance/07_110300-gov-booklet.pdf.

Chadwick, E. (1843). *Report on the sanitary conditions of the labouring population of Great Britain: A supplementary report on the results of a special inquiry into the practice of interment in towns. Made at the request of Her Majesty's principal secretary of state for the Home department.* London: W. Clowes and Sons.

Church, R. M. (1987). Pharmacy practice in the Indian Health Service. *American Journal of Hospital Pharmacy, 44*(4), 771–775.

Church, R. M. (1989). The expanded role of pharmacists in the public health service: An overview of a pharmacy practice model. *Hospital Formulary, 24*(9), 526–527, 530, 532.

Coleman, W. (1982). *Death is a social disease: Public health and political economy in early industrial France.* Madison: University of Wisconsin Press.

Committee on Assessing Health Care Reform Proposals. (1993). *Assessing health care reform.* Washington, DC: National Academy Press.

Committee on Assuring the Health of the Public in the 21st Century. (2002). *The future of the public's health in the 21st century.* Washington, DC: National Academies Press.

Committee on Public Health Strategies to Improve Health. (2011a). *For the public's health: Revitalizing law and policy to meet new challenges* (Vol. 2). Washington, DC: National Academies Press.

Committee on Public Health Strategies to Improve Health. (2011b). *For the public's health: The role of measurement in action and accountability* (Vol. 1). Washington, DC: National Academies Press.

Committee on Public Health Strategies to Improve Health. (2012). *For the public's health: Investing in a healthier future* (Vol. 3). Washington, DC: National Academies Press.

Council on Linkages Between Academia and Public Health Practice. (2014, June). *Core competencies for public health professionals.* Washington, DC: Council on Linkages Between Academia and Public Health Practice.

Doluisio, J. T. (1989). Positioning pharmacy for the 21st century. *DICP: The Annals of Pharmacotherapy, 23*(9), 706–710.

Ellis, E. T. (1903). The story of a very old Philadelphia drug store, 1729–1875 *American Journal of Pharmacy, 75,* 57–71.

England, J. W., & Kramer, J. E. (1922). *The first century of the Philadelphia College of Pharmacy, 1821–1921.* Philadelphia, PA: Philadelphia College of Pharmacy and Science.

Fee, E. (1992). The Welch-Rose report: Blueprint for public health education in America. In Delta Omega Honorary Public Health Society (Ed.), *The Welch-Rose report: A public health classic.* Baltimore, MD: Johns Hopkins University School of Hygiene and Public Health. Retrieved from http://www.deltaomega.org/documents/WelchRose.pdf.

Fischer, L., Ellingson, K., McCormick, K., & Sinkowitz-Cochran, R. (2014). The role of the public health analyst in the delivery of technical assistance to state health departments for healthcare-associated infection prevention. *Medical Care, 52*(2 Suppl. 1), S54–59. doi:10.1097/mlr.0000000000000055

Gibson, M. R. (1966). Public health in pharmacy curriculum: A syllabus. *American Journal of Pharmaceutical Education, 30*(1), 9–30.

Gibson, M. R. (1972a). Public-health education in colleges of pharmacy 1: Background and problem. *American Journal of Pharmaceutical Education, 36*(2), 189–204.

Gibson, M. R. (1972b). Public-health education in colleges of pharmacy 2: Survey of instruction. *American Journal of Pharmaceutical Education, 36*(4), 561–570.

Gibson, M. R. (1973). Public-health education in colleges of pharmacy 3: Testing, analysis of tests, conclusions, and recommendations. *American Journal of Pharmaceutical Education, 37*(1), 1–27.

Gorenflo, G. G., Klater, D. M., Mason, M., Russo, P., & Rivera, L. (2014). Performance management models for public health: Public health accreditation Board/Baldrige connections, alignment, and distinctions. *Journal of Public Health Management and Practice 20*(1), 128–134. doi:10.1097/PHH.0b013e3182aa184e

Griffenhagen, G. B. (2002). Great moments in pharmacy: Development of the Robert Thorn series depicting pharmacy's history. *Journal of the American Pharmaceutical Association, 42*(2), 170–182. doi:10.1331/108658002763508461

Hepler, C. D. (1988). Unresolved issues in the future of pharmacy. *American Journal of Hospital Pharmacy, 45*(5), 1071–1081.

Hill, E. K., Alpi, K. M., & Auerbach, M. (2010). Evidence-based practice in health education and promotion: A review and introduction to resources. *Health Promotion Practice, 11*(3), 358–366. doi:10.1177/1524839908328993

Ingram, R. C., Bender, K., Wilcox, R., & Kronstadt, J. (2014). A consensus-based approach to national public health accreditation. *Journal of Public Health Management and Practice, 20*(1), 9–13. doi:10.1097/PHH.0b013e3182a0b8f9

Institute of Medicine. (1988). *The future of public health: A consensus workshop.* Washington, DC: The National Academy Press. Retrieved from https://www.nap.edu/catalog/1091/the-future-of-public-health

Institute of Medicine. (2013). *Establishing transdisciplinary professionalism for improving health outcomes: Workshop summary.* Washington, DC: National Academies Press. Retrieved from http://www.nap.edu/catalog.php?record_id=18398.

Jacobson, D. M., & Teutsch, S. (2012). *An environmental scan of integrated approaches for defining and measuring total population health by the clinical care system, the government public health system, and stakeholder organizations.* Washington, DC: National Quality Forum.

Kindig, D., & Stoddart, G. (2003). What is population health? *American Journal of Public Health, 93*(3), 380–383.

Lemberger, A. P. (1988). Rho Chi lecture. The pharmaceutical sciences as academic disciplines. *Drug Intelligence & Clinical Pharmacy, 22*(10), 807–812.

Livingood, W. C., Sabbagh, R., Spitzfaden, S., Hicks, A., Wells, L., Puigdomenech, S., . . . Wood, D. L. (2013). A quality improvement evaluation case study: Impact on public health outcomes and agency culture. *American Journal of Preventive Medicine, 44*(5), 445–452. doi:10.1016/j.amepre.2013.01.011

Marshall, D., Pyron, T., Jimenez, J., Coffman, J., Pearsol, J., & Koester, D. (2014). Improving public health through state health improvement planning: A framework for action. *Journal of Public Health Management and Practice, 20*(1), 23–28. doi:10.1097/PHH.0b013e3182a5a4b8

Matthews, G. W., Markiewicz, M., & Beitsch, L. M. (2012). Legal frameworks supporting public health department accreditation: Lessons learned from 10 states. *Journal of Public Health Management and Practice, 18*(1), e8–e16. doi:10.1097/PHH.0b013e31822f62b0

Milne, T. J., & Johnson, R. E. (1979). *The role of the pharmacist in public health agencies.* Washington, DC: Pharmacy Services Committee, American Public Health Association.

National Association of County and City Health Officials. (2011). *2010 national profile of local health departments.* Washington, DC: Author.

National Indian Health Board. (2011). *2010 tribal public health profile: Exploring public health capacity in Indian country.* Washington, DC: Author. Retrieved from http://www.nihb.org/docs/07012010/NIHB_HealthProfile%202010.pdf.

National Public Health Performance Standards Program. (n.d.). *State public health system performance standards* Atlanta, GA: Centers for Disease Control and Prevention. Retrieved from http://www.cdc.gov/nphpsp/documents/statemodelstandardsonly.pdf.

Oddis, J. A. (1988). Future practice roles in pharmacy. *American Journal of Hospital Pharmacy, 45*(6), 1306–1310.

Penna, R. P. (1987). Pharmacy: A profession in transition or a transitory profession? *American Journal of Hospital Pharmacy, 44*(9), 2053–2059.

Public Health Emergency. (2017). National health security strategy. Retrieved from http://www. phe.gov/Preparedness/planning/authority/nhss/Pages/default.aspx.

Quanbeck, A. R., Madden, L., Edmundson, E., Ford, J. H. 2nd, McConnell, K. J., McCarty, D., & Gustafson, D. H. (2012). A business case for quality improvement in addiction treatment: Evidence from the NIATx collaborative. *The Journal of Behavioral Health Services & Research, 39*(1), 91–100. doi:10.1007/s11414-011-9259-6

Ravenel, M. P. (1921). The American Public Health Association: Past, present, future. In M. P. Ravenel (Ed.), *A half century of public health* (pp. 13–55). New York: American Public Health Association.

Robbins, J., Garman, A. N., Song, P. H., & McAlearney, A. S. (2012). How high-performance work systems drive health care value: An examination of leading process improvement strategies. *Quality Management in Health Care, 21*(3), 188–202. doi:10.1097/QMH. 0b013e31825e88f6

Rosen, G. (1958). *A history of public health*. Baltimore, MD: Johns Hopkins University Press.

Rosenberg, C. E. (1962). *The cholera years; the United States in 1832, 1849, and 1866.* Chicago: University of Chicago Press.

Roundtable on Population Health Improvement. (2013). *Population health implications of the Affordable Care Act: Workshop summary*. Washington, DC: National Academies Press. Retrieved from http://www.nap.edu/download.php?record_id=18546.

Shah, G. H., Leep, C. J., Ye, J., Sellers, K., Liss-Levinson, R., & Williams, K. S. (2014). Public health agencies' level of engagement in and perceived barriers to PHAB National Voluntary Accreditation. *Journal of Public Health Management and Practice*. Advance online publication. doi:10.1097/phh.0000000000000117

Smith, J. E. (1988). Leadership in a clinical profession. *American Journal of Hospital Pharmacy, 45*(8), 1675–1681.

Srinivasan, A., Craig, M., & Cardo, D. (2012). The power of policy change, federal collaboration, and state coordination in healthcare-associated infection prevention. *Clinical Infectious Diseases, 55*(3), 426–431. doi:10.1093/cid/cis407

Thielen, L., Dauer, E., Burkhardt, D., Lampe, S., & VanRaemdonck, L. (2014). An examination of state laws and policies regarding public health agency accreditation prerequisites. *Journal of Public Health Management and Practice, 20*(1), 111–118. doi:10.1097/PHH.0b013e3182a505c9

Thielen, L., Leff, M., Corso, L., Monteiro, E., Fisher, J. S., & Pearsol, J. (2014). A study of incentives to support and promote public health accreditation. *Journal of Public Health Management and Practice, 20*(1), 98–103. doi:10.1097/PHH.0b013e31829ed746

Turnock, B. J., & Barnes, P. A. (2007). History will be kind. *Journal of Public Health Management and Practice, 13*(4), 337–341.

U.S. Census Bureau. (2012). *American FactFinder: American Indian and Alaska Native (AIAN) alone or in any combination by selected tribal groupings*. Washington, DC: Author.

Victora, C. G., Habicht, J. P., & Bryce, J. (2004). Evidence-based public health: Moving beyond randomized trials. *American Journal of Public Health, 94*(3), 400–405.

Weir, E., d'Entremont, N., Stalker, S., Kurji, K., & Robinson, V. (2009). Applying the balanced scorecard to local public health performance measurement: Deliberations and decisions. *BMC Public Health, 9*, 127. doi:10.1186/1471-2458-9-127

Welch, W. H., & Rose, W. (1915). *Institute of Hygiene: Being a report by Dr. William H. Welch and Wickliffe Rose to the General Education Board Rockefeller Foundation*. New York: Rockefeller Foundation.

Winslow, C.-E. A. (1920). The untilled field of public health. *Modern Medicine, 2*, 183–191.

World Health Organization. (1948). *Preamble to the Constitution of the World Health Organization as adopted by the International Health Conference, New York, 19–22 June, 1946; signed on 22 July 1946 by the representatives of 61 states (Official Records of the World Health Organization, no. 2, p. 100) and entered into force on 7 April 1948.* Geneva: Author.

Worthen, D. B. (1928). Andrew Craigie, the first apothecary general of the United States. *Journal of the American Pharmacists Association, 42*(5), 811–813.

Ziobro, P. (2014, September 3). CVS renames itself CVS Health as it ends sale of tobacco products. *The Wall Street Journal Online, Business.*

2

Framing Public Health and Pharmacy

ARDIS HANSON, BRUCE LUBOTSKY LEVIN, AND PETER D. HURD

Charles-Edward Amory Winslow (1920), a pioneer in public health practice in America, saw public health as

> the science and the art of preventing disease . . . and the development of the social machinery which will ensure to every individual in the community a standard of living adequate for the maintenance of health; organizing these benefits in such fashion as to enable every citizen to realize his birthright of health and longevity. (pp. 6–7)

The World Health Organization (WHO; 1948, p. 100) defines health as "a state of complete physical, mental, and social well-being and not merely an absence of disease or infirmity." These definitions of health are mirrored by many nations today.

Historically, health is multidisciplinary in its approach to patient-care and services delivery. Its focus is *the* patient, singular, with a current emphasis on evidence-based practice that leads to the best patient outcomes. It draws upon a wide variety of health professionals in daily practice, across allopathic and osteopathic medicine, including physicians, nurses, dentists, and other health services professionals, such as physical therapists, occupational therapists, pharmacists, physician assistants, nurse practitioners, social workers, psychologists, nutritionists, rehabilitation counselors, health educators, health administrators, and health managers.

The field of public health utilizes a multidisciplinary approach in its examination of health problems in at-risk populations. However, unlike health, public health has a population-based focus. It draws heavily from the areas of biostatistics and epidemiology, environmental and occupational health, health policy and management, community and family health, global health, and, increasingly, public health genomics. Its professionals include nurses, physicians, epidemiologists, statisticians, health educators, environmental health specialists, industrial hygienists, sanitarians, food and drug inspectors, toxicologists, laboratory technicians, environmental scientists, crisis and disaster management workers, veterinarians, economists, social scientists, attorneys, nutritionists, dentists, behavioral health professionals, administrators, and managers. At times, many of these professionals are referred to as public health professionals.

Although pharmacy is considered the branch of the health/medical sciences that deals with the preparation, dispensing, and proper utilization of drugs, we see pharmacy as the bridge between the disciplines of health/medicine and public health, particularly within the area of community pharmacy. Within community pharmacy, the individual patient *and* the community in which the patient resides are equally important in the practice of community or public health pharmacy.

International, Regional, and National Perspectives

This second edition of *Introduction to Public Health in Pharmacy* is different from the original edition since we are incorporating a number of global perspectives of public health and pharmacy, including international perspectives (e.g., WHO, macro-level), regional perspectives (e.g., the European Union, meso-level), and perspectives mostly from the United States (e.g., country, micro-level). We feel this will help to provide readers of this second edition with a more comprehensive understanding of how issues in public health and pharmacy are framed and reframed as we move from a national understanding of public health and pharmacy to broader regional and global perspectives. We hope this additional global perspective will also help to demonstrate that, wherever one may reside, there are commonalities as well as significant differences in the practice, education, and research in the disciplines and careers of public health and pharmacy.

GLOBAL PERSPECTIVES

At the international level, the WHO is perhaps the best-known organization that collects, analyzes, and disseminates reports in the areas of public health research, education, and practice. As the directing and coordinating authority for health within the United Nations, the WHO is comprised of 193 countries and two associate members. It meets annually at the World Health Assembly to set policy and to approve the annual operating budget. A 34-member Executive Board, elected by the Assembly, provides support to membership. With headquarters in Geneva, WHO operates six regional offices and more than 150 offices throughout the world. The WHO and its member "states" play a key role in global health, working with a wide variety of stakeholders, including United Nations agencies, donors, nongovernmental organizations (NGOs), WHO collaborating centers, and the public and private sectors.

The six core functions of WHO are (a) providing technical support and building capacity, (b) providing leadership, (c) setting norms and standards, (d) shaping the research agenda, (e) articulating policy options, and (f) monitoring health and health trends (Taskforce on the Roles and Functions of the Three Levels of WHO, 2013). Each of these functions has obligations at the level of the country offices, the regional offices, and the WHO headquarters. The WHO works with its member states to set priorities for global public health within a number of categories: (a) communicable and noncommunicable diseases; (b) promoting health throughout the life course; (c) health systems; and (d) preparedness, surveillance, and response.

The WHO creates and maintains a number of authoritative sources, such as the *International Classification* series (WHO, 1994, 2001) and the *International Health Regulations* (WHO, 2005) that act as de facto standards for its members. In 1974, the WHO created the *Expanded Programme on Immunization* so all children would have access to basic vaccines to eradicate disease (WHO, 2007). In 1975, the Assembly introduced the concepts of "essential drugs" and "national drug policy." Two years later, the WHO published the *Essential Medicines List*. Over 156 countries now have national lists of essential medicines. In 1978, at its International Conference on Primary Health Care, the WHO set the goal of "health for all," which is an essential public health concept and was again ratified in 1998 for the 21st century (WHO Executive Board, 1998).

The WHO also has been a leader in the prevention, control, and eradication of diseases, ranging from yaws, smallpox, polio, and severe acute respiratory syndrome (SARS). It has expanded its prevention efforts regarding tobacco, nutrition, obesity, and disasters (WHO, 2007). The *WHO Framework Convention on Tobacco Control* attempts to reduce tobacco-related deaths. The *Global Strategy on Diet, Physical Activity, and Health* attempts to increase nutrition and reduce obesity. The WHO also has increased its emphasis on the consequences to health from natural and manmade disasters (e.g., South Asia tsunami and conflicts in Africa and the Middle East; WHO, 2007).

The WHO has also rethought the scope of the public's health from a global perspective, concluding a broader-based approach that encompasses environmental and biopsychosocial models. In 2005, WHO Director-General Lee Jong-Wook established a commission to address social factors leading to ill health and health inequities (Commission on Social Determinants of Health, 2007). The Social Determinants of Health Inequities (SDHI) conceptual framework, shown in Figure 2-1, encompasses three areas: (a) a socioeconomic and political context, (b) structural determinants of health inequities, and (c) intermediary determinants of health. Although many researchers have contributed to the SDHI, a special acknowledgement is given to the work by Finn Diderichsen (Diderichsen, Evans, & Whitehead, 2001; Diderichsen & Hallqvist, 1998; Marmot & Wilkinson, 1999).

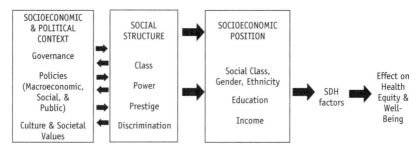

Figure 2-1. Social Determinants of Health Inequities (Solar & Irwin, 2010).

The 2011 WHO World Conference on Social Determinants of Health (Rio de Janeiro, Brazil) provided a global platform for dialogue among member states regarding the recommendations of the Commission on Social Determinants of Health (2008). After the culmination of a series of meetings, first with the member states and then with informal consultations attended by representatives of Permanent Missions, the Assembly (on October 21, 2011) adopted the Rio Political Declaration on Social Determinants of Health, with final endorsement on 26 June 2012.

The Rio Declaration was a global political commitment to implement the social determinants of health (SDH) approach to reduce health inequities and to achieve other WHO global priorities. The intent of the SDH approach is to inspire countries to develop dedicated national action plans and strategies with an emphasis on monitoring progress and increasing accountability.

We see the SDH model reflected at all levels of governments, across NGOs, and in public–private collaborations. The fact that WHO formally resolved and ratified the SDH model to reduce health inequities is significant. Using a common framework, language, and definitions, countries reconceptualize and measure health by establishing viable outcomes for their underserved populations, improving accessibility, enhancing quality of care, and establishing accountability to meet national goals.

REGIONAL PERSPECTIVES

To consider regional perspectives on health, there are a number of ways to conceptualize regions. Regions can be geographic (e.g., continents, subcontinental areas, or self-declared regions); socioeconomic areas, which may be self- or externally defined; or administrative areas (e.g., city, county, or agency districts). Each of these regions and regional perspectives may affect what elements of health a nation surveils, reviews, measures, treats, or legislates.

Within WHO, there are six regions: (a) Africa, (b) the Americas, (c) Southeast Asia, (d) Europe, (e) Eastern Mediterranean, and (f) Western Pacific. Each region has a regional office and a website providing information on its countries, programs, publications, and data, as well as a media center, events, and resources.

Europe

When we think of administrative regions, the European Union (EU) immediately is one center of our attention. The EU has a combined population of over 500 million inhabitants (7.3% of the world population). Essentially a political and economic organization, the EU is comprised of 28 member states and governed by the member states and seven supranational organizations. These organizations include (a) the European Parliament,(b) the European Council, (c) the Council of the European Union, (d) the European Commission, (e) the Court of Justice of the European Union, (f) the European Central Bank, and (g) the European Court of Auditors. The Parliament and the Council, for example, jointly adopt and amend legislative proposals, supervise the work of the Commission and other EU bodies, solicit input from other national parliaments, and decide on the EU budget.

However, the EU is not the only regional body that creates and adopts policies affecting public health and pharmacy practice, education, and research. The WHO European Region (ER) is also a major player. With 53 member states, the WHO ER has its main office in Copenhagen, Denmark, in addition to three technical centers and country offices in 29 member states. Like the EU, there are early meetings for representatives of its member states, which also result in regional policy. In addition to the Regional Committee, there is also a Standing Committee of the Regional Committee (SCRC), a subcommittee of the WHO Regional Committee for Europe. The SCRC is comprised of representatives from 12 countries, with each member elected for a three-year term. In addition, there are 290 collaborating centers in 34 countries in the WHO European region; this is over a third (36%) of the 800 WHO collaborating centers globally.

Now that we have examined two regional bodies that influence public health and pharmacy, we next look at an example of collaboration between the WHO Regional Office and its regional/national partners.

THE EUROPEAN OBSERVATORY ON HEALTH SYSTEMS AND POLICIES

The European Observatory on Health Systems and Policies examines the dynamics of health systems in Europe to promote evidence-based health policymaking. The Observatory is a partnership between the WHO Regional Office for Europe and the governments of Belgium, Finland, Ireland, the Netherlands, Norway, Slovenia, Spain, Sweden, and the Veneto region of Italy. Additional members include the European Commission, the European Investment Bank, The World Bank, the French National Union of Health Insurance Funds, the London School of Economics and Political Science, and the London School of Hygiene & Tropical Medicine. The Observatory conducts a number of studies on the economic and financial impact of population health, from assessing chronic disease management across European health systems to the economic impacts of integrated care. Its quarterly journal, *Eurohealth*, provides reports on emerging policy issues as well as on research and practice.

EUROPEAN POLICY FRAMEWORK: HEALTH 2020

Health 2020 is a "value- and evidence-based health policy framework" for the WHO European region (WHO Regional Office for Europe, 2013, p. 3). It clearly establishes that health is not only a major societal resource but also an asset that reifies the SDH frame of the Rio Declaration. The member states agreed to six broad goals. The sixth goal specifically encourages member states to set national goals and targets related to health issues in their respective nations (WHO Regional Office for Europe, 2013). This allows member states to determine health priorities, identify evidence-based practices, and address implementation facilitators and barriers. It also addresses the varying capacities across nations, targeted strategic initiatives, and increased monitoring and evaluation of population health.

Member states also selected four priority areas for policy action: (a) lifecourse approach to health; (b) noncommunicable and communicable diseases; (c) strengthening people-centered public health systems and emergency preparedness, surveillance, and response; and (d) creating resilient communities (Opolski & Wysocki, 2013). If the aim of public health and public health pharmacy is to improve the health of communities and improve the health of populations, then Health 2020 should provide a strong framework for the improvement of both across Europe.

UNITED STATES AND HEALTHY PEOPLE

In the United States, we see the incorporation of the WHO's definition of health across the federal and state Healthy People initiatives, most recently in *Healthy People 2020*. The *Healthy People 2020* framework is the product of a collaborative process among a number of stakeholders, including the U.S. Department of Health and Human Services (USDHHS), other federal health agencies, public stakeholders, and the *Healthy People 2020* advisory committee.

Building upon the WHO focus on ecological and SDH, the United States established the overarching goals and foundation health measures into its next 10-year national plan (Figure 2-2).

To examine how well the nation is achieving these goals requires measurement. The *Healthy People 2020* health measures examine general health status, health-related quality of life and well-being, determinants of health, and disparities. Measures of general health status include Life Expectancy (with international comparison), Healthy Life Expectancy, Years of Potential Life Lost (with international comparison), Physically and Mentally Unhealthy Days, Self-Assessed Health Status, Limitation of Activity, and Chronic Disease Prevalence. Health-related quality of life and well-being measures include Patient Reported Outcomes

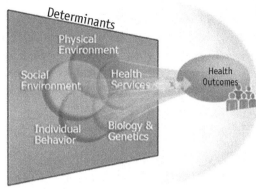

Figure 2-2. Graphic model of *Healthy People* 2020.

Measurement Information System, Global Health Measure (Hays, Bjorner, Revicki, Spritzer, & Cella, 2009), well-being measures, and participation measures (USDHHS, 2010).

Determinants of health measures emphasize an ecological approach to disease prevention and health promotion with foci on both individual-level and population-level determinants of health and interventions. They examine the relationship between health status and biology, individual behavior, health services, social factors, and policies (Secretary's Advisory Committee on National Health Promotion and Disease Prevention Objectives for 2020, 2010). *Healthy People 2020* defines a health disparity as "a particular type of health difference that is closely linked with social, economic, and/or environmental disadvantage." A disparity measure determines whether a health outcome exists in a greater or lesser extent between populations. Factors that may impact disparities in health outcomes include age, disability, geographic location, race or ethnicity, sex, sexual identity, and socioeconomic status (Secretary's Advisory Committee on National Health Promotion and Disease Prevention Objectives for 2020, 2010).

The Role of Pharmacy in Public Health

As we stated earlier in this chapter, the importance of public health in pharmacy, particularly the community, cannot be overstated. However, from a global perspective, there are great disparities in the distribution of pharmacies and pharmacists; in low-income countries, the density of pharmacies is greater than the density of pharmacists, which suggests that there are issues in access to and supply of medicines, finding a skilled workforce, and appropriate supervision of pharmaceutical services.

INTERNATIONALLY

Founded in 1912, the International Pharmaceutical Federation (Fédération Internationale Pharmaceutique [FIP]) is a NGO representing over 3 million pharmacists and pharmaceutical scientists globally (International Pharmaceutical Federation, 2008). In 1948, the FIP established an official relationship with the WHO. The FIP's strategic plan, *2020 Vision*, provides a mission to "improve global health by advancing pharmacy practice and science to enable better discovery, development, access to and safe use of appropriate, cost-effective, quality medicines worldwide" (International Pharmaceutical Federation, 2008, p. 14). The *FIP/WHO Guidelines on Good Pharmacy Practice: Standard for Quality of Pharmacy Services* (International Pharmaceutical Federation & WHO, 2011) examined the national standards for pharmacy practice in 37 countries and consulted with all 120 national member associations, the WHO, and additional experts.

As FIP describes the evolution of the role of the pharmacist from a product focus to a patient focus, promoting wellness, and preventing disease, collaborating in disease management programs become important areas for pharmacy practice, education, and policy at national and global levels. Its handbook, *Developing Pharmacy Practice—A Focus on Patient Care*, reflects this transition to a more patient-centered approach (e.g., pharmaceutical care; Wiedenmayer, Summers, Mackie, Gous, & Everard, 2006). It incorporates the Pharmacy Practice Activity Classification (PPAC) developed by the American Pharmacists Association to create a common language and framework that can help in assessing comparative studies, particularly important in today's patient-centered outcomes research studies. The PPAC also is incorporated in data collection on activities of licensed, practicing pharmacists, from traditional dispensing to health systems management (see Box 2-1).

The FIP also has been active in developing the role of pharmacists in areas such as maternal, newborn, and child health. Its statement of policy on improving maternal outcomes incorporates the *FIP/WHO Guidelines on Good Pharmacy Practice: Standard for Quality of Pharmacy Services* and is complemented by earlier FIP policies, such as the *Quality of Medicines for Children* (2008) and *The Pharmacist's Responsibility and Role in Teaching Children and Adolescents about Medicines* (2001). The FIP frames maternal health as including both the clinical and social aspects of health care, a good connection to the SDH framework that the WHO uses in developing its policy statements. FIP recommends that individual pharmacists take a greater role in maternal, newborn, and child health within their individual practices as well as within their nationally defined scopes of practice. It also recommends that FIP member organizations develop specific standards of practice within a national framework (International Pharmaceutical Federation, 2013).

In addition, FIP addresses issues for pharmacy workforce development and standards, including pharmacists and pharmacy support staff. Its 2012 *Global Pharmacy Workgroup Report* (International Pharmaceutical Federation, 2012) correlated

---

Box 2-1 **The Pharmacy Practice Activity Classification**

A. Ensuring appropriate therapy and outcomes
    A.1 Ensuring appropriate pharmacotherapy
    A.2 Ensuring patient's understanding/adherence to his or her treatment plan
    A.3 Monitoring and reporting outcomes
B. Dispensing medications and devices
    B.1 Processing the prescription or medicine order
    B.2 Preparing the pharmaceutical product
    B.3 Delivering the medication or device
C. Health promotion and disease prevention
    C.1 Delivering clinical preventive services
    C.2 Surveillance and reporting of public health issues
    C.3 Promoting safe medication use in society
D. Health systems management
    D.1 Managing the practice
    D.2 Managing medications throughout the health system
    D.3 Managing the use of medications within the health system
    D.4 Participating in research activities
    D.5 Engaging in interdisciplinary collaboration

---

responses from 90 countries and territories that responded to the survey, with descriptive data covering around 2.5 million pharmacists and 1.4 million pharmacy technicians. The FIP suggests that there may be a relationship between spending on health and pharmacist availability to the level of economic development in nations and territories. The FIP report also found that, globally, 55% of pharmacists work in community pharmacies, 18% work in hospitals, 10% work in industry, 5% work in research and academia, and 5% work in regulation. The European region had the highest number of community pharmacists (almost 70%).

The global report had several key messages for pharmacy practice. These include emphasizing access to and supply of quality medicines, improving workforce performance focusing on patient care and interprofessional collaboration, and continuing investment in professional education at all levels (pharmacists and support staff). In addition, it stressed the importance of creating and implementing a needs-based pharmacy educational system to address local system issues and communities.

European Pharmacy Practice and Education from a Public Health Perspective
Many European countries follow a universal health care model. As to be expected, there are differences in models of services delivery, payers, programs, prescription

coverage, quality of care, and assessment. The United Kingdom has a strong centralized National Health Service (Boyle, 2011). The Netherlands has a corporatist social health insurance system (Schafer et al., 2010). Italy has a federal regionalized national health system (Ferre et al., 2014). Other countries, such as Switzerland, have a compulsory health care model by which all citizens must purchase basic care private health insurance (Busato, Matter, Kunzi, & Goodman, 2012). Hence, depending upon the type of plan a country may have, and/or the extent of private insurance, there may be significant differences in pharmacy practices.

Regulations affecting pharmacy practice also affect pharmacy education, as each country has its own standards for licensing and credentialing graduates of professional schools. The Bologna Declaration of 1999 was the start of the European Higher Education Area, which now encompasses 47 countries (European Commission, Education, Audiovisual and Culture Executive Agency, & Eurydice, 2015). Now known as the Bologna Process, the Declaration created a transparent system of comparable degrees and system of credits that would promote employability of European citizens; ensure quality of education across national borders; and promote curricular development, interinstitutional co-operation, and integrated academic/research programs (European Commission et al., 2015).

The Public Health Education and Training in the Context of an Enlarging Europe (PHETICE; 2008) project was a collaborative endeavor to create a common European construct of public health which was funded by the European Commission Directorate of General Health and Consumer Protection during 2005–2008. PHETICE used the Bologna Process (see previous paragraph) as a model to determine core educational and pedagogical strategies as well as how to address jurisdictional issues between the European Commission and national authorities to develop common curricula and accreditation standards. PHETICE developed five European Master Programs in Public Health (with foci in epidemiology, gerontology, health promotion, public health, and public health nutrition) with the intent to expand them into central and eastern Europe (PHETICE, 2008).

As shown in Figure 2-3, the cyclical nature of structure, process, and outcome would allow PHETICE to meet the needs of different public health practitioners across varying levels of proficiency and national priorities (PHETICE, 2008). Concurrently, Skills for Health (2008) was defining the UK health sector competencies required within the field of public health across nine levels of career development, and the Association of Schools of Public Health in the European Region had created its own European Public Health Core Competencies Program for public health education (Birt & Foldspar, 2011).

The Galway Conference is another example of international collaboration on the development of core competencies for health promotion and health education that applies to all members of the health professions (Barry, Allegrante, Lamarre, Auld, & Taub, 2009). In June 2008, the International Union for Health Promotion

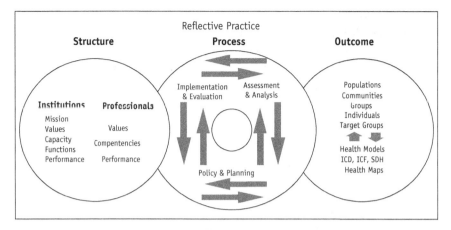

Figure 2-3. A model of public health and promotion competencies.

and Education, the Society for Public Health Education, and the Centers for Disease Control and Prevention created core values and principles, common definitions, and eight domains of core competencies for health promotion workforce development in Europe (Allegrante et al., 2009; Battel-Kirk, Barry, Taub, & Lysoby, 2009). The CompHP Core Competencies Framework for Health Promotion across the US member states and candidate countries' consists of 11 core domains and 68 core competency statements (Barry, Battel-Kirk, & Dempsey, 2012).

Created using a Delphi process that involved policymakers, practitioners, and academics from 34 countries (including EU member states, candidate countries, European Economic Area countries, and Switzerland; Barry et al., 2012), the development of competencies, standards, and accreditation is intended to assure quality in performance of all those who contribute to health promotion, such as community and population health pharmacists. The competencies are based on the core concepts and principles of health promotion outlined in the Ottawa Charter (WHO, 1986) and successive WHO charters and declarations on health promotion (e.g., Nairobi, Adelaide, Sundsvall, Jakarta, Mexico, Bangkok, and Helsinki; see www.who.int/healthpromotion/conferences/en/). Since the long-range plans include different levels of accreditation for varying levels and different fields of practice, developing a pan-European accreditation system will be a significant challenge but one that continues to build on previous pan-European successes (Santa-Maria Morales et al., 2009).

While standards for education and accreditation are critical, it is equally important to have congruence between professional organizations and government priorities. Anderson (2007), for example, describes a two-pronged approach from the UK pharmacy professionals to incorporate public health as a key area for future development, which coincided with state recognition of the need to draw a broader range of health professionals into public health activities. UK pharmacy was not only able to re-establish its earlier traditional advisory role but was able to redevelop it with a stronger tie-in to public health. To do so, however, it addressed a number of policy and professional factors, including (a) changes to national policy, (b) formal recognition by pharmacy's professional bodies, (c) incentives for community pharmacists, and (d) support from the public health professional community.

PHARMACISTS AND PHARMACY PRACTICE IN THE UNITED STATES FROM A PUBLIC HEALTH PERSPECTIVE

In the United States, the national objectives for public health embed pharmacists and pharmacy practice in public health. An examination of *Healthy People 2020* provides glimpses into the many ways pharmacists contribute to community and population health. Within the topic "Public Health Infrastructure," for example, pharmacists are a part of a capable and qualified workforce that is adept at assessing and responding to public health needs using up-to-date data and information systems. "Access to health services" requires (a) that an individual can access the appropriate provider and receive needed services at a health care location and (b) that the patient can communicate and trust the health care provider. The continued evolution of pharmacy practice in the community makes this a natural extension of current pharmacy practice.

In the "Educational and Community-Based Programs" section of *Healthy People 2020,* pharmacists are involved in the quality, availability, and effectiveness of educational and community-based programs designed to prevent disease and injury, improve health, and enhance quality of life. Addressing "Health Care-Associated Infections," pharmacists can provide guidance on the correct use of medical devices, antibiotic use, and use of syringes and needles. Finally, under "Social Determinants of Health," pharmacists can play a critical role in access to community-based health promotion and wellness programs and clinical and preventive care.

Other areas in which pharmacists can contribute as health providers include disease prevention and management, including immunization and infectious diseases. Pharmacists also play a role in health promotion, which encompasses injury and violence prevention; maternal, infant, and child health; nutrition and weight status; oral health; substance abuse; and tobacco use. See Table 2-1 for all the topical areas in *Healthy People 2020* and take a moment to consider the many ways pharmacists can contribute in each area.

While the Affordable Care Act (2010) and the Health Care and Education Reconciliation Act (2010) have incorporated pharmacists as a vital member of health care teams, neither act has given formal health care provider status to pharmacists. Without that status, pharmacists cannot receive direct reimbursement for health-related services, and they continue to face liability issues. However, bipartisan legislation introduced in 2016, the Pharmacy and Medically Underserved Areas Enhancement Act (H.R. 592 [2016a] and S. 314 [2016b]), would amend section 1861(s)(2) of the Social Security Act to include pharmacists on the list of recognized health care providers. However, the bill restricts pharmacists to the provision of services restricted to patients in medically underserved communities and to services that are consistent with the specific state scope of practice laws.

Table 2-1 **Topical Areas in *Healthy People 2020***

Access to Health Services	Healthcare-Associated Infections	Nutrition and Weight Status
Adolescent Health		
Arthritis, Osteoporosis, and Chronic Back Conditions	Health Communication and Health Information Technology	Occupational Safety and Health
Blood Disorders and Blood Safety	Health-Related Quality of Life and Well-Being	Older Adults
Cancer	Hearing, Other Sensory, or Communication Disorders	Oral Health
Chronic Kidney Disease		Physical Activity
Dementias, Including Alzheimer's Disease	Heart Disease and Stroke	Preparedness
Diabetes	HIV	Public Health Infrastructure
Disability and Health	Immunization and Infectious Diseases	Respiratory Diseases
Early and Middle Childhood	Injury and Violence Prevention	Sexually Transmitted Diseases
Educational and Community-Based Programs	Lesbian, Gay, Bisexual, and Transgender Health	Sleep Health
Environmental Health	Maternal, Infant, and Child Health	Social Determinants of Health
Family Planning	Medical Product Safety	Substance Abuse
Food Safety	Mental Health and Mental Disorders	Tobacco Use
Genomics		Vision
Global Health		

Implications for Public Health and Pharmacy Practice

Collaborative and complementary practice, policy, and research agendas could generate systems-wide changes in public health. In 2014, the U.S. Institute of Medicine's (IOM) Roundtable on Population Health Improvement examined "spread, scale, and sustainability" in population health. One of the first areas of business was to have workshop participants share how they each understood these terms within the contexts of their own work (IOM, 2015). Workshop participants responded that a number of actions could help spread improvement in public health. These include relationships, communication, addressing inequities, encouraging community leadership to create a culture and environment of health, developing policy and incentives to implement population health practices, and incorporating public health frameworks into training and education. Scaling up requires strong metrics that show tangible and demonstrable effects of value related to rewards and incentives, clear communication, engaged shared leadership, and a good grasp of the logistics to scale a program successfully. Achieving sustainability requires aligning incentives, planning for long-term financial management, establishing clear strategies to achieve goals, choosing the correct infrastructure to permit spread and scaling of a program, and encouraging community buy-in (IOM, 2015).

Innovative payment and service delivery models and strategies, such as incentives or accountable health communities, may help to improve population health (IOM, 2015). However, evaluation methods will also need to capture more data than just if the program achieved its desired outcomes; data should also address factors such as the length of time for implementation, relative costs, and costs of the demonstration project. Hence, local and relevant data are essential to defining targets and planning.

A "health in all policies" (HiAP) approach, such as those taken by *Health 2020* and *Healthy People 2020*, requires us to understand that mandates of all those involved in the provision of health care may have very different agendas. Accordingly, we need to create a shared language that can further communication at the proverbial "table of dialogue." It also requires us to have data on policy-relevant questions that demonstrate health has significantly improved and that we have achieved outcomes people prioritize. This demonstrates the importance of using both quantitative and qualitative studies that can clearly delineate improved economic, clinical, and patient outcomes.

How we work within an increasingly global community also will require us to be aware of the challenges involved in creating a public health or a HiAP approach that successfully integrates public health and pharmacy. There are a number of issues to consider with the implementation of a HiAP framework to ensure its six goals are met: (a) establish the need and priorities for HiAP; (b) frame planned action; (c) identify supportive structures and processes; (d) facilitate assessment and engagement; (e) ensure monitoring, evaluation and reporting; and (f) build capacity (WHO, 2014). While national governments authorize policy recommendations, public health authorities at all levels and across all professions are key individuals in intergovernmental, multilateral, bilateral, and regional agencies and networks who provide significant support to implement multisectoral actions to achieve public health outcomes in all national, regional, or global policies. It promises to be an exciting time, from policy and practice perspectives, to continue to be involved in strengthening the interactions between public health and pharmacy.

References

Allegrante, J. P., Barry, M. M., Airhihenbuwa, C. O., Auld, M. E., Collins, J. L., Lamarre, M. C., . . . Mittelmark, M. B. (2009). Domains of core competency, standards, and quality assurance for building global capacity in health promotion: the Galway consensus conference statement. *Health Education & Behavior, 36*(3), 476–482. doi:10.1177/1090198109333950

Anderson, S. (2007). Community pharmacy and public health in Great Britain, 1936 to 2006: How a phoenix rose from the ashes. *Journal of Epidemiology & Community Health, 61*(10), 844–848. doi:10.1136/jech.2006.055442

Barry, M. M., Allegrante, J. P., Lamarre, M. C., Auld, M. E., & Taub, A. (2009). The Galway Consensus Conference: International collaboration on the development of core competencies for health promotion and health education. *Global Health Promotion, 16*(2), 5–11. doi:10.1177/1757975909104097

Barry, M. M., Battel-Kirk, B., & Dempsey, C. (2012). The CompHP core competencies framework for health promotion in Europe. *Health Education & Behavior, 39*(6), 648–662. doi:10.1177/1090198112465620

Battel-Kirk, B., Barry, M. M., Taub, A., & Lysoby, L. (2009). A review of the international literature on health promotion competencies: Identifying frameworks and core competencies. *Global Health Promotion, 16*(2), 12–20. doi:10.1177/1757975909104100

Birt, C., & Foldspar, A. (2011). *European Core Competences for Public Health Professionals (ECCPHP)* (ASPHER Pub. No. 5). Brussels, Belgium: Association of Schools of Public Health in the European Region. Retrieved from http://aphea.net/docs/research/ECCPHP.pdf

Boyle, S. (2011). United Kingdom (England): Health system review. *Health Systems in Transit, 13*(1), 1–483, xix–xx.

Busato, A., Matter, P., Kunzi, B., & Goodman, D. (2012). Geographic variation in the cost of ambulatory care in Switzerland. *Journal of Health Services Research & Policy, 17*(1), 18–23. doi:10.1258/jhsrp.2011.010056

Commission on Social Determinants of Health. (2007, April). *A conceptual framework for action on the social determinants of health: Discussion paper for the Commission on Social Determinants of Health: Draft.* Geneva, Switzerland: World Health Organization.

Commission on Social Determinants of Health. (2008). *Closing the gap in a generation: Health equity through action on the social determinants of health.* Geneva, Switzerland: World Health Organization.

Diderichsen, F., Evans, T., & Whitehead, M. (2001). The social basis of disparities in health. In T. Evans, M. Whitehead, F. Diderichsen, A. Bhuiya, & M. Wirth (Eds.), *Challenging inequities in health* (pp. 13–23). New York, NY: Oxford University Press.

Diderichsen, F., & Hallqvist, J. (1998). Social inequalities in health: Some methodological considerations for the study of social position and social context. In B. Arve-Parès (Ed.), *Inequality in health: A Swedish perspective* (pp. 25–39). Stockholm, Sweden: Swedish Council for Social Research.

European Commission, Education, Audiovisual and Culture Executive Agency, & Eurydice. (2015). *The European Higher Education Area in 2015: Implementation report.* Luxembourg: Publications Office of the European Union. Retrieved from http://www.ehea.info/Uploads/SubmitedFiles/5_2015/132824.pdf

Ferre, F., de Belvis, A. G., Valerio, L., Longhi, S., Lazzari, A., Fattore, G., . . . Maresso, A. (2014). Italy: Health system review. *Health Systems in Transit, 16*(4), 1–168.

Hays, R. D., Bjorner, J. B., Revicki, D. A., Spritzer, K. L., & Cella, D. (2009). Development of physical and mental health summary scores from the Patient-Reported Outcomes Measurement Information System (PROMIS) global items. *Quality of Life Research, 18*(7), 873–880. doi:10.1007/s11136-009-9496-9

Health Care and Education Reconciliation Act, Pub. L. No. 111–152, 124 Stat. 1029 Stat. (2010). Retrieved from https://www.gpo.gov/fdsys/pkg/PLAW-111publ152/pdf/PLAW-111publ152.pdf

Institute of Medicine. (Ed.). (2015). *Spread, scale, and sustainability in population health: Workshop summary.* Washington, DC: National Academies Press.

International Pharmaceutical Federation. (2008). *2020 vision: FIP's vision, mission and strategic plan.* The Hague: The Netherlands: Author. Retrieved from http://www.fip.org/files/fip/strategic%20plan%20no%20annexes.pdf

International Pharmaceutical Federation. (2012). *2012 FIP global pharmacy workforce report.* The Hague, The Netherlands: Author. Retrieved from http://www.fip.org/static/fipeducation/2012/FIP-Workforce-Report-2012/data/FIP%20workforce%20Report%202012.pdf

International Pharmaceutical Federation. (2013). *FIP statement of policy: The effective utilization of pharmacists in improving maternal, newborn and child health (MNCH).* The Hague: The Netherlands: Author. Retrieved from http://www.fip.org/www/uploads/database_file.php?id=343&table_id=

International Pharmaceutical Federation, & World Health Organization. (2011). *FIP/WHO guidelines on good pharmacy practice: Standard for quality of pharmacy services.* The Hague, The Netherlands: International Pharmaceutical Federation. Retrieved from http://www.fip.org/www/uploads/database_file.php?id=331&table_id=

Marmot, M. G., & Wilkinson, R. G. (Eds.). (1999). *Social determinants of health.* Oxford: Oxford University Press.

Opolski, J. T., & Wysocki, M. J. (2013). Health 2020—new framework for health policy. Part II. *Przeglad epidemiologiczny, 67*(4), 647–650.

Patient Protection and Affordable Care Act, Pub. L. No. 111-152, 124 Stat. 1029–1084 Stat. (2010). Retrieved from https://www.gpo.gov/fdsys/pkg/PLAW-111publ148/pdf/PLAW-111publ148.pdf

Pharmacy and Medically Underserved Areas Enhancement Act H.R.592 (2016a). Retrieved from https://www.congress.gov/bill/114th-congress/house-bill/592

Pharmacy and Medically Underserved Areas Enhancement Act S.314 (2016b). Retrieved from https://www.congress.gov/bill/114th-congress/senate-bill/314

Public Health Education and Training in the Context of an Enlarging Europe. (2008). *A guide towards a more effective, comparable and mobile workforce across Europe.* Stockholm, Sweden: Author.

Retrieved from https://web.archive.org/web/20160315152140/http://www.phetice.org/docs/phetice_guide.pdf

Santa-Maria Morales, A., Battel-Kirk, B., Barry, M. M., Bosker, L., Kasmel, A., & Griffiths, J. (2009). Perspectives on health promotion competencies and accreditation in Europe. *Global Health Promotion, 16*(2), 21–31. doi:10.1177/1757975909104101

Schafer, W., Kroneman, M., Boerma, W., van den Berg, M., Westert, G., Deville, W., & van Ginneken, E. (2010). The Netherlands: Health system review. *Health Systems in Transition, 12*(1), v–xxvii, 1–228.

Secretary's Advisory Committee on National Health Promotion and Disease Prevention Objectives for 2020. (2010). *Healthy People 2020: An opportunity to address societal determinants of health in the U.S.* Washington, DC: U.S. Department of Health and Human Services.

Skills for Health. (2008, April). *Public Health Skills and Career Framework: Multidisciplinary/multi-agency/multi-professional.* Bristol, UK: Author. Retrieved from https://web.archive.org/web/20150319070415/http://www.sph.nhs.uk/sph-files/PHSkills-CareerFramework_Launchdoc_April08.pdf

Social Security Act Amendments of 1965, Pub. L. 89–97, 42 USC Title 42 §§1395 to 1395lll (1965). Retrieved from https://www.gpo.gov/fdsys/pkg/USCODE-2011-title42/html/USCODE-2011-title42-chap7-subchapXVIII.htm

Solar, O., & Irwin, A. (2010). *A conceptual framework for action on the social determinants of health: Debates, policy & practice, case studies.* (Social Determinants of Health Discussion Paper 2). Geneva, Switzerland: World Health Organization. Retrieved from http://apps.who.int/iris/bitstream/10665/44489/1/9789241500852_eng.pdf?ua=1&ua=1

Taskforce on the Roles and Functions of the Three Levels of WHO. (2013). *Report of the Taskforce on the Roles and Functions of the Three Levels of WHO.* Geneva, Switzerland: World Health Organization.

U.S. Department of Health and Human Services. (2010). *Healthy People 2020: Foundation health measure report: Health-related quality of life and well-being* Washington, DC: Author.

Wiedenmayer, K., Summers, R. S., Mackie, C. A., Gous, A. G. S., & Everard, M. (2006). *Developing pharmacy practice: A focus on patient care.* Geneva, Switzerland, and The Hague, The Netherlands: World Health Organization and International Pharmaceutical Federation. Retrieved from http://www.who.int/medicines/publications/WHO_PSM_PAR_2006.5.pdf?ua=1

Winslow, C.-E. A. (1920). The untilled field of public health. *Modern Medicine, 2,* 183–191.

World Health Assembly. (2011). *Rio political declaration on social determinants of health.* Rio de Janeiro, Brazil: Author. Retrieved from http://www.who.int/sdhconference/declaration/Rio_political_declaration.pdf?ua=1

World Health Organization. (1986). *The Ottawa Charter for Health Promotion.* Geneva, Switzerland: Author. Retrieved from http://www.who.int/healthpromotion/conferences/previous/ottawa/en/index.html

World Health Organization. (1948, June). *Official records of the World Health Organization, no. 2.* Geneva, Switzerland: Author.

World Health Organization. (1994). *International classification of diseases* (10th ed.). Geneva, Switzerland: Author.

World Health Organization. (2001). *International classification of functioning, disability and health.* Geneva, Switzerland: Author.

World Health Organization. (2005). *International health regulations* (2nd ed.). Geneva, Switzerland: Author.

World Health Organization. (2007). *Working for health: An introduction to the World Health Organization.* Geneva: Author.

World Health Organization. (2014). Health in All Policies (HiAP) framework for country action. *Health Promotion International, 29*(Suppl. 1), i19–i28. doi:10.1093/heapro/dau035

World Health Organization Executive Board. (1998). *Health-for-all policy for the twenty-first century*. Geneva, Switzerland: World Health Organization. Retrieved from http://apps.who.int/gb/archive/pdf_files/EB101/pdfangl/angr22.pdf

World Health Organization Regional Office for Europe. (2013). *Health 2020. A European policy framework and strategy for the 21st century*. Copenhagen, Denmark: Author. Retrieved from http://www.euro.who.int/__data/assets/pdf_file/0011/199532/Health2020-Long.pdf?ua=1

3

Global Health

ARDIS HANSON, PETER D. HURD, AND BRUCE LUBOTSKY LEVIN

Introduction

Around the world, tuberculosis (TB) continues to be a significant cause of death despite the fact that the disease is preventable and often curable if contracted. The history of TB goes back to the ancient Greeks, with Aristotle and Galen both writing of the contagious nature of *phthisi* (Shorstein Lecture, 1922). In 1882, Robert Koch found the tubercle bacillus that causes this infectious disease, an achievement that won him the Nobel Prize in Medicine (Tuberculosis Control Division, 1982). Tests to detect TB developed in the late 1800s and 1900s. Particularly of note are the development of the acid-fast staining test in 1892, X-rays in1895, and the tuberculin skin test 1907 (Tuberculosis Control Division, 1982). Drugs to treat this disease were available in the 1940s. Yet today, TB is still prevalent around the world, especially in developing countries (World Health Organization, 2015b).

TB has both a "global" public health story and a "drugs" public health story, both providing insights about the role of public health in disease prevention. The symptoms of active TB include coughing, blood in sputum, weakness, and weight loss. Coughing and spitting can spread the disease to others. There are simple tests to detect if a person has been infected with TB bacteria in humans, as mentioned earlier, the Mantoux tuberculin skin test is still in use as are TB blood tests known as interferon-gamma release assays (IGRAs). The US Food and Drug Administration (FDA) approved the QuantiFERON®–TB Gold In-Tube test (QFT-GIT) and the T-SPOT®TB test (T-Spot). However, to confirm TB as an active disease, chest X-rays and sputum samples are necessary. Some treatments of TB include active monitoring by health care workers, who observe and confirm that patients take the medications as directed, both to assure a disease cure and to reduce the chances that resistant strains will evolve.

Today, when people think of TB, they think of the drugs that can treat the disease. However, before effective drugs were developed, public health practices were decreasing the incidence of the disease. These practices included the pasteurization

41

of milk, rules against spitting in public, and isolation of those persons infected with active TB. These practices led to a reduction in people with the disease. Deaths declined from 190 deaths per 100,000 in 1900 to about 40 deaths per 100,000 in the 1940s, when drugs, such as streptomycin, were first used, followed by isoniazid in 1950, which was more effective (Centers for Disease Control and Prevention [CDC], 1999). TB continues to decline, and today the death rate is closer to less than 10 per 100,000 in the United States.

The key public health lesson is the explanation of the disease decline prior to the marketing of effective drugs that treated the disease. This helps highlight the role that public health has played in the fight against many diseases and the improvement of the health of society. However, the drug side of the story continues because now there are drug-resistant strains of TB to the drugs that worked so well previously. These strains developed partially because patients would stop taking the drug too early and the bacteria that remained became resistant to the drug.

From a global public health perspective, both the incidence of TB and the deaths from TB are higher in countries with lower income levels, with Africa, Southeast Asia, and the Western Pacific the most affected regions of the world (Henry K. Kaiser Family Foundation, 2016). The effects from social determinants of health (SDH) are seen in global health, where the relationship between poverty and poor health is an important concept to help understand TB from a global public health perspective.

Public Health in Global Health

Global public health includes the essentials of a healthy environment, such as drinkable water, food that is plentiful and safe to eat, and waste disposal that keeps the population safe. But global health also focuses on the prevention of disease, the promotion of healthy lifestyles, and the early detection of health problems. While these issues were once critical local problems, diseases like TB illustrate the importance of a global perspective of the health of our world population. Similarly, national health issues not only affect a state or nation, but they also have effects on regions of the world and globally.

HAITI: A CASE STUDY

Haiti is the poorest country in the Americas and one of the poorest in the world. According to the World Bank (2016a), more than 6 million (59%) Haitians live below the national poverty line ($2.42 per day) and over 2.5 million (24%) live below the national extreme poverty line ($1.23 per day). On January 12, 2010, a 7.0 magnitude earthquake devastated Haiti. The earthquake killed 220,000 people, injured over 300,000 people, and seriously damaged the health infrastructure; eight hospitals were totally destroyed and 22 hospitals were seriously damaged in the three regions most affected by the earthquake (Pan American Health Organization [PAHO], 2010a). Approximately $8 billion dollars of damages and losses occurred in Haiti (The World Bank, 2016a). This led to a global effort to restore the health of this developing country located in the Caribbean.

Imagine the difficulties of one of the poorest of countries in attempting to cope with this disaster. An estimated 1.5 million people were displaced internally due to the destruction of thousands of homes and entire neighborhoods. The aftermath of the storm left a severe shortage of health care facilities. There was a lack of resources to bury the dead, with thousands of bodies being buried in mass graves. There was a near-failure of telephone communication systems. Impassable roads were covered by debris for months and even years after the quake. The airport was too small to handle all the relief planes that needed to land, and the control tower was severely damaged. The ocean port needed major repairs before ships could dock and unload safely.

There was a lack of national resources, long delays in clearing rubble from devastated areas, and language problems since many residents of Haiti speak only Kreyol (with limited French and English speakers). Thus one can start to appreciate the magnitude of this kind of disaster. Food, water, and medical supplies were priorities for the aftermath. Then, 10 months later, in October 2010, Haiti suffered the largest cholera epidemic in modern history, with more than 8,000 people dead by 2013 (Gelting, Bliss, Patrick, Lockhart, & Handzel, 2013; Schuller & Levey, 2014).

During 2010, causes of death in Haiti differed from that of the more developed world, with 66% of deaths related to the disaster itself, 5% to stroke, 3% to cancer, and 2% to ischemic heart disease (Institute for Health Metrics and Evaluation, 2015). In developed countries, such as the United States, heart disease, cancer, and stroke are among the leading causes of death (National Center for Health Statistics, 2016).

Prior to the earthquake, Haiti had numerous public health problems, including significant water and sanitation problems, with approximately 8 million people lacking access to water and/or sanitation (PAHO, 2010b). Acute diarrheal disease was highly prevalent, and tuberculosis had the highest incidence in the Americas and was the seventh leading cause of death. There was a 30% coinfection rate for TB and HIV; malaria, dengue, lymphatic filariasis, other vector-borne diseases, respiratory and intestinal infections, anemia, diabetes, and hypertension all contributed to a very high morbidity and mortality rate in Haiti. Accidents and assaults, particularly violence against women, were common, with women five times more likely than men to be killed in assaults (PAHO, 2010b). In addition, approximately 50% of the population lack access to general health care, and most often seek traditional healers. Immunization rates are extremely low for measles, diphtheria, pertussis and tetanus, and polio in children under one year, with neonatal tetanus a major public health problem (PAHO, 2010b).

After the earthquake, the CDC collaborated with the Haitian Ministry of Health, Catholic Relief Services—AIDSrelief, Partners in Health, and a local nongovernmental organization (NGO), GHESKIO, to address immediate public health needs. These included

> 1) eliminate mother-to-child transmission of HIV; 2) eliminate the threat of cholera; 3) eliminate lymphatic filariasis; 4) ensure a robust, sustainable, self-correcting public health system; 5) reduce the under-five mortality rate from vaccine-preventable diseases by 35%; 6) reduce maternal mortality by 30%; and 7) reduce the prevalence of TB by 25%. (CDC, 2013, p. 1)

Prevention efforts also included HIV, cholera, and water supply.

Six years later, rubble still litters some of the streets in Haiti, rebuilding is still progressing, and only a portion of the funds that were dedicated to the recovery have been spent. This underscores the hard reality of disaster throughout the world: recovery is difficult and can take huge amounts of time (e.g., nuclear disaster sites continue to be restricted areas in Chernobyl, and nuclear waste from World War II continues to haunt areas of the United States including Hanford Nuclear Reservation in the state of Washington and the city of Coldwater Creek, Missouri.

GLOBAL HEALTH AND HEALTH EQUITY

Global health has two main elements: (a) a focus on health from a worldwide perspective (as contrasted with multinational, national, or local) and (b) an overarching goal of health equity. The global disease burden and individual country disease burden can provide one perspective for global health; that is, what are the disease-specific problems that face the world and how do they differ from country to country? From a worldwide perspective, the leading causes of death are cardiovascular disease and cancer. However, these vary from country to country. Developing countries face additional challenges: high infant mortality rates, infectious diseases and sexually transmitted diseases, chronic diseases, aging populations, and a lack of infrastructure to address all of these challenges. With an increasingly mobile global population, infectious and communicable diseases can spread across the world before detection.

Simply stated, the lower an individual's socioeconomic status, the worse his or her health will be. Hence, the simplest definition of health equity is the "absence of systematic disparities in health (or in the major SDH) between social groups who have different levels of underlying social advantage/disadvantage" (Braveman & Gruskin, 2003, p. 254). To achieve health equity means that all individuals, regardless of social standing, have equal access to health care, good nutrition, healthy living environments, and effective disease prevention strategies. Therefore, health inequities are disparities in health (or its social determinants) that favor more advantaged socioeconomic groups. Health disparities (or health inequities) refer to differences between social groups, regional populations, and racial and ethnic groups. The notion of health disparity means the health of one group is worse in comparison with another group.

In discussing health inequities, people tend to try to fix these differences. Disparities focus more on health outcomes that differ, and perhaps a better focus is on health inequity. In any event, these terms have been used in a variety of ways, usually referring to factors that could be more equal, resulting in better health outcomes. However, figuring out health inequities requires monitoring health (i.e., health status) and health care (i.e., health services, resource allocation, financing, utilization, and quality). Hence, "monitoring equity" requires ongoing assessment of how different social groups fare in absolute terms and identifying the size of gaps between groups (Braveman, 1998, 2003), a sort of early warning system to bring attention to the effectiveness of health and health care services and policies. One could argue the national (U.S.) *Healthy People* and regional (European) *Health 2020* plans are monitoring equity, as the objectives of both initiatives are to improve population health and reduce health care disparities.

In 2005, the World Health Organization (WHO) established the Commission on Social Determinants of Health to promote health equity through a global agenda. To do so, the Commission determined key areas and necessary actions to address daily living conditions and the underlying structural, social, economic, and political drivers. The Commission (2008, p. 2) offered three basic principles and a framework to (a) improve the conditions of daily living; (b) tackle the inequitable distribution of power, money, and resources; and (c) measure and understand the problem and assess the impact of actions taken. Figure 3-1 offers an example of Diedrichsen et al.'s (2001) social production of disease model, upon which the SDH are based.

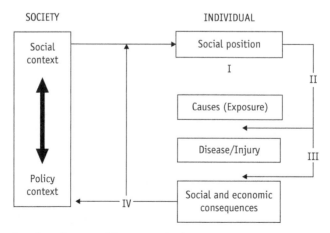

Figure 3-1. Social production of disease model (Diderichsen, Evans, & Whitehead, 2001).

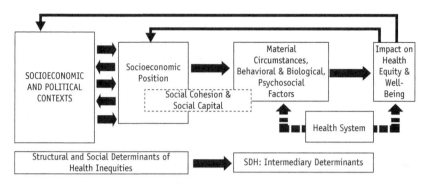

Figure 3-2. Committee on the Social Determinants of Health Final Framework (2007).

In 2016, the *2030 Agenda for Sustainable Development* was adopted by the United Nations, building upon the Millennium Development Goals of addressing extreme poverty (including income poverty, hunger, disease, lack of adequate shelter, and exclusion) and promoting gender equality, education, and environmental sustainability. Supported by the WHO (2016), the 17 Sustainable Development Goals and 169 targets of the agenda will address economic, social, and environmental actions over the next 15 years to end poverty, take action on climate change, and foster peaceful, just, and inclusive societies (United Nations General Assembly, 2015). As an example, the first three goals—(a) end poverty in all its forms everywhere; (b) end hunger, achieve food security and improved nutrition, and promote sustainable agriculture; and (c) ensure healthy lives and promote well-being for all at all ages—closely align with the focus of the SDH. Figure 3-2 offers a closer look at the factors involved in SDH and provides a way to visualize the social production of disease model and its relationships with the 17 Sustainable Development Goals and the SDH.

Although population based health promotion and disease prevention approaches are critical elements in creating, implementing, and sustaining global, regional, and national policy, these types of approaches may be very difficult to initiate, particularly in developing or resource-poor nations. The lack of comprehensive health information systems and the human resources to collect and operate such systems make it difficult for resource-poor countries to identify epidemiological profiles. However, epidemiological modeling approaches, such as burden of disease and risk factor analysis, have proven useful for developing countries (Bui et al., 2013; Nguyen et al., 2011).

Specific Problem Areas in Global Health

Global health includes broad categories that help to focus efforts on improving health. Maternal health, including pregnancy, childbirth, and maternal/perinatal nutritional issues would be one such category. Across all age groups, however, the reduction of specific diseases found worldwide, such as drug-resistant TB, malaria, polio, smallpox, and HIV/AIDS are examples of global health initiatives. Tobacco use and substance abuse would be other worldwide public health foci. As people live longer, chronic diseases become more prevalent as major public health issues.

INFANCY, CHILDHOOD, AND ADOLESCENCE

Malnutrition and suboptimum breastfeeding were the causes of 3.1 million child deaths, or 45% of all child deaths in 2011 (Black et al., 2013). Malnutrition, which includes fetal growth restriction, stunting, wasting, and vitamin and mineral deficiencies (e.g., vitamins A and D, iodine, iron, and zinc), increases the risk of neonatal deaths and increases the effect of every disease, including measles and malaria. Hence, one of the many public health issues in maternal and infant health is the emphasis on breastfeeding to avoid specific health risks from early weaning or the appeal of already prepared infant formula (Office of the Surgeon General, 2011). The WHO (2002a) recommends that mothers exclusively breastfeed their infants for the first six months of life, followed by "nutritionally adequate and safe complementary foods" while breastfeeding for up to two years of age or beyond. Early weaning can adversely affect the baby's immune system and may result in postpartum depression or failure to bond on the part of the mother. Formula feeding and early weaning are associated with poorer infant health, such as malnutrition (undernutrition) and increases in common childhood infections (e.g., diarrhea and ear infections).

Many childhood deaths are due to diarrheal diseases, respiratory tract infections, and malaria (Kyu et al., 2016). Mortality and Disability-Adjusted Life Year rates for lower respiratory tract infections and diarrheal diseases rank among the top five causes for deaths both in younger and older children in 2013 (Kyu et al., 2016). Five countries (India, Democratic Republic of the Congo, Pakistan, Nigeria, and Ethiopia) accounted for half of childhood deaths globally from diarrheal diseases. Lower respiratory tract infections, malaria, and diarrheal diseases were the leading causes of death in sub-Saharan countries (Kyu et al., 2016). These diseases are both preventable and treatable, yet they are part of the global health burden. Indeed, most of the 8 million deaths of children and adolescents in 2013 were avoidable (Kyu et al., 2016).

However, children and adolescents also suffer from Years Lost due to Disability (YLD) caused by disease. Iron deficiency anemia, for example, affected 619 million children and adolescents globally during 2013. Other major causes of YLDs were skin diseases, depressive disorders, low neck and back pain, conduct disorder, sense organ diseases, diarrheal diseases, anxiety disorders, migraine, and hemoglobinopathies (e.g., sickle cell anemia and thalassemia; Kyu et al., 2016). Diseases not treated during childhood and adolescence persist into adulthood and are causes of increased morbidity and mortality, as well creating more severe illnesses and more difficult to treat populations, as these children age into adulthood.

POLIOMYELITIS

In 1988, the WHO began its campaign to eradicate polio worldwide. More than 125 countries still had outbreaks of polio and an estimated 350,000 children were paralyzed annually by the disease (Aylward & Tangermann, 2011). By 2000, three WHO regions were certified polio-free (the Americas, the Western Pacific, and Europe).

During 2005 to 2011, in India, Nigeria, Pakistan, and Afghanistan, where eradication efforts had effectively stalled, a number of factors played a role in the continued transmission of polio. These included poor management of polio campaigns, less than effective polio vaccine effectiveness due to the high prevalence of diarrheal and non-polio enteroviruses, rumors that the vaccine induced sterility, migratory populations, the spread to previously polio-free countries, and the presence of continued conflict in some nations (Aylward & Tangermann, 2011).

The international community developed a number of strategies to overcome the final hurdles to eradication. One such strategy was the large-scale use of bivalent oral polio vaccine in supplementary immunization activities tailored to specific immunity thresholds within the infected areas, better planning for the polio campaigns, campaigns targeted to known routes of the polio transmission, and plans to address migrant and underserved populations (Aylward & Tangermann, 2011). By 2012, *wild polio* virus transmission was found only in Afghanistan and Nigeria. Then, in 2014, over 350 cases of *wild polio* virus in nine countries were reported, causing the WHO to call the spread of the *wild polio* virus "a public health emergency of international concern" (Hagan et al., 2015, p. 527).

In 2016, the Nigerian government confirmed that a circulating vaccine-derived polio virus type 2 (cVDPV2) was found in Maiduguri Municipal Council, Borno State, a security-compromised area in northeastern Nigeria (Etsano et al., 2016). Genetic variants of the vaccine viruses with the potential to cause paralysis, VDPVs are spread easily in areas with low population immunity. The Nigeria National Polio Emergency Operations Center initiated a number of emergency response measures. These included mass immunization campaigns for all children five years of age and under, increased surveillance for flaccid paralysis (AFP), and enhanced environmental surveillance for areas where cVDPV2 may flourish (e.g., sewage effluent sites, etc.). Over a million children were immunized and an additional 13 cases of AFP were identified (Etsano et al., 2016).

This is just one illustration of the public health issues that can occur in war-torn areas of a country, exposing limitations of existing surveillance systems, documenting low population immunity, and acknowledging risk of international contagion.

Solutions, such as targeted supplemental immunization activities and re-establishment of effective routine immunization activities to increase vaccination coverage, may be difficult to implement due to internal and cross-border conflicts, disruption of existing infrastructure, and lack of personnel. As with any infectious disease program, there should be a renewed focus on polio legacy planning, supporting routine immunization, introducing new vaccines, and strengthening national health infrastructure and services to reduce the possibility of new polio epidemics.

While finding the resources to vaccinate children around the world has been a challenge, the WHO continues to focus on the eradication of polio and the spread of polio to polio-free countries. Nevertheless, some groups oppose the introduction of Western ideas, including polio vaccinations, and see this as a very real symbol of things to avoid (Khan et al., 2015; Warraich, 2009). Consequently, there is opposition to what many would think is simply a way to prevent disease and help children grow into contributing adults in their societies.

MEASLES

Around the world, measles affects more than 20 million people each year (WHO, 2016), causing blindness, encephalitis, severe diarrhea, dehydration, and severe respiratory infections (e.g., pneumonia). Further, measles is one of the leading causes of death in children under five, especially in developing countries, which would include many countries in Africa.

Measles and childhood vaccination can provide a very important example of prevalence, incidence, and the role of social factors in preventing disease in populations. Measles vaccinations can prevent millions of deaths around the world, and the incidence of measles has declined significantly since 2000 (Perry et al., 2015). However, the fight against measles also shows how important social forces are in disease prevention (Flaherty, 2011).

A discredited study that linked the measles vaccine to autism (by Wakefield in 1998, retracted by *The Lancet* ["Retraction—Ileal-Lymphoid-Nodular Hyperplasia, Non-Specific Colitis, and Pervasive Developmental Disorder in Children," 2010]) had a devastating impact on vaccination rates, which dropped from 90% to 54% after the article was published. The controversy, generated by the 1998 Wakefield study, became a major public health issue in the United Kingdom (UK). In some areas of the UK, population immunity dropped significantly below herd immunity, which is the threshold above which sustained transmission is unlikely (measles >90%, rubella >85%; Burgess, Burgess, & Leask, 2006).

Further, outbreaks of measles and mumps occurred throughout the UK, and similar concerns were raised among providers in Australia and New Zealand as to the safety of the vaccine. Vaccination coverage gaps contribute to recent measles outbreaks and may represent a serious barrier for countries to maintain measles elimination status. The measles vaccination, approved in the United States in 1963, virtually eliminated measles in the country by 2000. However, a recent outbreak in the state of California, linked to attendance at Disneyland, was attributed again to the lack of vaccinations (Burgess et al., 2006; Diau et al., 2015; Scott et al., 2015; Wise, 2013).

Why the hesitancy to vaccinate? One explanation could be the public perception of risk, which is connected to two factors: hazard and outrage. Hazard is the scientific risk of morbidity or mortality; outrage is attributed to the factors surrounding an event that frighten, worry, or upset the public. The controversy surrounding the measles, mumps, and rubella (MMR) vaccine and autism is very similar to other scares, such as the pertussis vaccine controversy during the 1970s and 1980s that also occurred in Great Britain (Baker, 2003) The pertussis vaccine scare also resulted in a series of epidemics (whooping cough) across Britain, Europe, Japan, the United States, Russia, and Australia. Media exploitation exaggerated the vaccine's potential for harm and soft-pedaled the dangers of whooping cough itself. Parents became convinced that neurological damage would occur if their children were vaccinated. Prior to the routine vaccinations in the 1950s, an estimated 60% to 70% of British children had whooping cough, and over 9,000 infants and children died (Baker, 2003). Hence, between the public and the media, it took a significant amount of time and health education to address the safety of the pertussis and MMR vaccines and to bring the level of population immunity to previous levels.

Other reasons for the hesitancy to vaccinate may be religious or cultural beliefs that lead to exemptions from immunizations, lack of a national immunization program that reaches to all areas of a country, or failure to receive booster vaccinations. Any of these may be a factor when visiting a foreign country and/or entering into one's home country. There may be a lag between the time of infection and the subsequent presentation of symptoms. For those countries where infectious diseases, such as whooping cough or more recently Ebola, are not common, physicians may not recognize the symptoms as a specific disease until it is too late for the patient to receive appropriate countermeasures or the disease becomes a pandemic. On a final note, consider the balance between individual freedoms and the health of a population. Determining such a balance at a national or global level can present difficult choices.

TOBACCO CESSATION

Of all the potential ways to improve the health of a country, prevention of smoking in adolescents, encouraging the cessation of tobacco use as a secondary intervention, and using social forces such as prohibiting sale to those under 21 or increasing the locations that are smoke-free (including restaurants) could have a major impact on the health of the world. To do so requires both national and global plans. Resolution WHA48.11, adopted by the Forty-eighth World Health Assembly (1995), was the first instance of creating an international declaration on tobacco control. Eight years later, the WHO (2003) unanimously endorsed the Framework Convention on Tobacco Control (FCTC), which addressed both demand reduction strategies and supply-side concerns.

A number of international and regional organizations and NGOs were also developing prioritized agendas for global tobacco control (Baris et al., 2000; Stillman, Wipfli, Lando, Leischow, & Samet, 2005) with a population health focus. Developing national, regional, or global tobacco control research agendas that converge with a global goal of reducing tobacco use is extremely difficult. Such agendas must address infrastructure to address the issue, empirical evidence to substantiate the claim that tobacco cessation is central to improving national health outcomes, and the expertise and leadership skills to create a plan of action, determine a lead government agency for tobacco control, establish best practices and workforce development criteria, and prioritize a research agenda. The WHO endorses the *U.S. Public Health Service Guideline (PHS Guideline) on Treating Tobacco Use and Dependence* (Fiore et al., 2008). This meta-analysis of over 6,000 studies provides compelling evidence that tobacco cessation programs can increase smoking abstinence rates significantly, particularly the 5 As—asking all patients about tobacco use, advising smokers to quit, assessing readiness, providing assistance (e.g., counseling), and arranging follow-up—have been found to be very effective (Fiore et al., 2008).

Vietnam has one of the highest smoking rates in the world. Approximately 48% of the male adults smoke cigarettes (The World Bank, 2016b), and 28% of household food expenditures is spent on tobacco. Hoang Anh et al. (2014) estimate the total economic cost of smoking in 2011 was approximately 0.97% of the 2011 gross domestic product (24,679.9 billion Vietnamese dong [VND], equivalent to US$1,173.20). They further estimated the direct costs of inpatient at $9,896.2 billion VND (US$470.4 million) and outpatient care at $2,567.20 billion VND (US$122.0 million). Indirect costs (productivity loss due to morbidity and mortality) represent about 49.5% of the total costs of smoking ($2,652.9 billion VND [US$126.1 million] and $9,563.50 billion VND [US$454.60 million], respectively). Almost 6% of the 2011 government health care budget was spent on addressing these costs, approximately $4,534.3 billion VND (US$215.5 million; Hoang Anh et al., 2014).

To address its smoking as "epidemic," Vietnam adopted the FCTC in 2003, one of the first countries in the region to do so. A number of measures were adopted (Higashi, Khuong, Ngo, & Hill, 2011). By 2011, the Ministry of Health had drafted the Tobacco Harm Prevention Law using population-level interventions, including increases in excise taxes, warning labels on tobacco products, mass media campaigns, and legislatively mandated smoke-free areas (Higashi et al., 2011). The Reduce Smoking in Vietnam Partnership Project continued to build national tobacco control capacity in Vietnam, with four components of tobacco control that were key to the success of the project: (a) organizational structure/infrastructure, (b) leadership and expertise, (c) partnerships and networks, and (d) data and evidence from research (Stillman, David, Kibria, & Phan, 2014).

However, services to treat tobacco dependence are not readily accessible to smokers. In a survey of health care providers, including pharmacists, working in 23 community health centers in Vietnam, 23% of providers reported screening patients for tobacco use, 33% offered advice on how to quit, but less than 10% offered assistance to 50% or more of their patients during the past three months (Shelley, Nguyen, Pham, VanDevanter, & Nguyen, 2014).

As shown in this section, it is difficult to capture all of the factors that may affect population health, and it is even more difficult at times to issue blanket statements as to the role of pharmacists in the community and in health facilities. However, population and public health also are exacerbated by the SDH. Many of these forces often are beyond a simple solution, particularly as we examine the effects and forces of four areas: (a) aging, (b) poverty, (c) urbanization, and (d) globalization.

SOCIAL FORCES OF AGING, POVERTY, URBANIZATION

As the problem areas of global health change, some social forces will take on increasing importance while others will continue to play important roles in the public health picture. Poverty and lower socioeconomic status will continue to be associated with poorer health and increased health problems. This association can be found from early recorded history to today's health demographics (Lawrence, 1948; Stockwell, 1961; Warren & Hernandez, 2007). The aging world population is also changing world health to one of greater chronic diseases. As the population of the world continues to grow in the major cities, urbanization presents new challenges to the public health infrastructure and the provision of health care services, particularly with economic variability food insecurity, continued climate change, and the rise of chronic diseases (World Health Organization, 2010). Globalization also will lead to greater and more instantaneous access to information about the impact of medication use because of the larger numbers of technology adopters. However, globalization will also lead to an increase in the transmission of diseases due to increases in migration and immigration.

Aging
Over the past 100 years, we have seen an increasingly older population, with the significant rise in life expectancy in almost all regions of the world. Population aging may well be one of the most important social transformations of the 21st century and will affect many sectors of society, including housing, employment, health care delivery, infrastructure, and safety. The United Nations Department of Economic and Social Affairs Population Division (2015) estimates that by the year 2050, the global population of older persons will almost double in size to nearly 2.1 billion

persons. In addition, the number the "oldest old" (population above the age of 80 years) will number 434 million by 2050, triple the number of the oldest old in 2015 (125 million).

Further, the aging population has been greatly affected by industrialization and urbanization. The increasing prevalence of chronic diseases and their sequelae is becoming more common in developing countries, where the increase in the relative and absolute number of older persons has occurred more rapidly than in developed nations (United Nations Department of Economic and Social Affairs Population Division, 2015). For developing nations to adequately address the transition, an increasingly aged population will require a significant focus on primary prevention and adequate resource allocation. Many persons who survive to old age live in poverty. In the United States, almost 15% of adults ages 65 and older lived in poverty in 2014 (DeNavas-Walt & Proctor, 2015).

Poverty

Globally, approximately 13% (1 billion) of people lived in extreme poverty in 2012, roughly estimated at 551 million in Asia, 436 million in Africa, 15 million in South America, 5.9 million in North America, 0.3 million in Europe, and 50,000 in Oceania (The World Bank Group, 2016). Concurrently, the Food and Agriculture Organization of the United Nations (FAO, 2015) estimated that approximately one in nine persons suffered from chronic malnourishment across the globe during 2014–2016 (795 million people of 7.3 billion people). Of those, 780 million people (12.9%) who are malnourished live in developing countries; 11 million people who are malnourished live in developed countries (FAO, 2015).

The need for social protection programs is critical to address health and social issues that contribute to poverty and hunger. Social protection programs include social assistance (e.g., cash transfers, school meals, food stamps, and other targeted food assistance), social insurance and labor market programs (e.g., disability and/or old-age pensions, unemployment insurance, skills training, and wage subsidies), and supported housing and transportation. Although these programs account for only a small number of persons, ranging from 10% in low-income countries to 21% in lower middle income countries to 37% in upper middle income countries, these programs have been more successful in alleviating poverty than eliminating hunger.

The SDH literature suggest a number of reasons for the relationship(s) between disease and socioeconomic status, including poor nutrition, poor living environments, greater stress, fewer health care opportunities, and decreased access to health care services. Promoting health equity to reduce disparities and preventable deaths requires us to follow the WHO's lead to (a) improve the conditions of daily living; (b) tackle the inequitable distribution of power, money, and resources; and (c) measure and understand the problem and assess the impact of actions taken (Commission on Social Determinants of Health, 2008). Eliminating poverty, for example, brings significant challenges for society in the context of public health. Those with fewer resources are often less able to provide the public health environment they need. Similarly, deciding to use one's resources to improve the health of a nation requires an enlightened understanding of the value of public health.

Urbanization

The WHO (2010, p. 2) describes as "alarming" the growth of urban centers with heavily concentrated pockets of poverty. As people flock to major cities, governments have been unable to create and maintain essential infrastructures (e.g., health, education, housing, transportation, and safety) to make life livable for increasingly large numbers of urban residents who often bring untreated diseases and disabilities from rural and frontier areas. Slums and squatter settlements are overcrowded, unsafe, unsanitary, built in areas that are prone to natural disasters (e.g., floods, landsides, waste sites), and have increased health risks from environmental hazards, violence and crime, injuries, infectious diseases, and mental illnesses.

The WHO (2010) estimates that 32% of urban dwellers in developing countries lack access to improved sanitation (sewer, septic, compost or covered pit), and many poor urban dwellers may have shared sanitation or access only in public areas (Heijnen, Rosa, Fuller, Eisenberg, & Clasen, 2014).

Even though over 90% of urban dwellers in developing countries have access to a source of water within 1 kilometer of their dwelling, there remains concern over water storage and supply practices (WHO, 2010), especially with use of spring water, tap water, surface water, and grey water from contaminated ground soil (Katukiza, Ronteltap, van der Steen, Foppen, & Lens, 2014). Further, vector-borne and zoonotic pathogens, especially rodent-borne, are common among urban homeless and marginalized people, in the United States and Europe, as well as in developing countries (Leibler, Zakhour, Gadhoke, & Gaeta, 2016).

Finally, there are health inequities for urban dwellers, with intraurban differences that encompass more than life expectancy and child mortality. In Glasgow, Scotland, males will live on average almost 30 years longer (82 years) if they live in Lenzie, East Dunbartonshire rather than in Carlton (54 years; Commission on Social Determinants of Health, 2008). In Nairobi, Kenya, the mortality rate for children who live in the Embakasi slum is 254 per 1,000; the average mortality rate for Nairobi is 62 per 1,000 (Knowledge Network on Urban Settings, 2008).

Both rural and urban areas provide public health challenges. Rural areas, whether in the United States or elsewhere, continue to have challenges with access to care. The clinic is a long walk from home, the medications that can be dispensed are limited in choice and quantity, and the providers may be visitors rather than local residents. Nevertheless, the growth of urban public health concerns continues to be one of the cornerstones of public health around the world. Placing many people together creates (safe) drinking water issues, waste disposal challenges, and the potential for the rapid spread of infectious diseases. As the world shrinks in terms of time/travel, these urban issues are global, creating public health problems all of us must address.

Globalization

Globalization is not a new concept. Scholte (2000, pp. 15–17) argues there are at least five broad definitions of the term. Within the context of internationalization, globalization describes cross-border relations between countries, which encourage international exchange and interdependence. Globalization also can be seen as a loosening of government-imposed restrictions on movements between countries to create a more open or borderless world economy, such as we see in the creation of the European Union (EU). Globalization is often seen as universalization, such as radio, television, and now the Internet spreads knowledge, experiences, and objects across the world. Globalization is seen as Westernization or modernization where certain social or political structures are spread throughout the world. Finally, globalization is "supraterritoriality," where the notion of transworld or transborder relations brings home the concept of globalization. Within these many definitions of globalization, issues of public health and population health are found, as in the case of Ebola.

CASE STUDY: EBOLA

The challenges of Ebola control in West Africa, and the impact of this disease internationally, is one example of how global health both affects and is affected by the consequences of national and global policies. Control of travel, fear of disease, use of quarantine, lack of resources, and media are just a few elements that play out in this case study.

In 1976, cases of Ebola were first reported in Zaire, Gabon, and the Sudan, Africa (CDC, 2016c). In the UK, there was a reported case (no fatality) of Ebola due to a contaminated needle stick in a laboratory. In 1989, the *Reston ebolavirus*, a form of Ebola not lethal to humans, was introduced into the United States by macaques imported from the Philippines. Almost 20 years later, in 1995, Ebola broke out again in the Democratic Republic of the Congo, and one death from Ebola was reported in a Russian lab.

During 2000–2004, outbreaks were reported in Gabon, the Republic of the Congo, South Sudan, and Uganda (CDC, 2016b). By 2007, a new strain of Ebola was reported in Uganda, and Ebola was again reported in the Democratic Republic of the Congo and Uganda in 2012. In 2014, Ebola was again reported in the Democratic Republic of the Congo and in West Africa (CDC, 2016b).

Until then, the largest number of cases reported in any one outbreak was 424, with the largest number of deaths at 280. However, the outbreak in West Africa was the largest outbreak in history, with over 28,639 suspected, probable, and confirmed cases and over 11,316 deaths across the countries of Guinea, Liberia, and Sierra Leone, with additional cases reported in Nigeria, Senegal, Mali, Spain, the

United Kingdom, Italy, and the United States (WHO, 2015a). More than 17,300 children were estimated to be orphaned due to the Ebola outbreak (CDC, 2016a).

There were 881 confirmed health care professional infections reported in Guinea, Liberia, and Sierra Leone, with 513 reported deaths (WHO, 2015a). Of the doctors, nurses, and midwives lost to Ebola, Guinea lost 1% (78), Liberia lost 8% (83), and Sierra Leone lost 7% (79; Evans, Goldstein, & Popova, 2015). Due to the loss of these health care professionals, The World Bank estimates that maternal mortality alone will increase by 38% in Guinea, 74% in Sierra Leone, and as much as 111% in Liberia, with over 4,000 women estimated to die per year World Bank Group (2014). When combined with the estimated mortality of infants (6,700) and children under the age of five (14,100), an additional 24,900 people could die as a consequence of Ebola (Evans et al., 2015).

The Ebola epidemic also affected access to health care across Guinea, Liberia, and Sierra Leone for other infectious and communicable diseases. It is estimated an additional 10,600 lives were lost to persons with HIV, tuberculosis, and malaria (Parpia, Ndeffo-Mbah, Wenzel, & Galvani, 2016). Routine vaccinations for infectious and communicable diseases were reduced as much as 30% as efforts were redirected to address the Ebola epidemic, which may increase morbidity and mortality from other diseases (Takahashi et al., 2015).

In addition to the impact of Ebola on the health care systems in Guinea, Liberia, and Sierra Leone, The World Bank (2014) projected an estimated $2.2 billion was lost in 2015 in the gross domestic product of the three countries.

Medication Safety and Pharmacovigilance

Pharmacovigilance (PV) is not only a global issue but has the global potential to improve health care considerably. The adverse effects of thalidomide that gained worldwide prominence in the late 1950s and early 1960s were considered the turning point regarding the need to monitor the effects of pharmaceuticals globally. The definition of PV spans public health, population health, and pharmacy practice (WHO, 2006). The WHO (2002b, 2006) uses the term to refer to the detection, assessment, understanding, and prevention of adverse effects or other drug-related problems. The International Pharmaceutical Federation/Fédération Internationale Pharmaceutique sees the foundation of PV as monitoring the use of medications, after initial approval, for safety and effectiveness (International Pharmaceutical Federation, 2006).

Why the emphasis on PV? The answer is simple: to reduce the number of adverse events that occur during any form of pharmaceutical treatment, whether they are serious reportable events (SRE), adverse drug events (ADE), or an adverse drug reaction (ADR). An SRE is a preventable, serious, and unambiguous *adverse event* that should never occur. An ADE is any unexpected medical occurrence that may present during treatment with a pharmaceutical product. An ADR is an unwanted, undesirable effect of a medication that occurs during usual clinical use. An ADE differs from an ADR in that the former may not be part of a causal relationship between the treatment and the drug, whereas an ADR is a causal effect. SREs often have ADEs and ADRs as a component of an adverse event, so reporting as much information as possible about the event is critical to improving patient care and outcomes. Since an SRE is clearly identifiable and measurable, information about an SRE is important to have in a reporting system. Because the risk of occurrence is more likely to occur based on a health care facility's policies and procedures, SREs are of interest to public and health care professionals and providers (National Quality Forum, 2011).

A systematic review of research on pharmacy dispensing errors, with data from Australia, Brazil, Denmark, Spain, and the UK, found the incidence of dispensing errors in community pharmacies ranged between 0.01% and 3.32% and the error incidence in hospital pharmacies ranged between 0.02% and 2.7% (James et al., 2009). The incidence of dispensing errors varied depending on the study setting, dispensing system, research method, and operational definitions (James et al., 2009). Other systematic reviews of medication errors in the Middle East and Asia report finding little literature on the topic or studies of poor quality (Alsulami, Conroy, & Choonara, 2013; Salmasi, Khan, Hong, Ming, & Wong, 2015), while reports from Africa indicate a growing use of PV with the need for better pediatric and geriatric pharmacovigilance as well as for herbal/traditional remedies (Isah, Pal, Olsson, Dodoo, & Bencheikh, 2012).

Further, the costs associated with adverse and preventable drug reactions adversely affect patients' lifespans and quality of life and reduce confidence in the ability of local, state, and national health care providers and systems to provide appropriate patient care.

UNITED STATES

Within the United States, preventable medication errors were estimated to affect more than 7 million patients, contribute to 7,000 deaths, cost nearly $21 billion in direct medical costs across all health care settings annually, and are the third leading cause of death in America. Injectable medications have among the highest risks for error by health personnel and result in the most severe harms for patients (Kale, Keohane, Maviglia, Gandhi, & Poon, 2012). In 2000, the Institute of Medicine estimated that one medication error occurred per patient per day in hospital care (Kohn, Corrigan, & Donaldson, 2000). More recent studies report that up to one of five medication doses are associated with an error and that between 3% and 7% of these errors are potentially harmful to patients (Poon et al., 2010), with half of patients experiencing one or more preventable adverse events that resulted in an extended hospital stay, permanent harm, a life-sustaining intervention, or death (Levinson, 2010).

In the United States, the FDA has responsibility for two postmarketing safety surveillance programs that allow for both voluntary and mandated reporting: the FDA Adverse Event Reporting System (FAERS) and the Vaccine Adverse Event Reporting System (VAERS). The FAERS surveils all approved drug and therapeutic biologic products submitted to the FDA; the VAERS is a vaccine safety surveillance program cosponsored by the CDC and the FDA. The Federal Food, Drug, and Cosmetic Act (21 U.S.C. §§355b) of 1938 and the National Childhood Vaccine Injury Act (42 U.S.C. §§300aa-1-aa-34) of 1986 requires health professionals and vaccine manufacturers to report to the U.S. Department of Health and Human Services all specific adverse events that occur after the administration of routinely recommended drugs, devices, and vaccines.

Certified as a Patient Safety Organization by the U.S. Agency for Healthcare Research and Quality, the Institute for Safe Medication Practices' National Medication Errors Reporting Program is a voluntary practitioner error-reporting program that annually receives hundreds of error reports from health care professionals. The National Coordinating Council for Medication Error Reporting and Prevention (NCC MERP), formed in 1995, manages the National Alert Network and the National Medication Errors Reporting Program. In addition, the NCC-MERP Index, a standard taxonomy that classifies an error according to the severity of the outcome, is used by a number of hospitals and health care providers as a decision algorithm.

In the United States, surprisingly, only 27 states (out of 50) and the District of Columbia have state adverse event reporting systems to collect information from hospitals and/or other health care facilities about adverse medical events resulting in patient death or serious harm (Hanlon, Sheedy, Taylor Kniffin, & Rosenthal, 2015). However, they use indicators from the National Quality Forum's (2011) *Serious Reportable Events in Healthcare* to facilitate uniform, comparable public reporting to improve patient safety and health systems. Two events pertain to pharmaceuticals that cause patient death or serious injury: Product or Device Events and Care Management Events. The first pertains to use of contaminated drugs, devices, or biologics; the second is associated with medication error (i.e., "wrong drug, wrong dose, wrong patient, wrong time, wrong rate, wrong preparation, or wrong route of administration"; National Quality Forum, 2011, p. 9).

EUROPEAN UNION

In the EU, legislation requires information on medication errors to be collected and reported through national PV systems. In addition, EU regulations ensure harmonization of safety standards on medicines licensed by EU members and establish fees for PV work on centrally approved products. Regulatory agencies and pharmaceutical companies participate in an EU-wide medicines regulatory network coordinated by the European Medicines Agency (EMA). EMA is responsible for the operation of the EudraVigilance system, which has analyzed information on suspected adverse reactions to medicines authorized in the European Economic Area since 2001. EMA's Pharmacovigilance Risk Assessment Committee manages the pharmacovigilance process through the use of periodic safety update reports (PSURs), postauthorization safety studies (PASS), and referrals (European Medicines Agency, 2016). PSURs are risk-benefit medicine evaluations submitted at stipulated intervals by drug companies. PASSs generally characterize safety hazards or describe the effectiveness of risk management activities. Referrals are conducted to resolve concerns about the benefit-risk balance of specific medicines or combinations of medicines when there are disagreements among members (EMA, 2016).

In 2015, the EMA and the Heads of Medicines Agencies endorsed a good practice guide to reduce medication errors. The practice guide is divided into two main parts. The first part clarifies specific issues related to recording, coding, reporting, and assessment of medication errors (EMA, 2015a). The second part examines key principles of risk management planning, describes the primary sources and categories of medication errors, and recommends actions to minimize the risk of these errors throughout the product life cycle (EMA, 2015b). In addition, the EMA coordinates the European Database of Suspected Adverse Drug Reaction Reports, which is publicly available through http://www.adrreports.eu/.

WORLD HEALTH ORGANIZATION

Since the formation of the WHO Programme for International Drug Monitoring in 1961, the WHO actively promotes PV at the country level with the intent to improve patient care and patient safety with regard to the use of medicines. The WHO also ensures local, state, national, and regional public health programs/systems have the resources and information they need to enhance population health (WHO, 2014). Since the Uppsala Monitoring Centre (UMC) has managed VigiBase®, the WHO's global individual case safety report (ICSR) database contains over 12 million records and entries from 123 countries (Lundin, 2016). In 2005, the World Alliance for Patient Safety (2005) published the *WHO Draft Guidelines for Adverse Event Reporting and Learning Systems* to help countries develop or advance reporting and learning systems for patient safety.

Since that time, a number of initiatives help nations develop, improve, and maintain PV systems. The UMC, for example, has been actively promoting the international ICSR standard exchange format, the International Conference on Harmonization E2B (ICH E2B), which contains all relevant data fields to allow for a comprehensive medical analysis of the data. However, for developing countries with limited resources who are entering the PV program, the UMC created an ICRS data management tool that allows these countries to use the ICH E2B format.

Another initiative was the 2009–2013 Monitoring Medicines project funded by the FP-7 EU framework with 11 consortium partners from Europe (Sweden, UK, Denmark, Netherlands, Switzerland), Africa (Ghana, Kenya, Morocco), and Asia (Philippines; Pal, Olsson, & Brown, 2015). Stakeholders included the WHO, drug regulators, pharmacovigilance centers, consumers, public health and disease specialists, and patient safety networks. Two of its objectives were to "support and strengthen consumer reporting of suspected ADRs" and "develop additional pharmacovigilance methods to complement data from spontaneous reporting systems" (Pal et al., 2015, p. 320). A prototype web-based consumer reporting tool, compliant with the ICH E2B standard format for electronic data exchange, was developed successfully and is available as a free add-on module for all current users of VigiFlow® ICSR management system (a component of VigiBase®) in more than 60 countries.

A second prototype interface was created to use a standard ADR terminology in the PV centers. This involved a reworking of the WHO-ART subject terms into new term classes (System Organs), a graphical display to allow searching by anatomical site, and the ability to map terms to lowest level terms in the Medical Dictionary for Regulatory Activities (MedDRA). MedDRA-preferred terms were selected to identify substandard or falsified medicines (Pal et al., 2015).

Participants also suggested the use of cohort event monitoring (CEM) and targeted spontaneous reporting (TSR) for long-term use in populations with specified diseases (Pal, Duncombe, Falzon, & Olsson, 2013). CEM requires the reporting of all adverse events within a cohort of patients identified as having received treatment with a specific drug. TSR captures adverse drug reactions in a well-defined group of patients on a specific long-term treatment regimen. Both are based on the premise that patients who receive repeated follow-ups at the same health facility during long-term treatment would be monitored routinely for suspected ADRs (Pal et al., 2013).

International Development of Pharmaceuticals, Drug Counterfeiting, and a Culture of Corruption

The international development of pharmaceuticals and the world market for medications of all types has led to counterfeiting of products, patent law failure, and a culture of corruption. The technology to make medications that appear identical to trade-name drugs is available around the world and is used to make drugs that may or may not contain the active ingredients advertised. In some of the countries with larger manufacturing capabilities, patents are ignored and the medication is copied and produced despite patents by the international drug company that has rights to the product. These drugs, too, can become part of the supply of counterfeit products.

In addition to this kind of illegal behavior, corruption in the international drug manufacturing industry is a significant and costly part of the global scene. With so much potential for profit, influence can be purchased for a price, drug research studies can be unreliable, and drug claims for success can be exaggerated or can ignore dangerous side effects. Placing this in perspective, the capability of an individual in a developing country who is purchasing medication on a tablet by tablet basis to make a careful analysis of the product that is being sold is minimal and the potential for abuse of this market is great.

Implications for Public Health and Pharmacy Practice

Global health is an integral part of the broader public health field. There will be an increasing need for pharmacists who understand both the local and global impact of public health on their individual health and the health of their communities. Public health pharmacists also can help to address health inequities and disparities, as the pharmacist may be the only resident health practitioner in his or her particular community.

From national, regional, and global perspectives, there are a number of recurrent themes that affect the development of public health policy. These include issues surrounding standardized and comparable data and adequate capacity for research in health and non-health related areas (e.g., policy, economics). Without adequate descriptive or analytic data, it is difficult to create a unifying public health and/or social agenda for identified public health concerns. Further, to build a comprehensive research agenda and internal and external partnerships requires a great deal of financial and human resources. As shown in the projects noted in this chapter, there are a number of models to develop national strategies, policies, and programs to address public health concerns.

We know that infectious and vaccine-preventable diseases among children and adolescents remain major challenges in developing nations. If the children survive to adulthood, the burden of disability and years lived with a disability increase substantially, resulting in significant economic costs to the individual, the public, and the nation, hence the need for strong prevention and intervention foci to establish and sustain effective public health and medical treatment.

We are also facing advances in medicine and pharmacy that can radically change public health practice. The growing acceptance of herbal and indigenous medicine as part of conventional practice is one such example, as are the expanding use of biogenetic drugs and DNA knowledge around the world. The continued focus on the importance of community-based pharmacists, especially as part of medical/patient-centered homes and as prevention/intervention practitioners, is reflected across the global literature.

The fundamental topics of public health have seemingly changed over time but actually they remain the same. Safe drinking water was important in England in the 1800s; infectious diseases are still problematic today. Chronic illnesses are on the rise due to development and unhealthy behaviors, and local health problems are now international health problems, such as AIDS, SARSs and H1N1. Trying to figure out what is next will take many more pages than we have available in this chapter. However, public health and pharmacy practice are central components of national, regional, and global policy and health practice.

References

Alsulami, Z., Conroy, S., & Choonara, I. (2013). Medication errors in the Middle East countries: A systematic review of the literature. *European Journal of Clinical Pharmacology*, 69(4), 995–1008. doi:10.1007/s00228-012-1435-y

Aylward, B., & Tangermann, R. (2011). The global polio eradication initiative: Lessons learned and prospects for success. *Vaccine*, 29(Suppl. 4), D80–D85. doi:10.1016/j.vaccine.2011.10.005

Baker, J. P. (2003). The pertussis vaccine controversy in Great Britain, 1974–1986. *Vaccine*, 21(25–26), 4003–4010.

Baris, E., Brigden, L. W., Prindiville, J., da Costa e Silva, V. L., Chitanondh, H., & Chandiwana, S. (2000). Research priorities for tobacco control in developing countries: A regional approach to a global consultative process. *Tobacco Control*, 9(2), 217–223.

Black, R. E., Victora, C. G., Walker, S. P., Bhutta, Z. A., Christian, P., de Onis, M., . . . Uauy, R. (2013). Maternal and child undernutrition and overweight in low-income and middle-income countries. *The Lancet*, 382(9890), 427–451. doi:10.1016/s0140-6736(13)60937-x

Braveman, P. (1998). *Monitoring equity in health: A policy-oriented approach in low- and middle-income countries* (WHO/CHS/HSS/98.1). Geneva, Switzerland: World Health Organization. Retrieved from http://apps.who.int/iris/bitstream/10665/65228/1/WHO_CHS_HSS_98.1.pdf

Braveman, P. (2003). Monitoring equity in health and healthcare: A conceptual framework. *Journal of Health, Population, and Nutrition*, 21(3), 181–192.

Braveman, P., & Gruskin, S. (2003). Defining equity in health. *Journal of Epidemiology & Community Health*, 57(4), 254–258.

Bui, L. N., Nguyen, N. T. T., Tran, L. K., Vos, T., Norman, R., & Nguyen, H. T. (2013). Risk factors of burden of disease: A comparative assessment study for evidence-based health policy making in Vietnam. *The Lancet*, 381, S23. doi:10.1016/S0140-6736(13)61277-5

Burgess, D. C., Burgess, M. A., & Leask, J. (2006). The MMR vaccination and autism controversy in United Kingdom 1998–2005: Inevitable community outrage or a failure of risk communication? *Vaccine*, 24(18), 3921–3928. doi:10.1016/j.vaccine.2006.02.033

Centers for Disease Control and Prevention. (1999). Achievements in public health, 1900–1999: Decline in deaths from heart disease and stroke—United States, 1900–1999. *MMWR: Morbidity and Mortality Weekly*, 48(30), 649–656.

Centers for Disease Control and Prevention. (2013). *CDC in Haiti*. Atlanta, GA: Author. Retrieved from http://www.cdc.gov/globalhealth/countries/haiti/pdf/haiti.pdf

Centers for Disease Control and Prevention. (2016a). *Cost of the Ebola epidemic.* Atlanta, GA: Author. Retrieved from http://www.cdc.gov/vhf/ebola/outbreaks/2014-west-africa/cost-of-ebola.html

Centers for Disease Control and Prevention. (2016b). *Ebola outbreaks 2000–2014.* Atlanta, GA: Author. Retrieved from http://www.cdc.gov/vhf/ebola/outbreaks/history/summaries.html

Centers for Disease Control and Prevention. (2016c). *Outbreaks chronology: Ebola virus disease.* Atlanta, GA: Author. Retrieved from http://www.cdc.gov/vhf/ebola/outbreaks/history/chronology.html

Commission on Social Determinants of Health. (2007). *A conceptual framework for action on the social determinants of health: Discussion paper for the Commission on Social Determinants of Health: Draft.* Geneva, Switzerland: World Health Organization.

Commission on Social Determinants of Health. (2008). *Closing the gap in a generation: Health equity through action on the social determinants of health.* Geneva, Switzerland: World Health Organization. Retrieved from http://apps.who.int/iris/bitstream/10665/43943/1/9789241563703_eng.pdf

DeNavas-Walt, C., & Proctor, B. D. (2015, September). *Income and poverty in the United States: 2014* (Current Population Reports, P60-252). Washington, DC: U.S. Census Bureau. Retrieved from http://www.census.gov/content/dam/Census/library/publications/2015/demo/p60-252.pdf

Diau, J., Jimuru, C., Asugeni, J., Asugeni, L., Puia, M., Maomatekwa, J., . . . Massey, P. D. (2015). Measles outbreak investigation in a remote area of Solomon Islands, 2014. *Western Pacific Surveillance and Response Journal, 6*(3), 17–21. doi:10.5365/wpsar.2015.6.2.001

Diderichsen, F., Evans, T., & Whitehead, M. (2001). The social basis of disparities in health. In T. Evans, M. Whitehead, F. Diderichsen, A. Bhuiya, & M. Wirth (Eds.), *Challenging inequities in health* (pp. 13–23). New York, NY: Oxford University Press.

Etsano, A., Damisa, E., Shuaib, F., Nganda, G. W., Enemaku, O., Usman, S., . . . Wiesen, E. (2016). Environmental isolation of circulating vaccine-derived poliovirus after interruption of wild poliovirus transmission—Nigeria, 2016. *MMWR: Morbidity & Mortality Weekly Report, 65*(30), 770–773. doi:10.15585/mmwr.mm6530a4

European Medicines Agency. (2015a). *Good practice guide on recording, coding, reporting and assessment of medication errors* (EMA/762563/2014). London: Author. Retrieved from http://www.ema.europa.eu/docs/en_GB/document_library/Regulatory_and_procedural_guideline/2015/11/WC500196981.pdf

European Medicines Agency. (2015b). *Good practice guide on risk minimisation and prevention of medication errors* (EMA/606103/2014). London: Author. Retrieved from http://www.ema.europa.eu/docs/en_GB/document_library/Regulatory_and_procedural_guideline/2015/11/WC500196981.pdf

European Medicines Agency. (2016). *Pharmacovigilance.* London: Author. Retrieved from http://www.ema.europa.eu/ema/index.jsp?curl=pages/regulation/general/general_content_000258.jsp&mid=WC0b01ac05800241de

Evans, D. K., Goldstein, M., & Popova, A. (2015, July). *The next wave of deaths from Ebola? The impact of health care worker mortality.* New York, NY: World Bank Group.

Fiore, M., Jaén, C. R., Baker, T. B., Bailey, W. C., Benowitz, N. L., Curry, S. J., . . . Wewers, M. E. (2008). *Treating tobacco use and dependence: 2008 update.* Rockville, MD: U.S. Department of Health and Human Services, Public Health Service. Retrieved from http://www.ncbi.nlm.nih.gov/books/NBK63952/

Flaherty, D. K. (2011). The vaccine-autism connection: A public health crisis caused by unethical medical practices and fraudulent science. *The Annals of Pharmacotherapy, 45*(10), 1302–1304. doi:10.1345/aph.1Q318

Food and Agriculture Organization of the United Nations, International Fund for Agricultural Development, & World Food Program. (2015). *The state of food insecurity in the world*

2015: Meeting the 2015 international hunger targets: Taking stock of uneven progress. Rome, Italy: Authors. Retrieved from http://www.fao.org/3/a4ef2d16-70a7-460a-a9ac-2a65a533269a/i4646e.pdf

Forty-eighth World Health Assembly. (1995). WHA48.11: An international strategy for tobacco control. Geneva, Switzerland: World Health Organization. Retrieved from http://www.who.int/tobacco/framework/wha_eb/wha48_11/en/

Gelting, R., Bliss, K., Patrick, M., Lockhart, G., & Handzel, T. (2013). Water, sanitation and hygiene in Haiti: Past, present, and future. The American Journal of Tropical Medicine and Hygiene, 89(4), 665–670. doi:10.4269/ajtmh.13-0217

Hagan, J. E., Wassilak, S. G., Craig, A. S., Tangermann, R. H., Diop, O. M., Burns, C. C., & Quddus, A. (2015). Progress toward polio eradication: Worldwide, 2014–2015. MMWR: Morbidity & Mortality Weekly Report, 64(19), 527–531.

Hanlon, C., Sheedy, K., Taylor Kniffin, T., & Rosenthal, J. (2015, January). 2014 guide to state adverse event reporting systems. Portland, ME; Washington, DC: National Academy for State Health Policy. Retrieved from http://www.nashp.org/sites/default/files/2014_Guide_to_State_Adverse_Event_Reporting_Systems.pdf

Heijnen, M., Rosa, G., Fuller, J., Eisenberg, J. N., & Clasen, T. (2014). The geographic and demographic scope of shared sanitation: An analysis of national survey data from low- and middle-income countries. Tropical Medicine & International Health, 19(11), 1334–1345. doi:10.1111/tmi.12375

Henry K. Kaiser Family Foundation. (2016, March). The U.S. government and global tuberculosis efforts. Menlo Park, CA: Author. Retrieved from http://kff.org/global-health-policy/fact-sheet/the-u-s-government-and-global-tuberculosis-efforts/

Higashi, H., Khuong, T. A., Ngo, A. D., & Hill, P. S. (2011). Population-level approaches to universal health coverage in resource-poor settings: Lessons from tobacco control policy in Vietnam. MEDICC Review, 13(3), 39–42.

Hoang Anh, P. T., Thu, L. T., Ross, H., Quynh Anh, N., Linh, B. N., & Minh, N. T. (2014). Direct and indirect costs of smoking in Vietnam. Tobacco Control. doi:10.1136/tobaccocontrol-2014-051821

Institute for Health Metrics and Evaluation. (2015). GBD [Global Burden of Disease] compare: Table: Haiti, Both sexes, all ages, 2010, DALYS. Retrieved from: http://vizhub.healthdata.org/gbd-compare/

International Pharmaceutical Federation. (2006). FIP statement of policy: The role of the pharmacist in pharmacovigilance The Hague, The Netherlands: Author. Retrieved from http://fip.org/www/uploads/database_file.php?id=273&table_id=

Isah, A. O., Pal, S. N., Olsson, S., Dodoo, A., & Bencheikh, R. S. (2012). Specific features of medicines safety and pharmacovigilance in Africa. Therapeutic Advances in Drug Safety, 3(1), 25–34. doi:10.1177/2042098611425695

James, K. L., Barlow, D., McArtney, R., Hiom, S., Roberts, D., & Whittlesea, C. (2009). Incidence, type and causes of dispensing errors: A review of the literature. The International Journal of Pharmacy Practice, 17(1), 9–30.

Kale, A., Keohane, C. A., Maviglia, S., Gandhi, T. K., & Poon, E. G. (2012). Adverse drug events caused by serious medication administration errors. BMJ Quality & Safety, 21(11), 933–938. doi:10.1136/bmjqs-2012-000946

Katukiza, A. Y., Ronteltap, M., van der Steen, P., Foppen, J. W., & Lens, P. N. (2014). Quantification of microbial risks to human health caused by waterborne viruses and bacteria in an urban slum. Journal of Applied Microbiology, 116(2), 447–463. doi:10.1111/jam.12368

Khan, M. U., Ahmad, A., Aqeel, T., Salman, S., Ibrahim, Q., Idrees, J., & Khan, M. U. (2015). Knowledge, attitudes and perceptions towards polio immunization among residents of two highly affected regions of Pakistan. BMC Public Health, 15, 1100. doi:10.1186/s12889-015-2471-1

Knowledge Network on Urban Settings. (2008). Our cities, our health, our future. Report to the WHO Commission on Social Determinants of Health from the Knowledge Network on Urban Settings.

Kobe, Japan: WHO Centre for Health Development. Retrieved from http://www.who.int/social_determinants/resources/knus_final_report_052008.pdf

Kohn, L. T., Corrigan, J. M., & Donaldson, M. S. (Eds.). (2000). *To err is human: Building a safer health system.* Washington, DC: National Academies Press.

Kyu, H. H., Pinho, C., Wagner, J. A., Brown, J. C., Bertozzi-Villa, A., Charlson, F. J., . . . Vos, T. (2016). Global and national burden of diseases and injuries among children and adolescents between 1990 and 2013: Findings from the Global Burden of Disease 2013 study. *JAMA Pediatrics, 170*(3), 267–287. doi:10.1001/jamapediatrics.2015.4276

Lawrence, P. S. (1948). Chronic illness and socioeconomic status. *Public Health Reports, 63*(47), 1507–1521.

Leibler, J. H., Zakhour, C. M., Gadhoke, P., & Gaeta, J. M. (2016). Zoonotic and vector-borne infections among urban homeless and marginalized people in the United States and Europe, 1990–2014. *Vector Borne and Zoonotic Diseases, 16*(7), 435–444. doi:10.1089/vbz.2015.1863

Levinson, D. R. (2010November). *Adverse events in hospitals: National incidence among Medicare beneficiaries* (OEI-06-09-00090). Washington, DC: U.S. Department of Health and Human Services, Office of Inspector General. Retrieved from https://oig.hhs.gov/oei/reports/oei-06-09-00090.pdf

Lundin, T. (2016). Positive trends for Vigibase: 12 million reports & counting. *Uppsala Reports, 71*, 14–15. Retrieved from http://www.who-umc.org/graphics/34744.pdf.

National Center for Health Statistics. (2016). *Leading causes of death.* Atlanta, GA: Centers for Disease Control and Prevention. Retrieved from http://www.cdc.gov/nchs/fastats/leading-causes-of-death.htm

National Quality Forum. (2011). *Serious reportable events in healthcare: 2011 update: A consensus report.* Washington, DC: Author. Retrieved from https://www.qualityforum.org/Publications/2011/12/SRE_2011_Final_Report.aspx

Nguyen, N. T. T., Long, T. K., Linh, B. N., Vos, T., Anh, N. D., & Huong, N. T. (2011). *Vietnam burden of disease and injury study 2008.* (Vietnam Evidence for Health Policy [VINE] Project). Brisbane, Australia; Hanoi, Vietnam: School of Population Health, University of Queensland; Hanoi School of Public Health, Ministry of Health (VN). Retrieved from http://library.hsph.edu.vn/sites/library.hsph.edu.vn/files/Ganh%20nang%20benh%20tat%20va%20chan%20thuong%20o%20VN-Eng_0.pdf

Office of the Surgeon General. (2011). *The Surgeon General's call to action to support breastfeeding.* Rockville, MD: Author. Retrieved from http://www.ncbi.nlm.nih.gov/books/NBK52682/

Pal, S. N., Duncombe, C., Falzon, D., & Olsson, S. (2013). WHO strategy for collecting safety data in public health programmes: Complementing spontaneous reporting systems. *Drug Safety, 36*(2), 75–81. doi:10.1007/s40264-012-0014-6

Pal, S. N., Olsson, S., & Brown, E. G. (2015). The Monitoring Medicines Project: A multinational pharmacovigilance and public health project. *Drug Safety, 38*(4), 319–328. doi:10.1007/s40264-015-0283-y

Pan American Health Organization. (2010a). *Earthquake in Haiti—January 2010.* Washington, DC: Author. Retrieved from http://www.paho.org/disasters/index.php?option=com_content&view=article&id=1088&Itemid=1112&lang=en

Pan American Health Organization. (2010b). *Haïti: Population health assessment prior to the 2010 earthquake.* (Health Information & Analysis; Health Surveillance, Disease Control and Prevention). Retrieved from https://www.google.com/webhp?sourceid=chrome-instant&ion=1&espv=2&ie=UTF-8#q=Ha%C3%AFti%3A+Population+health+assessment+prior+to+the+2010+earthquake

Parpia, A. S., Ndeffo-Mbah, M. L., Wenzel, N. S., & Galvani, A. P. (2016). Effects of response to 2014–2015 Ebola outbreak on deaths from malaria, HIV/AIDS, and tuberculosis, West Africa. *Emerging Infectious Diseases, 22*(3), 433–441. doi:10.3201/eid2203.150977

Perry, R. T., Murray, J. S., Gacic-Dobo, M., Dabbagh, A., Mulders, M. N., Strebel, P. M., . . . Goodson, J. L. (2015). Progress toward regional measles elimination—worldwide, 2000–2014.

MMWR: Morbidity and Mortality Weekly Report, 64(44), 1246-1251. doi:10.15585/
mmwr.6444a4

Poon, E. G., Keohane, C. A., Yoon, C. S., Ditmore, M., Bane, A., Levtzion-Korach, O., . . . Gandhi,
T. K. (2010). Effect of bar-code technology on the safety of medication administration. *New
England Journal of Medicine, 362*(18), 1698–1707. doi:10.1056/NEJMsa0907115

Retraction—Ileal-lymphoid-nodular hyperplasia, non-specific colitis, and pervasive developmental disorder in children. (2010). *The Lancet, 375*(9713), 445. doi:10.1016/
s0140-6736(10)60175-4

Salmasi, S., Khan, T. M., Hong, Y. H., Ming, L. C., & Wong, T. W. (2015). Medication errors in the
Southeast Asian countries: A systematic review. *PLoS One, 10*(9), e0136545. doi:10.1371/
journal.pone.0136545

Scholte, J. A. (2000). *Globalization: A critical introduction*. New York, NY: St. Martin's Press.

Schuller, M., & Levey, T. (2014). Kabrit ki gen twop met: Understanding gaps in WASH services in
Haiti's IDP camps. *Disasters, 38*(Suppl. 1), S1–S24. doi:10.1111/disa.12053

Scott, N., Gabriel, S., Sheppeard, V., Peacock, A., Scott, C., Flego, K., . . . Seale, H. (2015). Responding
to a measles outbreak in a Pacific island community in western Sydney: Community inter-
views led to church-based immunization clinics. *Western Pacific Surveillance and Response
Journal, 6*(2), 51–57. doi:10.5365/wpsar.2014.5.3.004

Shelley, D., Nguyen, L., Pham, H., VanDevanter, N., & Nguyen, N. (2014). Barriers and facilitators to expanding the role of community health workers to include smoking cessation services in Vietnam: A qualitative analysis. *BMC Health Services Research, 14*, 606. doi:10.1186/
s12913-014-0606-1

Shorstein Lecture. (1922). The history of tuberculosis. *British Medical Journal, 2*(3229), 987–988.

Stillman, F. A., David, A. M., Kibria, N., & Phan, H. T. (2014). Building capacity for implementation
of the framework convention for tobacco control in Vietnam: Lessons for developing countries. *Health Promotion International, 29*(3), 442–453. doi:10.1093/heapro/dat005

Stillman, F. A., Wipfli, H. L., Lando, H. A., Leischow, S., & Samet, J. M. (2005). Building capacity
for international tobacco control research: The Global Tobacco Research Network. *American
Journal of Public Health, 95*(6), 965–968. doi:10.2105/ajph.2004.047183

Stockwell, E. G. (1961). Socioeconomic status and mortality in the United States. *Public Health
Reports, 76*, 1081–1086.

Takahashi, S., Metcalf, C. J., Ferrari, M. J., Moss, W. J., Truelove, S. A., Tatem, A. J., . . . Lessler, J.
(2015). Reduced vaccination and the risk of measles and other childhood infections post-
Ebola. *Science, 347*(6227), 1240–1242. doi:10.1126/science.aaa3438

The World Bank. (2016a). *Haiti*. Washington, DC: Author. Retrieved from http://www.worldbank.
org/en/country/haiti

The World Bank. (2016b). Smoking prevalence, males (% of adults): Vietnam 2012–2013 [Table].
Washington, DC: Author. Retrieved from http://databank.worldbank.org/data/reports.
aspx?source=2&series=SH.PRV.SMOK.MA&country=

The World Bank Group. (2014, October 7). *The economic impact of the 2014 Ebola epidemic:
Short and medium term estimates for West Africa*. New York, NY: Author. Retrieved from
http://documents.worldbank.org/curated/en/524521468141287875/pdf/912190WP0
see0a00070385314B00PUBLIC0.pdf

The World Bank Group. (2016). *World development indicators*. Washington DC: International
Bank for Reconstruction and Development/The World Bank. Retrieved from https://
openknowledge.worldbank.org/bitstream/handle/10986/23969/9781464806834.
pdf?sequence=2&isAllowed=y

Tuberculosis Control Division. (1982). Historical perspectives: Centennial: Koch's discovery of the
tubercle bacillus. *MMWR: Morbidity and Mortality Weekly Report, 31*(10), 121–123.

United Nations Department of Economic and Social Affairs Population Division. (2015).
World population ageing 2015 (ST/ESA/SER.A/390). New York, NY: Author. Retrieved

from http://www.un.org/en/development/desa/population/publications/pdf/ageing/WPA2015_Report.pdf

United Nations General Assembly. (2015). *70/1. Transforming our world: The 2030 Agenda for Sustainable Development* (A/RES/70/1). New York, NY: Author. Retrieved from http://www.un.org/ga/search/view_doc.asp?symbol=A/RES/70/1&Lang=E

Warraich, H. J. (2009). Religious opposition to polio vaccination. *Emerging Infectious Diseases, 15*(6), 978. doi:10.3201/eid1506.090087

Warren, J. R., & Hernandez, E. M. (2007). Did socioeconomic inequalities in morbidity and mortality change in the United States over the course of the twentieth century? *Journal of Health and Social Behavior, 48*(4), 335–351.

Wise, J. (2013). Largest group of children affected by measles outbreak in Wales is 10–18 year olds. *BMJ, 346,* f2545. doi:10.1136/bmj.f2545

World Alliance for Patient Safety. (2005). *WHO draft guidelines for adverse event reporting and learning systems: From information to action* (WHO/EIP/SPO/QPS/05.3). Geneva, Switzerland: Author. Retrieved from http://osp.od.nih.gov/sites/default/files/resources/Reporting_Guidelines.pdf

World Health Organization. (2002a). *Global strategy on infant and young child feeding* (WHA55 A55/15). Geneva, Switzerland: Author. Retrieved from http://apps.who.int/gb/archive/pdf_files/WHA55/ea5515.pdf?ua=1

World Health Organization. (2002b). *The importance of pharmacovigilance: Safety monitoring of medicinal products.* London: Author. Retrieved from http://apps.who.int/medicinedocs/en/d/Js4893e/

World Health Organization. (2003). *WHO Framework Convention on Tobacco Control.* Geneva, Switzerland: Author. Retrieved from http://www.who.int/tobacco/framework/WHO_FCTC_english.pdf

World Health Organization. (2006). *The safety of medicines in public health programmes: Pharmacovigilance an essential tool.* Geneva, Switzerland: Author. Retrieved from http://www.who.int/medicines/areas/quality_safety/safety_efficacy/Pharmacovigilance_B.pdf?ua=1

World Health Organization. (2010). *Why urban health matters.* Geneva, Switzerland: Author. Retrieved from http://www.who.int/world-health-day/2010/media/whd2010background.pdf

World Health Organization. (2014, October). *Reporting and learning systems for medication errors: the role of pharmacovigilance centres.* Geneva, Switzerland: Author. Retrieved from http://apps.who.int/iris/bitstream/10665/137036/1/9789241507943_eng.pdf?ua=1

World Health Organization. (2015a). *Ebola situation report.* Geneva, Switzerland: Author. Retrieved from http://apps.who.int/iris/bitstream/10665/192654/1/ebolasitrep_4Nov2015_eng.pdf?ua=1

World Health Organization. (2015b). *Global tuberculosis report 2015.* Geneva, Switzerland: Author. Retrieved from http://www.who.int/tb/publications/global_report/en/

World Health Organization. (2016, May 2). *Immunization, vaccines and biologicals: Measles.* Geneva, Switzerland: Author. Retrieved from http://www.who.int/immunization/diseases/measles/en/

4

Epidemiology

ARDIS HANSON AND BRUCE LUBOTSKY LEVIN

Basic Concepts and Principles in Epidemiology for Pharmacists

Epidemiology, a basic science of public health, is the study of the factors that determine the frequency and distribution of disease in human populations (MacMahon & Pugh, 1970). A quantitative discipline based upon probability, statistics, research methodologies, and disease etiology, epidemiology uses causal reasoning (i.e., hypotheses) to examine what factors cause, exacerbate, and/or prevent disease (morbidity) and death (mortality). Epidemiology encompasses the distribution of disease, factors that cause disease, and the attributes of disease in defined populations.

Epidemiology examines the incidence, frequency, and prevalence of endemic and epidemic outbreaks. Epidemiological surveys and estimates establish morbidity in specific geographic areas/regions and in specified populations. More formally, epidemiology is the study of the interrelationships of host (the organism harboring the disease), agent (cause of the disease), and environment (external factors that cause or allow disease transmission). These three factors determine the frequency, distribution, and control of disease in human populations. As such, epidemiology looks at characteristics of time, place, and people in determining the causes and occurrences of health-related events.

Epidemiology is descriptive in that it looks at the what, who, when, and where of health-related events. Epidemiology is also observational, experimental, and applied. Observational epidemiologists perform studies that observe the behaviors, characteristics, and outcomes of the populations being studied. Experimental epidemiologists conduct empirical studies where study participants receive treatments or interventions (Moore et al., 2007; Phimarn et al., 2013). They perform systematic evaluations of theory-driven hypotheses using, in the best case, randomized clinical trials to tease out small effects of pathogens or environmental variables. Applied epidemiology addresses public health issues, such as when

Table 4-1 **Differences between Descriptive and Analytic Epidemiology**

Descriptive Epidemiology	Analytic Epidemiology
Examines frequency and distribution of risk factors	Studies risk/protective factors of diseases
Searches for information/clues	Uses available information/clues
Formulates hypotheses	Tests hypotheses
No comparison groups	Uses comparison groups
Answers who, what, when, where, and how	Answers how and why

pharmacists monitor reports of communicable diseases in their communities (Forland et al., 2012) or when they determine the effectiveness and efficacy of a lifestyle awareness program, such as obesity or cholesterol awareness (Jordan & Harmon, 2015; Table 4-1).

Definition and Core Functions of Epidemiology

The term *epidemiology* comes from the Greek words *epi* (on or upon), *demos* (people), and *logos* (the study of); it roughly translates into "the study of what comes upon people." MacMahon and Pugh's classic definition of epidemiology has been expanded to "the study of the distribution and determinants of health-related states or events in specified populations, and the application of this study to the control of health problems" (Last, 2001, p. 61). It is relatively easy to see how these perspectives translate into the study of disease surveillance, comprised of events, populations, locations, chronologies, and transmissions. These elements help characterize epidemiologic events, such as measles outbreaks or the use of technology to prevent diseases. By understanding these factors, epidemiologists attempt to provide insight into what *causes* a disease to occur, determine *potential for further spread* of the disease in a community, and identify *interventions to prevent* additional cases or recurrences. Hence, epidemiology can inform larger public health, community-based actions, as well as discrete clinical practice and research.

Often, epidemiology is seen as a component of other disciplines, due to its emphases on quantitative analysis, disease/population surveillance, and interventions; however, epidemiology is its own discipline, with theoretical and epistemological frameworks, systematic methodologies, and unique technologies and tools. Core functions of epidemiology were identified during the 1990s as public health surveillance, field investigation, analytic studies, evaluation, linkages, and policy development (Rothman, 1993; Teret, 2001).

History of Epidemiology

Around 400 BCE., Hippocrates wrote "On Airs, Waters, and Places." In this work, he posited a relationship between environmental and lifestyle factors and development of disease (Hippocrates, 2008), a forerunner of the social determinants of health framework used internationally today. He also distinguished endemic from epidemic outbreaks: those diseases always present in an area versus a disease brought into the area from outside. So not only is Hippocrates the father of medicine, but he is also the first epidemiologist. However, the observations of Hippocrates were often dismissed in favor of other theories of disease causation, such as miasmatic theory ("bad" or night air; Last, 2001).

By the 1500s vital statistics collections started to appear in the Western world. The city of London established weekly death registries, known as *Bills of Mortality,* which recorded burials by number buried, the parish, the cause of death, and the gender of the deceased. In 1662, Captain John Graunt wrote the first *Natural and Political Observations Mentioned in a Following Index, and Made Upon the Bills of Mortality,* which was his analysis of the *Bills of Mortality.* A seminal work in epidemiology, Graunt provided a trend analysis that showed mortality rates exceeded the rate of births (based upon christenings). He described his method in Chapter 2, "In my Discourses upon the Bills I shall first speak of the Casualties, then give my Observations with reference to the Places, and Parishes comprehended in the Bills; and next of the Years, and Seasons" (Graunt, 2008, p. 37). His work, with others, contributed to the use of vital statistics data to monitor the health of a given population or area.

William Farr, a British epidemiologist and physician, began publishing annual reports on the causes of death in England when he worked as a statistician in the General Register Office in the 1830s. He established a standard for recording causes of death and for constructing national life tables. The resultant system allows researchers to compare mortality rates across populations. National life tables can determine trends in period life expectancy (i.e., the average number of years people will live beyond their current age) based on age and gender. Two of his more notable essays focus on statistical methodologies that became the cornerstones of modern epidemiology (Farr, 1837, 1862).

John Snow, another British physician, is considered the founder of public health in the United Kingdom and one of the founders of modern epidemiology. He played a pivotal role in determining the cause of the 1854 London cholera outbreak by determining the outbreak originated in the water supply from a household water supplier in SoHo. He literally walked door to door to determine which SoHo households had cholera outbreaks and identified their water supplier. Mapping each outbreak, he was able to backtrack the major source of contamination to the Southwark and Vauxhall Waterworks Company public water pump on Broad Street. His studies revealing the pattern of the spread of the disease and its connection to the water source persuaded the local city council to disable the pump. Snow's 1855 publication, *On the Mode of Communication of Cholera*, expanded further upon his earlier work that focused on the pathology of cholera (Snow, 1849).

EPIDEMIOLOGY IN THE UNITED STATES

The introduction of the field of microbiology into the United States in the last decades of the 19th century witnessed significant developments to the field of epidemiology. Lemuel Shattuck published the first report dealing with sanitation and public health issues in 1850. His report emphasized the need for the establishment of state and local boards of health, recommendations that standardized vital statistics be collected, health information be exchanged, sanitary inspections be scheduled, and research conducted on infectious diseases such as tuberculosis, which was then the leading cause of morbidity and mortality (Shattuck, 1850).

Subsequently, Austin Flint (1873) determined that "an extrinsic poison which patients bring with them . . . an intrinsic typhoid product—that is, a contagium" (p. 165) propagated by a contaminated well was the cause of the 1843 waterborne typhoid fever outbreak in North Boston.

Likewise, Wade Hampton Frost's research on the Buffalo poliomyelitis epidemic of 1912 led to a comprehensive characterization of the epidemiology of poliomyelitis, which identified transmission by healthy carriers and subclinical cases of the disease (Frost, 1976).

As interest in epidemiology grew, professional associations and schools were established. In 1918, the Johns Hopkins School of Hygiene and Public Health was the first school of public health established in the United States. The American Epidemiological Society and the Epidemiology Section of the American Public Health Association were established in 1923 and 1928, respectively. In 1940, the U.S. Public Health Service established the Malaria Control in War Areas, later known as the Communicable Disease Center, and now as the Centers for Disease Control and Prevention ([CDC]; Andrews, 1946; CDC, 2015).

EPIDEMIOLOGY AT THE INTERNATIONAL LEVEL

Globalization has significant implications for epidemiology, since it facilitates the spread of communicable diseases and associated risks due to increased movement of people and goods among nations. As a leader in global health and disease surveillance, the World Health Organization (WHO) has a critical interest in strengthening education, training, and research in public health. For over 80 years, the WHO's *Weekly Epidemiological Record* has collated and disseminated global epidemiological data for disease surveillance, emphasizing diseases and risk factors that threaten international health. Translated into more than 25 languages, its textbook,

Basic Epidemiology, uses examples from across the globe to illustrate epidemiologic frameworks and methodologies (Bonita, Beaglehole, & Kjellström, 2006).

The WHO maintains the Global Health Observatory and provides world health statistics through the Global InfoBase, an interactive repository of statistics on chronic diseases, and also supports the STEPwise approach to surveillance (STEPS). Its Global Reference List of 100 Core Health Indicators provides a concise review on national and global trends and situations (WHO, 2015a). The WHO also establishes international objectives, such as the previous Millennium Development Goals and the current Sustainable Development Goals (WHO, 2015b). Perhaps one of the WHO's greatest contributions has been the development of the Global Burden of Disease concept (Murray & López, 1994, 1996), which has significantly changed how disease and disability are viewed from global and national health, societal, and economic perspectives (Murray et al., 2012).

Although the United Nations (UN) is not actively involved in generating epidemiological data, it is involved in global health initiatives, working closely with the WHO. The 2011 UN High-Level Meeting on Non-Communicable Diseases (NCDs) focused world attention for the first time on premature death and preventable morbidity and disability from NCDs (i.e., heart disease, stroke, cancer, diabetes, and chronic respiratory disease; Beaglehole et al., 2011). At that meeting, the NCD Alliance, an organization of 2,000 organizations in more than 170 countries, proposed five priority interventions: (a) tobacco control, (b) salt reduction, (c) improved diet and physical activity, (d) reduction in hazardous alcohol intake, and (e) essential drugs and technologies, with the most urgent and immediate priority being tobacco control (Beaglehole, Bonita, Yach, Mackay, & Reddy, 2015). The WHO then formally adopted the UN's NCDs resolution at its 66th World Health Assembly (2013) and incorporated them into its 2013–2020 global action plan (WHO, 2013), and most recently integrated them into its 2015 Sustainable Development Goals (WHO, 2015b).

Subspecialties in Epidemiology

As we will see by the following examples, there are many subspecialty areas within epidemiology, ranging from pharmacoepidemiology and molecular epidemiology to very specific infectious and chronic disease epidemiology. Pharmacoepidemiologists study the effects of drugs used in large populations and the outcomes of drug therapies using data from clinical trials and epidemiological studies. The emphases of these studies center on drug-related adverse effects and patterns of drug utilization, postmarketing surveillance, the formulation and interpretation of regulatory guidelines, as well as cost-benefit analyses, risk assessment of drug therapy, cost-effectiveness, and efficacy of specific drugs (Council for International Organizations of Medical Sciences, 1992; Faich, Castle, & Bankowski, 1990). An international survey by the

International Society for Pharmacoepidemiology's Education Committee identified pharmacovigilance, analysis of exposure data, epidemiologic methods, and communication skills as essential categories with identified core competencies (Jones, Tilson, & Lewis, 2012).

Molecular, occupational, and environmental epidemiologists use biological markers to detect disease earlier, reduce misclassification of exposure and outcome, and understand disease mechanisms and etiologic pathways. They may, for example, examine changes and patterns of changes in DNA to determine a particular carcinogenic agent or see which persons (hosts) are at highest risk for a specific disease via molecular biomarkers. In their study on triple negative breast cancer, Newman and Kaljee (2017) suggested western, sub-Saharan African women may possess genetic components associated with higher hereditary susceptibility for specific patterns of mammary carcinogenesis than east African women or Caucasian women of American or European descent.

Specific infectious epidemiology can provide data on quality of life and care issues that may start new chains of enquiry for research and practice. For example, Homøe et al. (2017), in their otitis media epidemiological study, found new risk factors and comorbidities affected the quality of life for children and their families, such as weaker immunologic responses and tendency to obesity. Shim (2017) describes the cost-effectiveness analysis of a dengue vaccination program in Mexico that incorporated clinical cross-immunity and susceptibility enhancement upon secondary infection as important characteristics of dengue epidemiology. Peak and colleagues (2017) argue that the natural history of the infectious disease, its inherent transmissibility, and the intervention feasibility are critical elements when comparing the effectiveness of symptom monitoring to quarantine.

Clearly, these types of epidemiological studies can guide pharmacists, public health practitioners, and policymakers on the use of pharmaceutical and nonpharmaceutical interventions during an outbreak of an emerging pathogen or chronic disease. Hence, a basic understanding of epidemiology, as well as its vocabulary, measures, and methodology, are important tools for pharmacists in evaluation of the literature, the improvement of patient care, and engagement in public health policy initiatives.

The Vocabularies of Epidemiology

Since epidemiology is the study of the patterns, causes, and effects of health and disease conditions in set populations, language is important in determining theoretical frames, showing clinical relationships, and informing transdisciplinary practice from a causal perspective. Epidemiologic data identifies emerging problems and assesses the effectiveness of measures to control existing problems. Epidemiology may be said to be the language of population health, and that language encompasses a number of standard vocabularies. The *Dictionary of Epidemiology* (DoE), an authoritative source sponsored by the International Epidemiological Association, remains the central reference for epidemiology, biostatistics, public health, medicine, and affiliated fields.

Commonly used terms include *epidemic, endemic,* and *pandemic* and *incidence* and *prevalence*. An epidemic event occurs when a disease enters from outside a community; an endemic event occurs when a disease comes from within a population; and a pandemic is an epidemic that occurs over a large area. Examples include the cholera outbreak in Haïti, the measles outbreak at Disney World, and the H1N1 outbreak, respectively.

Incidence refers to the rate of occurrence of new cases of a disease or disorder in a given period in a specific population. Prevalence refers to frequency of existing cases in a defined population at a given point in time. Since epidemiologists utilize quantities of heterogeneous data from numerous sources and formats, standard nomenclatures and ontologies are critical to establish large-scale epidemiological models and effective model-based prediction methods. One way of managing the heterogeneity in data is through semantic interoperability via unambiguous concepts (metadata) to create ontologies to assist in the capture of medical information and knowledge (Hanson & Levin, 2013). Ontologies describe a domain of knowledge (i.e., concepts and their relationships) and establish standard specifications for each domain (e.g., diseases, geographical locations, or chronology). The relationships established within a domain of knowledge are an inference mechanism that enables pattern recognition. Ontologies also can map to Universal Resource Identifiers, assist in visualization, and query development, discovery, and surveillance.

There are ontologies that model transmission of infection, such as the Pathogen Transmission Ontology (Schriml et al., 2010), and diseases, such as the Disease Ontology (Schriml et al., 2012), Infectious Disease Ontology (Cowell & Smith, 2010), Symptom Ontology (Schriml et al., 2010), and Vaccine Ontology (He et al., 2014). In addition, there are epidemiologic ontologies for subspecialties that are more granular, such as the PREDOSE (PREscription Drug abuse Online Surveillance and Epidemiology), a semantic web platform for drug abuse epidemiology (Cameron et al., 2013). More recently, the emphases have been on addressing legacy terminologies and data with the development of crosswalks across multiple vocabularies and ontologies (Ceusters & Smith, 2010; Hanson & Levin, 2013).

To assist in standards development and interoperability of ontologies, the Open Biomedical Ontologies (OBO) consortium created the OBO Foundry guidelines, designed to enhance interoperability among families of ontologies (Smith et al., 2007). Another example is the Epidemiology Ontology (EPO), which models parameters for epidemiology, demography, transmission of infection processes, participants, and related procedures. Developed by Pesquita, Ferreira, Couto, and Silva (2014), the EPO utilizes the DoE and is part of the Network of Epidemiology Related Ontologies (NERO; Ferreira, Pesquita, Couto, & Silva, 2012). NERO contains 13 ontologies, including MeSH (Medical Subject Headings vocabulary) and the National Cancer Institute Thesaurus, and is itself integrated into the Epidemic Marketplace (Couto et al., 2012).

Resources, such as Otonbee (Ong et al., 2017), the National Center for Biomedical Computing BioPortal (Musen et al., 2012), and the Epidemic Marketplace (Couto et al., 2012), provide new opportunities for epidemiologists to work with naming conventions and standardizing vocabulary to customize data depending upon their intended uses. Just as pharmaceutical ontologies allow drugs to be described at multiple levels and link to multiple drug classification schemes and clinical issues, so do epidemiological ontologies provide other levels of linkages to surveillance, practice, and research.

Consider the role ontologies play in disease outbreak information extraction systems. To be aware of fast-breaking infectious diseases requires new ways of thinking about surveillance (Figure 4-1). International report-based monitoring systems, such as BioCaster, use specific ontologies and text mine outbreak-related textual data from the Internet and add geotemporal encoding of disease outbreaks (Collier et al., 2008). These early warning monitoring systems often are effective at country and province/state levels. The Global Health Monitor system, for example, captures and plots disease events over a selected time span, categorized into news genres, syndromes, and agents (Collier, 2012). New event-based Internet biosurveillance schemes to improve monitoring, such as spatiotemporal zoning, are important extensions of traditional surveillance systems (Choi, Cho, Shim, & Woo, 2016; O'Shea, 2017) and allow visualization of epidemics in process.

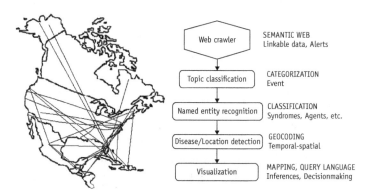

Figure 4-1. Visualizing disease monitoring and surveillance.

Measurement of Health Outcomes: Types of Measures

We measure epidemiology in many ways. We measure the frequency of disease and death, the impact on populations, and elements and patterns of disease transmission. Mortality and morbidity measure the frequency of the occurrence of deaths in a defined population and the incidence or prevalence of a disease in a population, respectively. Then there are disease phases (i.e., a measure of a time) including incubation, latency, and acute, decline, and convalescent periods. Then there are measures of effect, such as risk and odds, expressed as ratios.

Counts are the most basic of ways to measure. They refer to the number of cases of a disease or other health event under study. For example, if we know the documented number of cases of measles in Guangzhou, China, then that knowledge assists us in planning for current and future resources that may be necessary, such as medical personnel and amount of vaccine needed for that number of cases. However, counts do not reflect the total number of persons who may be affected by a disease. So we also use other measures, including proportions, ratios, and rates, which are mathematical equations with numerators and denominators.

Proportions examine all persons with the health event of interest (A, nominator) and all persons in the total population (A + B, denominator). Determining proportions provides a way to estimate the number of people who are at risk of developing diseases or specific health outcomes. Hence, proportions show probable relationships using probability theory. To make proportions easier to understand by the lay public, we multiply proportions by 100 to arrive at a percentage.

Unlike proportions, *ratios* also are a fraction (A:B, numerator/denominator) but are a relatively simple measure. Ratios state how much of one thing there is compared to another thing, such as of 300 cases of type 2 diabetes in persons aged 70 or older; 200 men had type 2 diabetes and 100 women had type 2 diabetes; the ratio of male to female cases is 2 to 1. Expressed mathematically, the ratio would look like this: A:B = male:female = 200:100 = 2:1.

Rates in epidemiology contain three elements, one in the nominator and two in the denominator. The nominator contains the *count* of health outcomes during a specific period of time, and the denominator contains the size of the population under study plus the time period of observation. The mortality rate in the United States, for example, is 8.2 deaths/1,000 population, which gives the average annual number of deaths during a year per 1,000 population. Counts, ratios, and rates then construct other epidemiologic measures, such as prevalence, incidence, and effects.

Prevalence and incidence are measures of disease frequency. The relationship between incidence and prevalence can be expressed as P = ID, where P = prevalence, I = incidence rate, and D = average duration of the disease. *Prevalence* measures existing cases of disease in a population at a specified point in time (point prevalence) or specified period of time (period prevalence). Expressed as a proportion, prevalence can quantify burden of disease, for example, of the 10,000 male residents living in Lutz, Florida, on March 15, 2017, 1,000 have diabetes, or 1,000/10,000 = 0.1 or 10%.

Incidence, on the other hand, measures new cases of disease in a previously disease-free or condition-free population (at risk) during a specific time. Simply said, incidence measures the transition from a state of health to a state of disease using proportions and rates. Incidence uses two main measures: *risk* (or cumulative incidence [CI]) and *rate* (person-time units). *Incidence risk* (IR) is the number of cases of disease in a specified time period divided by the number of disease-free persons at the beginning of that time period (cohort). IR assumes the entire population is at risk when the study period began; however, it is subject to variations within a cohort, as persons may refuse to participate, leave the area, die, or enter the study after it has already started. To account for these variances, the incidence rate is used. CI is most useful. If the research interest is on the probability that an individual will become ill over a specified period, the CI is used. If the research interest is on how fast new disease cases occur, then the IR calculation is preferred.

The *steady state* measure provides a functional relationship between incidence and prevalence. If the IR and the duration of disease are constant over time and the prevalence of the disease is low, then $P/1 - P = IR \times$ average duration of disease, where P is the number of persons with the disease in a population divided by the number of all persons in the population.

Measures of effect assess the strength of an association between a possible risk factor and the subsequent occurrence of a disease. To do this, we compare the incidence of disease in a group of persons exposed to a potential risk factor with the incidence in a group of persons not exposed to the potential risk factor. This is expressed commonly as a ratio of disease frequency for the two groups. We refer to these measures collectively as measures of relative risk, that is, the strength of an association between an exposure and disease to determine if there is a causal relationship between the observed associations. Table 4-2 provides equations for common epidemiologic measures of frequency and effect.

We also measure how diseases affect populations. *Burden of disease* addresses the total significance of disease on society, beyond the immediate cost of treatment (Murray & López, 1994). It measures years of life lost to ill health or the difference between total life expectancy and disability-adjusted life expectancy. A Disability-Adjusted Life Year (DALY) is a summary measure of the health of a population. One DALY represents one lost year of healthy life and estimates the gap between the current health of a population and the state of a population if that disease was not present.

The DALYS use measures of years of potential life lost (YPLLs) and years lived with disability (YLDs) to build its formula. YPLL measures the impact of premature mortality on a population. It is calculated as the sum of the differences between

Table 4-2 **Common Epidemiologic Measures**

Measures of Disease Frequency	Point Prevalence	# cases in population at one point in time
		# persons in population at the same period in time
	Incidence Risk	# cases of disease in a specified time period
		# disease-free persons at beginning of that time period
	Incidence Rate	# new cases of disease in a given time period
		Total person-time at risk during the study period
Measures of Effect	Risk Ratio	Risk (cumulative incidence) in exposed group
		Risk (cumulative incidence) in unexposed group
	Rate Ratio	Incidence rate in exposed group
		Incidence rate in unexposed group
	Odds Rate	Odds of disease in exposed group
		Odds of disease in unexposed group

some predetermined minimum (or desired lifespan) and the age of death for individuals who died earlier than that predetermined age. YLDs measure the number of years lived with a disability. When YLDs are added to the YLLs for a certain disease or disorder, the burden of disability associated with a disease or disorder can be reported as DALYs. Hence, mortality (YLLs) and morbidity (YLDs) are combined into a single, common metric.

The Global Burden of Disease (GBD) Disease and Injury Incidence and Prevalence Collaborators (GBD, 2016) quantify prevalence and incidence of the major sequelae for a comprehensive list of diseases and injuries globally. In 2015, upper respiratory infections (17.2 billion) and diarrheal diseases (2.39 billion) were the most prevalent diseases contributing to morbidity and mortality. However, there was a positive association between conflict and depression and anxiety, confirming that mental illnesses and substance use disorders contribute significantly to global disability (GBD, 2016). Emerging and re-emerging infectious diseases pose a persistent challenge to global health prevention, intervention, and surveillance due to the immediacy of emergence and the time lag between outbreak and decline. The GBD Collaborators were able to capture the Ebola virus disease outbreaks in Africa but were unable to capture chikungunya and Zika virus across the Americas (GBD, 2016). Hence, these epidemiological measures contribute to a better understanding of quality of life, cost effectiveness, cost efficacy, and comparative effectiveness research and outcomes in health and public health (Antioch, Drummond, Niessen, & Vondeling, 2017; Kislan, Bernstein, Fearrington, & Ives, 2016).

Methods in Epidemiology

Methods in epidemiology have developed rapidly over the past five decades to address numerous statistical and data issues, such as addressing confounding variables, challenges posed by the analysis of retrospective and longitudinal data, and the reduction of bias. Since epidemiology determines how exposures relate to outcomes, the focus is on what causes a specific disease event within a specific population. Unfortunately, standards of diagnosis, factors, and data recording often change over time or across nations, governments, and communities, so analyses are confounded or made more complicated. Since epidemiologists base conclusions on comparisons of disease rates in groups, identifying high-risk and priority groups rests on unbiased comparison of rates.

Two primary methods are descriptive and analytic epidemiology. Descriptive epidemiology depicts existing health problems and patterns of disease. These patterns often generate research hypotheses, which analytic epidemiology examines more formally. Important concepts include person, place, and time, and causality, chance, bias, and confounding.

In *descriptive epidemiology*, the characteristics of persons, places, and time frame the distribution of disease. Person characteristics include inherent characteristics (age, gender, race/ethnicity), acquired characteristics (educational level, marital status), activities/behaviors (occupation, leisure activities, use of medications/tobacco/drugs), or the conditions under which they live (socioeconomic status, access to medical care). Place attributes address geographic factors, from macro levels (country), meso levels (state), and micro levels (city, town) to place categories, such as urban or rural, domestic or foreign, and institutional or noninstitutional, to place of diagnosis. Climate, location, and other environmental factors associated with place, such as smog, can affect disease occurrence.

Occurrences are the most commonly described characteristics of time and patterns of time. Occurrences, for example, can be cyclic (e.g., influenza) or sporadic (cholera outbreaks). Monitoring disease occurrence or the effectiveness of public health interventions require an understanding of the patterns of disease occurrence by time. Three common views of time include secular trends, cyclic fluctuations, and point epidemics (Porta, 2016). A *secular trend* categorizes changes in disease occurrence over long periods in time, while *cyclic fluctuations* refer to shorter term increases and decreases in disease occurrence within a year (seasonal) or over a period of a few years (secular). *Point source epidemic* refers to increased disease occurrence among a group of people exposed almost simultaneously to some type of etiologic agent, such as a pathogen or contaminant.

Analytic epidemiology refers to the study of the *determinants* of health-related outcomes. Determinants are those factors that increase or decrease a person's risk of a specific health outcome, such as age, health-related behaviors, or interventions. Analytic epidemiology is hypothesis driven, in that the researcher identifies the variables of interest, formulates a relationship among the variables and population, and compares two groups of individuals (e.g., cases and controls) with respect to the variables. The challenge for analytic epidemiologists is to determine if their results are valid and represent a causal relationship between the variables. To do so, they examine chance, bias, and confounding.

Chance refers to the possibility that the apparent relationship between variables is spurious. When researchers conduct statistical analyses unguided by a priori hypotheses, they are more likely to produce statistically significant findings by chance. *Bias* refers to systematic error in the conduct of a study. Errors due to bias can occur in the design of and execution of the study or in the analysis and interpretation of the study data. There are many types of bias, including observer, referral, informational, and selection (Schwartz, Campbell, Gatto, & Gordon, 2015). *Confounding* occurs when an exposure-outcome relationship is distorted by a third factor that is not the intermediate in the causal pathway and can occur during both the study design and analysis phases (Maldonado, 2013).

Confounding by indication is a particular problem in in nonrandomized (observational) drug studies when characteristics of two groups taking two different drugs or two groups taking one drug versus no drug differ substantially. Consider the ongoing discussions of hypericum perforatum (St. John's wort), an over-the-counter medication, and fluoxetine, a prescription drug, for depression. Ioannidis (2008) argues that very large long-term trials and careful prospective meta-analyses of individual-level data may offer better evidence on the efficacy of each rather than biased selection of study populations and multiple, small randomized trials that offer selective and distorted reporting of results.

Clearly, judging causality is more complicated than the scope of this chapter; however, it is a critical component in any review of the literature to determine if exposure causally affects the health outcome of interest. Although Hill's (1965) nine criteria offer a framework by which to judge causality, there are always exceptions and reservations as new methodologies and epistemologies emerge (Ioannidis, 2016). Readers are encouraged to review Rothman, Greenland, and Lash (2015) for a more thorough discussion of these issues.

Types of Epidemiologic Studies

Different research study designs reflect different levels of evidence in the "evidence pyramid." At the bottom of the pyramid (lowest level) are case-controlled studies, case series, and case reports; followed by cohort studies, randomized clinical trials, critically appraised individual articles, critically appraised topics (evidence syntheses), and topped by systematic reviews and meta-analysis. A case study, for example, is clearly a strong design for assessing why or in which way an effect has occurred; a randomized clinical trial is best for clinical decision-making, while longitudinal cohort studies best address prognostic and etiologic questions. Therefore, levels of evidence are necessary because they allow us to interpret the reliability of information to formulate recommendations intended to improve specific events or actions in health care.

Analytic epidemiologists test hypotheses that a specific factor is the cause of a health effect. Other factors taken into consideration are characteristics of the exposure(s) and health outcome(s). Case-control, cohort, and cross-sectional studies are the most common types of analytic studies, although interventional studies and randomized clinical trials are also analytic studies.

CASE CONTROL STUDIES

Case control studies are observational studies that compare individuals with a disease (cases) to other individuals who do not have the disease (control subjects) from the same population. Also known as "retrospective studies" and "case-referent studies," case control studies are designed to estimate the odds of contracting the disease and retrospectively determine if there is a relationship to exposure to a specific risk factor in each group. Case control studies are good studies to examine rare conditions or diseases, since control subjects represent the expected exposure prevalence and cases represent incidence. They are also useful as initial studies to establish associations as a base for more rigorous studies. However, bias can influence data quality due to the reliance on memory and recall. They are also more prone to confounding when both exposure and outcome are strongly related to a third variable.

A simple example is oral cancer. The factor under examination is smokeless tobacco (e.g., chewing tobacco, naswar, snuff, snus, gutka, and topical tobacco paste). Depending on the type of smokeless tobacco he or she uses, a person may be at low, medium, or high risk for oral cancer. Consider the following example. The estimated burden of disease figures for smokeless tobacco use in 113 countries led to 1.7 million DALYs lost and 62,283 deaths due to cancers of mouth, pharynx, and esophagus (Siddiqi et al., 2015). Over 85% of this burden was in Southeast Asia, where over 250 million persons in South and Southeast Asia use smokeless tobacco.

However, building epidemiological evidence regarding some of its harmful effects is difficult. Recent meta-analyses have shown relationships between smokeless tobacco, chronic oral lesions, and oral cancer (Khan et al., 2016) and a manifold increased risk of esophageal squamous-cell carcinoma among persons who chewed both areca nut and smokeless tobacco (Akhtar, 2013). However, there is the need for more powerful studies that quantify dose-response relationships (Gupta & Johnson, 2014).

Pharmacoepidemiologists use case-control studies also for postmarketing surveillance. Yang and colleagues (2014) report on the measles vaccine effectiveness in Guangzhou, southern China from 1951 to 2012. Using test-negative cases as controls, they determined a significant overall decline in the incidence of measles in the measles-vaccinated population of children between 8 months to 14 years of age. They found that two doses of measles vaccine were more effective than one dose in preventing measles and recommended giving the vaccine to transient and other non-vaccine targeted populations (Yang et al., 2014).

COHORT STUDIES

Cohort studies compare health outcomes between different groups of people stratified by exposure status (i.e., the presence or absence of a particular exposure). Since participants in cohort studies are allocated to comparison groups based upon whether they meet exposure requirements, cohort studies permit researchers to observe and evaluate possibly harmful exposures in a natural setting. Cohort studies may be prospective or retrospective.

In *prospective studies*, both exposed and unexposed participants are followed over time to determine the initial occurrence of the health outcome(s) under study. By determining the temporal relationship between exposure and outcome, cohort studies allow direct measurement and comparison of incidence between the exposure groups (using the risk ratio). Prospective studies are good to examine emerging, new exposures. Several notable prospective cohort studies are the Framingham Heart Study, which has defined cardiovascular disease risk factors and prevention guidelines over the past five decades (Tsao & Vasan, 2015), and the Medication Use Patterns, Treatment Satisfaction, and Inadequate Control of Osteoporosis Study that examined gastrointestinal symptoms and association with medication for osteoporosis in Europe and Canada (Modi et al., 2016). A twist on the cohort study, the Monitoring Medicines project, a European Union study, used cohort event monitoring to support and strengthen pharmacovigilance reporting from a larger public health perspective (Pal, Olsson, & Brown, 2015).

In the retrospective cohort study, both the exposure(s) and health outcome(s) of interest have already occurred. Investigators go back to a point in time after outcomes have already occurred and try to establish the exposure status. Retrospective studies are good for studies that examine long latency events (events that occur many times over the years) or for studies examining rare or unusual exposures that may be natural or manmade. Pharmacoepidemiologists often use cohort studies for postmarketing surveillance and phase IV studies to assess the safety and efficacy of an approved compound or medical device and in specific disease management.

CROSS-SECTIONAL STUDIES

Cross-sectional studies, also known as prevalence surveys, *simultaneously* assess exposure and health outcomes of interest and are often used in national studies, such as the studies conducted by the CDC's National Center for Health Statistics. Many cross-sectional studies are a blend of descriptive and analytical analyses.

Descriptive cross-sectional studies assess the frequency and distribution of a particular disease in a defined population. In their cross-sectional study of 220 Kuwaiti community pharmacies, Awad and Waheedi (2012) examined the frequency of counseling, comfort level, and perceived effectiveness of obesity management services offered by local pharmacists. Although a majority of pharmacists counseled patients on ways to lose weight, the pharmacists felt that patients not only lacked awareness about pharmacists' expertise in counseling, but obese patients lack willpower and are nonadherent to weight reduction intervention (Awad & Waheedi, 2012).

Analytical cross-sectional studies often attempt to investigate the association between a putative risk factor and a health outcome. Schistosomiasis, a chronic parasitic disease caused by blood fluke, was reported to be in Shan State, Myanmar; however, there had been neither serological studies to detect it or any associated factors among the residents (Soe, Oo, Myat, & Maung, 2017). Significant factors for seropositivity were being male, geographical location within four selected rural health center areas, and educational levels. In addition, the ELISA test showed satisfactory sensitivity and specificity levels for use. The authors recommend that Myanmar place schistosoma infection in its list of Diseases under National Surveillance and monitor prevalence testing (Soe et al., 2017).

There are benefits and challenges to using cross-sectional studies. Cross-sectional studies are good for developing descriptive analyses and generating hypotheses. They are relatively quick and easy to conduct since researchers collect data on all variables one time, allowing them to study multiple outcomes and exposures. Hence, cross-sectional studies can help describe magnitude and distribution of an event or outcome under study. However, cross-sectional studies are prone to bias. Since they simultaneously assess exposure and outcome, antecedent-consequence bias asks the question if the exposure preceded the outcome or was a consequence. Survival bias must be careful not to associate of duration of disease with exposure status.

RANDOMIZED CONTROLLED TRIAL

The randomized control trial (RCT) is the apex of the evidence pyramid for clinical decision-making research studies (Parfrey & Ravani, 2015). The random assignation of subjects to a particular exposure group, an experimental group (new intervention or drug) versus comparison or control (a standard practice intervention or placebo), ensures that the respective groups will be similar based on the distribution of all of their other characteristics. Researchers or clinicians then compare the subsequent health experiences of the exposure groups using risk or rate ratios to determine the effectiveness of the intervention.

However, there are a number of challenges in conducting an RCT. The researcher must define clearly the RCT protocol (hypothesis, patients, interventions, controls, outcomes, measures, and methods) that comprise the study to satisfy the rigorous review by the institutional review board to ensure compliance with federal regulations for human subject research. RCT protocols must include an hypothesis of an anticipated association between one or more predictor and outcome variables contrasted with a null hypothesis of no association and subjected to statistical evaluation at a predetermined significance level. Predictor and outcome variables are carefully selected for their theoretical association and defined prior to the study. In addition to choosing an appropriate (representative) sample of the population from which to recruit, there may be delays and challenges to recruiting enough participants to randomize the participants into two (or more) comparison groups. Randomized, double-blinded studies ensure that the investigator(s) do not know which group is receiving what intervention until after the data is collected or unless there are untoward side effects in participants. Participants must provide informed consent and data collection, and researchers must adhere to strict quality control measures that ensure patient privacy and confidentiality. Each step has consequences for the internal validity of the trial; however, a well-designed, methodologically sound RCT provides strong evidence of a cause-effect relation if one exists.

The Consolidated Standards for Reporting Trials (CONSORT) are recommendations for improving the quality of reports of RCTs (Moher et al., 2012). Not only do these types of reporting guidelines provide researchers with minimum criteria for reporting, these guidelines can increase the transparency and quality of biomedical publications (Hutton, Wolfe, Moher, & Shamseer, 2017). In pharmacological studies, for example, many RCTs assess the *efficacy* of different interventions and therapies under ideal or close to ideal conditions, unlike real-world studies, which measure *effectiveness*. Hence, pharmacists need to review carefully and thoroughly subsequent RCTs that examine off-label use of prescription medications or to patient subgroups not included in the original RCTs that led to approval of a particular medication (Kip & Quilliam, 2008). Appropriate use of CONSORT guidelines for articles in medical journals will assist pharmacists in their review of the literature on the efficacy of drugs or medical devices (Mills et al., 2004).

Screening

Screening is a common health care practice that has its roots in epidemiology and public health. Screening devices are readily available in many pharmacies with or without a prescription, such as colorectal cancer screening kits, diabetic testing lists, and pregnancy tests. Understanding the basic principles of screening can assist pharmacists in their interactions with patients regarding use of or results of a screening test. Screening is the "examination of asymptomatic people in order to classify them as likely or unlikely to have the disease that is the object of screening" (Morrison, 1985, p. 3). Based upon the definition, screening focuses on persons who are subclinical (i.e., they may have a particular disease but are unaware of having the disease). Hence, screening helps identify those individuals who may need additional diagnostic workup for serious diseases, individuals who are treated more effectively before symptoms occur, or when the prevalence of disease in the subclinical stage is relatively high.

One such example is phenylketonuria (PKU). Hospitals now routinely conduct PKU screening after the birth of a child to determine if the infant is able to convert phenylalanine to tyrosine, amino acids needed for normal growth and development (Paul & Brosco, 2013). Without that conversion enzyme, infants suffer seizures, brain damage, and intellectual disability. Female children diagnosed with PKU require lifelong follow-up to prevent maternal PKU, and both male and female children with PKU often experience behavioral problems, psychiatric distress, and executive function impairment through their lifecycle (Burton et al., 2013; de Baulny, Abadie, Feillet, & de Parscau, 2007; Jahja et al., 2013). In this case, although PKU is relatively rare, the long-term consequences and costs of care are significant for the individual throughout his or her lifetime.

Screening tests should be reliable and valid. Reliable screenings give consistent results with repeated tests across multiple settings and multiple administrations to individuals. Valid screenings indicate which individuals have the disease and which do not and have high sensitivity and specificity. *Sensitivity* is the test's ability to designate a subject correctly with the disease as positive. *Specificity* is the test's ability to designate a subject correctly without the disease as negative. The more sensitive the test, the fewer false positive results are displayed; the more specific the test, the fewer false negative results. A false positive result indicates a subject without the disease has the disease based on the screening test. A false negative result indicates a subject with the disease does not the disease based on the screening test.

The ideal case is to have a test that is both highly sensitive and highly specific. A 2 × 2 table, also known as a contingency table, is a useful tool to compare the performance of a screening test to the gold standard (diagnostic) test since it categorizes all test results as either positive or negative and test characteristics represented by sensitivity and specificity (Table 4-3).

As with all tests, the most important clinical questions remain the same. If the test is positive, what is the chance the patient really has disease? If the test is negative, what is the chance the patient does not have the disease? For a fuller review of the principles in this section, see Kip and Quilliam (2008) or Weiss (2016).

Table 4-3 **2 × 2 Comparison Table**

	+ (present)	Disease	– (absent)
Gold Standard Test	a + c (all people with the disease)		b + d (all people without the disease)
A Screening Test +	a (true positives)		b (false positives)
–	c (false negatives)		d (true negatives)

Implications for Pharmacists and Pharmacy Practice

Epidemiology can increase our understanding of at-risk populations, meet selected needs for addressing specific disease states or physical/mental/substance use disorders, identify services utilization, and potentially drive policy. Pharmacy data can be a valuable source of drug information in epidemiological studies. Hence, a basic understanding of the principles and applications of epidemiological vocabulary, methods, and theoretical frameworks is essential for the practicing pharmacist. Without a working knowledge of epidemiology, it is all too easy to be confused by presentations of the pharmacological management of a particular disease state, whether at professional conferences, pharmacy and therapeutics committees, or in the media (Kip & Quilliam, 2008). As clinical decision-making becomes more complex, the volume of the medical literature expands exponentially, with numerous studies utilizing different levels of evidence to make their cases as to best practice, changes in policy, and research funding. Hence, a working knowledge of epidemiology can provide important information in patient care as well as keep one current with the field.

References

Akhtar, S. (2013). Areca nut chewing and esophageal squamous-cell carcinoma risk in Asians: A meta-analysis of case-control studies. *Cancer Causes & Control, 24*(2), 257–265. doi:10.1007/s10552-012-0113-9

Andrews, J. M. (1946). The United States Public Health Service Communicable Disease Center. *Public Health Reports, 61,* 1203–1210.

Antioch, K. M., Drummond, M. F., Niessen, L. W., & Vondeling, H. (2017). International lessons in new methods for grading and integrating cost effectiveness evidence into clinical practice guidelines. *Cost Effectiveness and Resource Allocation, 15,* 1. doi:10.1186/s12962-017-0063-x

Awad, A., & Waheedi, M. (2012). Community pharmacists role in obesity treatment in Kuwait: A cross-sectional study. *BMC Public Health, 12,* 863. doi:10.1186/1471-2458-12-863

Beaglehole, R., Bonita, R., Horton, R., Adams, C., Alleyne, G., Asaria, P., . . . Watt, J. (2011). Priority actions for the non-communicable disease crisis. *The Lancet, 377*(9775), 1438–1447. doi:10.1016/s0140-6736(11)60393-0

Beaglehole, R., Bonita, R., Yach, D., Mackay, J., & Reddy, K. S. (2015). A tobacco-free world: A call to action to phase out the sale of tobacco products by 2040. *The Lancet, 385*(9972), 1011–1018. doi:10.1016/s0140-6736(15)60133-7

Bonita, R., Beaglehole, R., & Kjellström, T. (2006). *Basic epidemiology.* Geneva, Switzerland: World Health Organization. Retrieved from http://apps.who.int/iris/bitstream/10665/43541/1/9241547073_eng.pdf

Burton, B. K., Leviton, L., Vespa, H., Coon, H., Longo, N., Lundy, B. D., . . . Bilder, D. (2013). A diversified approach for PKU treatment: Routine screening yields high incidence of psychiatric distress in phenylketonuria clinics. *Molecular Genetics and Metabolism, 108*(1), 8–12. doi:10.1016/j.ymgme.2012.11.003

Cameron, D., Smith, G. A., Daniulaityte, R., Sheth, A. P., Dave, D., Chen, L., . . . Falck, R. (2013). PREDOSE: A semantic web platform for drug abuse epidemiology using social media. *Journal of Biomedical Informatics, 46*(6), 985–997. doi:10.1016/j.jbi.2013.07.007

Centers for Disease Control and Prevention. (2015, July 22). Our history—our story. Retrieved from https://www.cdc.gov/about/history/ourstory.htm

Ceusters, W., & Smith, B. (2010). A unified framework for biomedical terminologies and ontologies. *Studies in Health Technologies and Informatics, 160*(Part 2), 1050–1054.

Choi, J., Cho, Y., Shim, E., & Woo, H. (2016). Web-based infectious disease surveillance systems and public health perspectives: A systematic review. *BMC Public Health, 16*(1), 1238. doi:10.1186/s12889-016-3893-0

Collier, N. (2012). Uncovering text mining: A survey of current work on web-based epidemic intelligence. *Global Public Health, 7*(7), 731–749. doi:10.1080/17441692.2012.699975

Collier, N., Doan, S., Kawazoe, A., Goodwin, R. M., Conway, M., Tateno, Y., . . . Taniguchi, K. (2008). BioCaster: Detecting public health rumors with a web-based text mining system. *Bioinformatics, 24*(24), 2940–2941. doi:10.1093/bioinformatics/btn534

Council for International Organizations of Medical Sciences. (1992). Basic requirements for the use of terms for reporting adverse drug reactions. *Pharmacoepidemiology and Drug Safety, 1*(1), 39–45. doi:10.1002/pds.2630010109

Couto, F. M., Ferreira, J. D., Zamite, J., Santos, C., Posse, T., Graça, P., . . . Silva, M. J. (2012). The Epidemic Marketplace Platform: Towards semantic characterization of epidemiological resources using biomedical ontologies. In R. Cornet & R. Stevens (Eds.), *Proceedings of the 3rd International Conference on Biomedical Ontology (ICBO 2012)* (Vol. 897, pp. 1–2). Graz, Austria: International Conference on Biomedical Ontology. Retrieved from http://ceur-ws.org/Vol-897/demo_1.pdf.

Cowell, L. G., & Smith, B. (2010). Infectious disease ontology. In V. Sintchenko (Ed.), *Infectious disease informatics* (pp. 373–395). New York: Springer.

de Baulny, H. O., Abadie, V., Feillet, F., & de Parscau, L. (2007). Management of phenylketonuria and hyperphenylalaninemia. *Journal of Nutrition, 137*(6 Suppl. 1), 1561S–1563S; discussion 1573S–1575S.

Faich, G. A., Castle, W., & Bankowski, Z. (1990). International reporting on adverse drug reactions: The CIOMS Project. CIOMS ADR Working Group. *International Journal of Clinical Pharmacology, Therapy, and Toxicology, 28*(4), 133–138.

Farr, W. (1837). On a method for determining the danger and the duration of diseases at every period of their progress. *British Annals of Medicine, 1*, 72–79.

Farr, W. (1862). A method of determining the effects of systems of treatment in certain diseases. *BMJ, 2*, 193–195.

Ferreira, J. D., Pesquita, C., Couto, F. M., & Silva, M. J. (2012). Bringing epidemiology into the semantic web. In R. Cornet & R. Stevens (Eds.), *Proceedings of the 3rd International Conference on Biomedical Ontology (ICBO 2012), KR-MED Series* (pp. 1–5). Graz, Austria: Medical University of Graz. Retrieved from http://ceur-ws.org/Vol-897/session1-paper02.pdf.

Flint, A. (1873). Relations of water to the propagation of fever. *Public Health Papers & Reports, 1*, 164–172.

Forland, F., De Carvalho Gomes, H., Nokleby, H., Escriva, A., Coulombier, D., J., G., & Jansen, A. (2012). Applicability of evidence-based practice in public health: Risk assessment on Q fever under an ongoing outbreak. *European Surveillance, 17*(3), 20060.

Frost, W. H. (1976). Some conceptions of epidemics in general by Wade Hampton Frost. *American Journal of Epidemiology, 103*(2), 141–151.

GBD 2015 Disease and Injury Incidence and Prevalence Collaborators (2016). Global, regional, and national incidence, prevalence, and years lived with disability for 310 diseases and injuries, 1990–2015: A systematic analysis for the Global Burden of Disease Study 2015. *The Lancet, 388*(10053), 1545–1602. doi:10.1016/s0140-6736(16)31678-6

Graunt, J. (1662). *Natural and political observations mentioned in a following index: and made upon the bills of mortality*. Oxford: William Hall.

Graunt, J. (2008). Natural and political observations mentioned in a following index, and made upon the bills of mortality (Abridged). In D. Schneider & D. E. Lilienfeld (Eds.), *Public health: The development of a discipline: Vol. 1. From the age of Hippocrates to the progressive era* (pp. 28–72). Brunswick, NJ: Rutgers University Press.

Gupta, B., & Johnson, N. W. (2014). Systematic review and meta-analysis of association of smokeless tobacco and of betel quid without tobacco with incidence of oral cancer in South Asia and the Pacific. *PLoS One, 9*(11), e113385. doi:10.1371/journal.pone.0113385

Hanson, A., & Levin, B. L. (2013). *Mental health informatics*. New York, NY: Oxford University Press.

He, Y., Racz, R., Sayers, S., Lin, Y., Todd, T., Hur, J., . . . Xiang, Z. (2014). Updates on the web-based VIOLIN vaccine database and analysis system. *Nucleic Acids Research, 42*, D1124–D1132. doi:10.1093/nar/gkt1133

Hill, A. B. (1965). The environment and disease: Association or causation? *Proceedings of the Royal Society of Medicine, 58*, 295–300.

Hippocrates. (2008). On airs, waters, and places. In D. Schneider & D. E. Lilienfeld (Eds.), *Public health: The development of a discipline: Vol. 1. From the age of Hippocrates to the progressive era* (pp. 7–24). New Brunswick, NJ: Rutgers University Press.

Homøe, P., Kværner, K., Casey, J. R., Damoiseaux, R. A., van Dongen, T. M., Gunasekera, H., . . . Weinreich, H. M. (2017). Panel 1: Epidemiology and diagnosis. *Otolaryngology: Head & Neck Surgery, 156*(4 Suppl.), S1–S21. doi:10.1177/0194599816643510

Hutton, B., Wolfe, D., Moher, D., & Shamseer, L. (2017). Reporting guidance considerations from a statistical perspective: Overview of tools to enhance the rigour of reporting of randomised trials and systematic reviews. *Evidence-Based Mental Health*. Advance online publication. doi:10.1136/eb-2017-102666

Ioannidis, J. P. (2008). Effectiveness of antidepressants: An evidence myth constructed from a thousand randomized trials? *Philosophy, Ethics, and Humanities in Medicine, 3*, 14. doi:10.1186/1747-5341-3-14

Ioannidis, J. P. (2016). Exposure-wide epidemiology: Revisiting Bradford Hill. *Statistics in Medicine, 35*(11), 1749–1762. doi:10.1002/sim.6825

Jahja, R., Huijbregts, S. C., de Sonneville, L. M., van der Meere, J. J., Bosch, A. M., Hollak, C. E., . . . van Spronsen, F. J. (2013). Mental health and social functioning in early treated Phenylketonuria: The PKU-COBESO study. *Molecular Genetics and Metabolism, 110*(Suppl.), S57–S61. doi:10.1016/j.ymgme.2013.10.011

Jones, J. K., Tilson, H. H., & Lewis, J. D. (2012). Pharmacoepidemiology: Defining the field and its core content. *Pharmacoepidemiology & Drug Safety, 21*(7), 677–689. doi:10.1002/pds.3198

Jordan, M. A., & Harmon, J. (2015). Pharmacist interventions for obesity: Improving treatment adherence and patient outcomes. *Integrated Pharmacy Research and Practice, 4*, 79–89. doi:10.2147/IPRP.S72206

Khan, Z., Khan, S., Christianson, L., Rehman, S., Ekwunife, O., & Samkange-Zeeb, F. (2016). Smokeless tobacco and oral potentially malignant disorders in South Asia: A systematic review and meta-analysis. *Nicotine & Tobacco Research.* Advance online publication. doi:10.1093/ntr/ntw310

Kip, K. E., & Quilliam, B. J. (2008). Applied epidemiology for pharmacists: Basic concepts and principles. In B. L. Levin, P. D. Hurd, & A. Hanson (Eds.), *Introduction to public health in pharmacy* (pp. 17–54). Sudbury, MA: Jones & Bartlett.

Kislan, M. M., Bernstein, A. T., Fearrington, L. R., & Ives, T. J. (2016). Advanced Practice Pharmacists: A retrospective evaluation of the efficacy and cost of ClinicaL Pharmacist PractitionErs managing ambulatory Medicare patients in North Carolina (APPLE-NC). *BMC Health Services Research, 16*(1), 607. doi:10.1186/s12913-016-1851-2

Last, J. M. (Ed.) (2001). *Dictionary of epidemiology* (4th ed.). New York, NY: Oxford University Press.

MacMahon, B., & Pugh, T. E. (1970). *Epidemiology: Principles and methods.* Boston, MA: Little, Brown.

Maldonado, G. (2013). Toward a clearer understanding of causal concepts in epidemiology. *Annals of Epidemiology, 23*(12), 743–749.

Mills, E., Loke, Y. K., Wu, P., Montori, V. M., Perri, D., Moher, D., & Guyatt, G. (2004). Determining the reporting quality of RCTs in clinical pharmacology. *British Journal of Clinical Pharmacology, 58*(1), 61–65. doi:10.1111/j.1365-2125.2004.2092.x

Modi, A., Sen, S., Adachi, J. D., Adami, S., Cortet, B., Cooper, A. L., . . . Sajjan, S. (2016). Gastrointestinal symptoms and association with medication use patterns, adherence, treatment satisfaction, quality of life, and resource use in osteoporosis: Baseline results of the MUSIC-OS study. *Osteoporosis International, 27*(3), 1227–1238. doi:10.1007/s00198-015-3388-3

Moher, D., Hopewell, S., Schulz, K. F., Montori, V., Gotzsche, P. C., Devereaux, P. J., . . . Altman, D. G. (2012). CONSORT 2010 explanation and elaboration: Updated guidelines for reporting parallel group randomised trials. *International Journal of Surgery, 10*(1), 28–55. doi:10.1016/j.ijsu.2011.10.001

Moore, T. A., Buchanan, R. W., Buckley, P. F., Chiles, J. A., Conley, R. R., Crismon, M. L., . . . Miller, A. L. (2007). The Texas Medication Algorithm Project antipsychotic algorithm for schizophrenia: 2006 update. *Journal of Clinical Psychiatry, 68*(11), 1751–1762.

Morrison, A. S. (1985). *Screening in chronic disease.* New York, NY: Oxford University Press.

Murray, C. J., & López, A. D. (1994). Quantifying disability: Data, methods and results. *Bulletin of the World Health Organization, 72*(3), 481–494.

Murray, C. J., & López, A. D. (1996). *The global burden of disease: A comprehensive assessment of mortality and disability from diseases, injuries, and risk factors in 1990 and projected to 2020.* Cambridge, MA: Harvard School of Public Health.

Murray, C. J., Vos, T., Lozano, R., Naghavi, M., Flaxman, A. D., Michaud, C., . . . Memish, Z. A. (2012). Disability-adjusted life years (DALYs) for 291 diseases and injuries in 21 regions, 1990–2010: A systematic analysis for the Global Burden of Disease Study 2010. *The Lancet, 380*(9859), 2197–2223. doi:10.1016/s0140-6736(12)61689-4

Musen, M. A., Noy, N. F., Shah, N. H., Whetzel, P. L., Chute, C. G., Story, M. A., & Smith, B. (2012). The National Center for Biomedical Ontology. *Journal of the American Medical Informatics Association, 19*(2), 190–195. doi:10.1136/amiajnl-2011-000523

Newman, L. A., & Kaljee, L. M. (2017). Health disparities and triple-negative breast cancer in African American Women: A review. *JAMA Surgery.* Advance online publication. doi:10.1001/jamasurg.2017.0005

O'Shea, J. (2017). Digital disease detection: A systematic review of event-based Internet biosurveillance systems. *International Journal of Medical Informatics, 101*, 15–22. doi:10.1016/j.ijmedinf.2017.01.019

Ong, E., Xiang, Z., Zhao, B., Liu, Y., Lin, Y., Zheng, J., . . . He, Y. (2017). Ontobee: A linked ontology data server to support ontology term dereferencing, linkage, query and integration. *Nucleic Acids Research, 45*(D1), D347–d352. doi:10.1093/nar/gkw918

Pal, S. N., Olsson, S., & Brown, E. G. (2015). The Monitoring Medicines Project: A multinational pharmacovigilance and public health project. *Drug Safety, 38*(4), 319–328. doi:10.1007/s40264-015-0283-y

Parfrey, P. S., & Ravani, P. (2015). On framing the research question and choosing the appropriate research design. *Methods in Molecular Biology 1281*, 3–18. doi:10.1007/978-1-4939-2428-8_1

Paul, D. B., & Brosco, J. P. (2013). *The PKU paradox: A short history of a genetic disease.* Baltimore, MD: Johns Hopkins University Press.

Peak, C. M., Childs, L. M., Grad, Y. H., & Buckee, C. O. (2017). Comparing nonpharmaceutical interventions for containing emerging epidemics. *Proceedings of the National Academy of Sciences of the United States of America.* Advance online publication. doi:10.1073/pnas.1616438114

Pesquita, C., Ferreira, J. D., Couto, F. M., & Silva, M. J. (2014). The epidemiology ontology: An ontology for the semantic annotation of epidemiological resources. *Journal of Biomedical Semantics, 5*(1), 4. doi:10.1186/2041-1480-5-4

Phimarn, W., Pianchana, P., Limpikanchakovit, P., Suranart, K., Supapanichsakul, S., Narkgoen, A., & Saramunee, K. (2013). Thai community pharmacist involvement in weight management in primary care to improve patient's outcomes. *International Journal of Clinical Pharmacy, 35*(6), 1208–1217. doi:10.1007/s11096-013-9851-3

Porta, M. S. (2016). *Dictionary of epidemiology* (6th ed.). New York, NY: Oxford University Press.

Rothman, K. J. (1993). Policy recommendations in epidemiology research papers. *Epidemiology, 4*(2), 94–99.

Rothman, K. J., Greenland, S., & Lash, T. L. (2015). *Modern epidemiology* (3rd ed.). Philadelphia, PA: Wolters Kluwer Health.

Schriml, L. M., Arze, C., Nadendla, S., Chang, Y. W., Mazaitis, M., Felix, V., . . . Kibbe, W. A. (2012). Disease ontology: A backbone for disease semantic integration. *Nucleic Acids Research, 40*, D940–D946. doi:10.1093/nar/gkr972

Schriml, L. M., Arze, C., Nadendla, S., Ganapathy, A., Felix, V., Mahurkar, A., . . . Hall, N. (2010). GeMInA, Genomic Metadata for Infectious Agents, a geospatial surveillance pathogen database. *Nucleic Acids Research, 38*, D754–D764. doi:10.1093/nar/gkp832

Schwartz, S., Campbell, U. B., Gatto, N. M., & Gordon, K. (2015). Toward a clarification of the taxonomy of "bias" in epidemiology textbooks. *Epidemiology, 26*(2), 216–222. doi:10.1097/ede.0000000000000224

Shattuck, L. (1850). *Report of a general plan for the promotion of public and personal health, devised, prepared and recommended by the commissioners appointed under a resolve of the Legislature of Massachusetts, relating to a sanitary survey of the state.* Boston, MA: Dutton & Wentworth.

Shim, E. (2017). Cost-effectiveness of dengue vaccination in Yucatan, Mexico using a dynamic dengue transmission model. *PLoS One, 12*(4), e0175020. doi:10.1371/journal.pone.0175020

Siddiqi, K., Shah, S., Abbas, S. M., Vidyasagaran, A., Jawad, M., Dogar, O., & Sheikh, A. (2015). Global burden of disease due to smokeless tobacco consumption in adults: analysis of data from 113 countries. *BMC Medicine, 13*, 194. doi:10.1186/s12916-015-0424-2

Smith, B., Ashburner, M., Rosse, C., Bard, J., Bug, W., Ceusters, W., . . . Lewis, S. (2007). The OBO Foundry: Coordinated evolution of ontologies to support biomedical data integration. *Nature Biotechnology, 25*(11), 1251–1255. doi:10.1038/nbt1346

Snow, J. (1849). *On the pathology and mode of communication of cholera.* London: John Churchill.

Snow, J. (1855). *On the mode of communication of cholera* (2nd ed.). London: John Churchill.

Soe, H. Z., Oo, C. C., Myat, T. O., & Maung, N. S. (2017). Detection of schistosoma antibodies and exploration of associated factors among local residents around Inlay Lake, Southern Shan State, Myanmar. *Infectious Diseases of Poverty, 6*(1), 3. doi:10.1186/s40249-016-0211-0

Teret, S. (2001). Policy and science: Should epidemiologists comment on the policy implications of their research? *Epidemiology, 12*(4), 374–375.

Tsao, C. W., & Vasan, R. S. (2015). Cohort profile: The Framingham Heart Study (FHS): Overview of milestones in cardiovascular epidemiology. *International Journal of Epidemiology, 44*(6), 1800–1813. doi:10.1093/ije/dyv337

Weiss, N. S. (2016). *Exercises in epidemiology: Applying principles and methods* (2nd ed.). New York, NY: Oxford University Press.

World Health Assembly. (2013, May 27). Follow-up to the Political Declaration of the High-level Meeting of the General Assembly on the Prevention and Control of Non-communicable Diseases. Rio de Janeiro, Brazil: Author. Retrieved from http://apps.who.int/gb/ebwha/pdf_files/WHA66/A66_R10-en.pdf?ua=1

World Health Organization. (2013). *Global action plan for the prevention and control of noncommunicable diseases 2013–2020*. Geneva, Switzerland: Author. Retrieved from http://www.who.int/iris/bitstream/10665/94384/1/9789241506236_eng.pdf?ua=1

World Health Organization. (2015a). *Global reference list of 100 core health indicators, 2015*. Geneva, Switzerland: Author. Retrieved from http://apps.who.int/iris/bitstream/10665/173589/1/WHO_HIS_HSI_2015.3_eng.pdf?ua=1

World Health Organization. (2015b). *Health in 2015: From MDGs, Millennium Development Goals to SDGs, Sustainable Development Goals*. Geneva, Switzerland: Author. Retrieved from http://apps.who.int/iris/bitstream/10665/200009/1/9789241565110_eng.pdf?ua=1

Yang, Z., Xu, J., Wang, M., Di, B., Tan, H., He, Q., . . . Fu, C. (2014). Measles epidemic from 1951 to 2012 and vaccine effectiveness in Guangzhou, southern China. *Human Vaccines & Immunotherapeutics, 10*(4), 1091–1096.

5

Disease Prevention and Health Promotion

PETER D. HURD, JUSTINNE GUYTON, AND ARDIS HANSON

Introduction

When people think of public health, they often think of the development of epidemiology and the eonian public health story about John Snow in 1854. Snow plot mapped the cholera cases in London and talked with the people to determine links between their behaviors and the disease. Using this epidemiologic approach, he determined that people who drank the water from the Broad Street pump were more likely to contract cholera. Closing the pump was effective in stopping the spread of the disease (Cockerham, 2004). Ever since John Snow removed the pump handle from the cholera-infected well in London, heralding the start of a population-based approach to public health, the world has struggled with the realities of health promotion and disease prevention.

While over a century and a half separates us from that event, cholera continues to be a public health concern. After Hurricane Matthew devastated much of Haïti's southern coast (a Category 4 storm on October 4, 2016), water was once again contaminated by the bacteria causing cholera, adding to the problems of this small, poor country (Ferreira, 2016). The World Health Organization (WHO) pledged to send 1 million doses of cholera vaccine to Haïti ([Staff], 2016). In a country like Haïti, the challenges for young children are much more than the risk of cholera; risks include malnutrition, lack of health facilities or access to them, and simply having a dry, safe place to sleep.

Cholera was unknown in Haïti until 2010 (a massive earthquake in Haïti that year that led to a worldwide response to help; see Chapter 3 in this volume) when United Nations peacekeepers improperly disposed of waste from their base, which spread disease throughout the river system that was also used for drinking water. Roughly 10,000 people have died from cholera since 2010. The fact that a hurricane can exacerbate the impact of cholera on those trying to help following an earthquake underlines the complexities of worldwide public health efforts in health promotion and disease prevention. Today, a cholera vaccine that is effective and affordable (Desai et al., 2016) can help the 1.3 billion people at-risk for cholera, reduce the estimated 2.86 million cholera cases annually, and decrease the estimated 95,000 deaths annually from cholera (Ali, Nelson, Lopez, & Sack, 2015). The availability of a vaccination for cholera is one of many ways that public and private payers are offering an array of prevention and wellness programs.

In the United States, Medicare offers preventive screenings, employer-based payers offer gym memberships and nutrition classes, and patient self-management programs are reining in the costs and deleterious effects of chronic illnesses, offering a significant return on investment. Consumer-directed care places patients and consumers in the driver's seat of their personal health delivery systems. The current fascination with health and wellness may be the very catalyst we need for making individuals take greater ownership of their own health care, realizing the personal benefits that are gained and the benefits that can accrue to society for individual action. Time will tell if these approaches will steer consumers and patients down the same road that led John Snow to that Broad Street pump.

The unsustainable nature of our current health care delivery systems is awakening many payers, employers, health care providers, policy analysts, individual consumers, and patients to the benefits of improving behaviors that negatively affect their health and the health of populations. Nevertheless, what programs are most needed and most beneficial in changing behaviors? A basic tool of public health programs, community needs assessment, is key to effective community health promotion. Other components of health care delivery systems also are looking at the health needs of local and regional populations. Organized pharmacy is a part of this focus on community engagement and public health. Pharmacy educators and pharmacy practitioners are exploring public health pathways, with many schools of pharmacy actively engaged in public health projects. Some examples of this kind of collaboration between schools of pharmacy and various public health initiatives in the community are described in this chapter.

Pharmacy educators and pharmacy practitioners are exploring public health pathways, with many schools actively engaged in public health projects. This chapter provides some examples of this kind of collaboration between schools of pharmacy and various public health initiatives in local communities.

Campbell University School of Pharmacy

Through the Campbell University School of Pharmacy's Wellness Institute (2017), North Carolinians take a more active role in their health and wellness and gain access to health care providers. The Wellness Institute focuses on public health education approaches that can lead to healthy lifestyles for individuals. The Institute's outreach includes health fairs and health screenings at Campbell and in the surrounding counties, health and wellness presentations by faculty and students, diabetes education, and continuing education for health care providers. The program also runs a Diabetes Care Project for Campbell University employees and their dependents. Enrollees meet with clinical pharmacists on a regular basis in this project. The Institute recognizes that lifestyle choices made early in life have a long-term effect upon our health in later years. The Campbell University College of Pharmacy and Health Sciences (2017) offers a master's of science degree in public health, which can be combined with the doctor of pharmacy (PharmD) degree. This option is part of the various efforts to integrate pharmacy and other health professions at Campbell University.

Duquesne University Mylan School of Pharmacy

Duquesne University's Mylan School of Pharmacy operates a number of centers, some of which have direct links to public health. The Center for Pharmacy Care, established in 2002, is part of the Academic Partners Program and provides disease prevention and disease management services (Center for Pharmacy Care, 2017; Mylan School of Pharmacy, 2017). Outreach opportunities include a Health and Wellness Fair in downtown Pittsburgh, educational programs at high schools and elementary schools, and collaboration with the county health department on such topics as opioid abuse (Mylan School of Pharmacy, 2017).

University of California at San Francisco School of Pharmacy

Utilizing the *U.S. Public Health Service Clinical Guideline for Treating Tobacco Use and Dependence* as a model, the University of California at San Francisco School of Pharmacy faculty created a turnkey tobacco cessation program that prepares both students and practitioners to help patients quit smoking. Originally designed to improve clinician-assisted tobacco cessation counseling skills in health care education as a train the trainer approach, the program is now widely used across many health professions with its blend of pharmacotherapy and tailored behavioral counseling interventions (Corelli, Fenlon, Kroon, Prokhorov, & Hudmon, 2007). The program, Rx for Change, is regularly updated and available online following a free registration (University of California at San Francisco School of Pharmacy, 2017). Since the American Association of Colleges of Pharmacy recognizes that tobacco cessation education should be a required component of pharmacy curricula, programs such as these teach pharmacists the requisite skills to deliver evidence-based interventions to their patients (McBane et al., 2013).

Virginia Commonwealth University School of Pharmacy

The Virginia Commonwealth University School of Pharmacy (2017), in conjunction with the University's public health program, offers a PharmD/master's of public health (MPH) degree program. With this combination of degrees, students focus on both pharmaceutical care, with more of a patient focus, and on the health of populations. Because this degree combines pharmacy faculty and Department of Family Medicine and Population Health, Division of Epidemiology faculty, the student has an opportunity to combine research skills, patient care, and population health. Similarly, this program combines experiential learning in public health and pharmacy. With strong ties to the Virginia Department of Health, this degree offers many hands-on and applied opportunities (Virginia Commonwealth University School of Pharmacy, 2017).

Samford University McWhorter School of Pharmacy

The McWhorter School of Pharmacy also offers a joint PharmD/MPH degree program. For the student interested in a more international focus, Samford also has a number of international experiences available to pharmacy students. Creating this kind of combination could provide for a very valuable educational package. Clinics located in local health departments provide Samford University McWhorter School of Pharmacy faculty and students the opportunity to work directly with patients and health department staff, including through the Jefferson Department of Health. Making pharmacotherapy recommendations, participating in travel clinics, encouraging flu shots, and operating smoking cessation clinics help to develop important population-based knowledge in pharmacy students as well as provide patients with prevention and wellness messages from faculty and students. In 2005, the Samford program developed a service-oriented and internationally focused residency program located in local public health departments (Hogue, 2005). Students can work in clinical sites in 14 states and 10 countries; on average, 100 students work abroad performing mission work, taking classes in London, or engaging in four-year practice experiences (McWhorter School of Pharmacy, 2017).

University of Southern California School of Pharmacy

In addition to its combined PharmD/MPH program, the FUENTE initiative is an example of the integration of health promotion and health management into the curriculum at the University of Southern California (USC) School of Pharmacy (Globe, Johnson, Conant, & Frausto, 2004). This initiative combined didactic and experiential education tools to teach pharmacy students public health and management concepts. Students conducted two service-learning opportunities to provide health promotion and disease prevention messages to elementary school students through health fairs and poison prevention programs. Because of the curriculum, USC pharmacy students were able to develop and implement subsequent health promotion programs. The USC School of Pharmacy continues to do health screenings and programs for senior citizens. The California Department of Public Health Medical Officer was the School of Pharmacy's commencement speaker in 2017, suggesting the long-term and continuing relationships with public health and the community (University of Southern California School of Pharmacy, 2017).

Northeastern University Bouvé School of Pharmacy

An interdisciplinary approach to public health that provides both services to patients and education for students is the approach used at the Bouvé College of Health Sciences at Northeastern University (Bouvé College of Health Sciences, 2017). Students have the opportunity to participate in full-time practical experiences that also count as part of the Introductory Pharmacy Practice Experience (IPPE) required for graduation. Students also may obtain a dual degree in public health (PharmD/MPH). Courses count in both programs, and students have various options to complete the MPH degree requirements after they have finished their PharmD degree.

St. Louis College of Pharmacy

The St. Louis College of Pharmacy invests in health literacy and wellness as part of its introductory pharmacy practice experience for third-year pharmacy students. During the course of an academic year, students collect medical and medication histories, perform screening assessments, and assess medication adherence, as well as conduct household safety checks and provide general recommendations to residents of local independent-living senior apartments (Grice et al., 2014). This has evolved into annual health promotion and screening efforts. These "wellness visits," led by a clinical pharmacist, target patients in a comprehensive assessment, including through risk assessment for cognitive impairment, psychosocial risks, behavioral risks, ability to perform activities of daily living, fall risk, hearing impairment risk, and home safety. At the end of the visit, patients receive education, referrals for further testing, and a personalized prevention plan, which is like a checklist of future screenings, immunizations, and other preventative services.

The St. Louis College of Pharmacy also partners with the St. Louis County Department of Public Health (2017) to provide clinical learning sites for pharmacy students and residents. One site provides patients with diabetes personalized care plans based upon the results of activation assessment and health literacy screening. Education also includes group diabetes classes, which provide patients with access to resources written to support those with low health literacy.

Health Behavior, Prevention, and Promotion

Many of the activities that individuals and populations pursue will have a direct effect upon their health, while other behaviors have a more indirect effect. While some behaviors might have little noticeable direct influence upon health, it is difficult to think of behaviors that would have little or no potential to influence health outcomes. Simple things, such as drinking safe water, breathing clean air, and eating uncontaminated food, have potential health outcomes. Clearly, health behaviors can mitigate or exacerbate chronic diseases, such as heart disease, cancer, diabetes, and stroke. Human behaviors can also affect the resurgence of infectious diseases (e.g., tuberculosis) and the emergence of new infectious diseases (e.g., HIV/AIDS, hepatitis C, and human papillomavirus [HPV]). Other behavioral factors, such as tobacco use, diet, exercise, alcohol consumption, sexual behavior, and avoidable injuries, contribute prominently to mortality. One of the current emphases in prevention and promotion programming is the relationship among behavior change and the social determinants of health (Commission on Social Determinants of Health, 2008; Marmot, Allen, Bell, Bloomer, & Goldblatt, 2012; Rowlands, Shaw, Jaswal, Smith, & Harpham, 2015; World Health Organization, 2016). This is particularly critical if one is looking at prevention of and/or changes to incidence of long-term chronic disease due to unhealthy and at-risk behaviors or programming to concurrently address multiple risk factors.

HEALTH BEHAVIOR

Health behavior can be defined as "the activity undertaken by individuals for the purpose of maintaining or enhancing their health, preventing health problems, or achieving a positive body image" (Cockerham, 2004, p. 94). This definition can include both the activities of people with no identified disease and those who are taking positive steps that might include diet and/or exercise. Another definition of health behavior includes more of an attitude component: "those personal attributes such as beliefs, expectations, motives, values, perceptions, and other cognitive elements; personality characteristics, including affective and emotional states and traits; and overt behavior patterns, actions, and habits that relate to health maintenance, to health restoration, and to health improvement" (Gochman, 1982, p. 169).

For pharmacists working in the field of public health, an expanded categorization of health behavior may be more applicable: preventive health behavior, illness behavior, and sick-role behavior (Kasl & Cobb, 1966a, 1966b). A healthy individual engages in *preventive health behavior* when he or she engages in any activity for the purpose of preventing or detecting illness in an asymptomatic state (Kasl & Cobb, 1966b). An ill individual engages in *illness behavior* when he or she engages in activity to first define the state of health and then to discover a suitable remedy (Kasl & Cobb, 1966b). Ill individuals also engage in *sick-role behavior* when he or she engages in activities with the intent of getting well (Kasl & Cobb, 1966a). Kasl and Cobb's definitions support O'Donnell's updated definition adopted by the *American Journal of Health Promotion*:

> Health Promotion is the art and science of helping people discover the synergies between their core passions and optimal health, enhancing their motivation to strive for optimal health, and supporting them in changing their lifestyle to move toward a state of optimal health. Optimal health is a dynamic balance of physical, emotional, social, spiritual, and intellectual health. Lifestyle change can be facilitated through a combination of learning experiences that enhance awareness, increase motivation, and build skills and, most important, through the creation of opportunities that open access to environments that make positive health practices the easiest choice. (O'Donnell, 2009, pp. iv–v)

Since pharmacists work with individuals ranging from healthy to different levels of sickness, Kasl and Cobb's categories are more appropriate in determining behavior patterns and information needs.

Measuring Health Behaviors
In the United States, the federal *Healthy People* initiative began as a 10-year strategy to improve the health of the nation, with an emphasis on the prevention of major chronic illnesses, injuries, and infectious diseases. *Healthy People 2000: Final Review* tracked the 10-year progress between 1990 and 2000 on a variety of national objectives, including a number of health behaviors (National Center for Health Statistics, 2001). The report substantiated prevention efforts in the United States toward the goal of reducing health disparities for more than half the objectives identified in

Healthy People 2000 (U.S. Department of Health and Human Services [USDHHS], 1990). The monitoring and assessment goals of *Healthy People 2010* (USDHHS, 2000) were even more ambitious than the *2000* goals. For example, the *2000* goal to *reduce* health disparities was strengthened in *2010* to focus on *eliminating* health disparities. *Healthy People 2020* continues this trend, including many topics appropriate for pharmacy: decreasing adverse drug events, improving communications to empower patients, building health skills, counseling from prescribers and pharmacists, and decreased disparities (USDHHS, 2010). Some of the new areas in *Healthy People 2020* include social determinants of health, dementias including Alzheimer's disease, and health care–associated infections.

Tracking *Healthy People 2020* will assist local, state, and national programs in the production of and use of health data to meet the goals of *2020*. A set of 26 leading health indicators (LHIs) were identified based upon their importance as public health issues and the availability of data to measure their progress (10 LHIs in 2010). Using two conceptual frameworks, Health Determinants and Health Outcomes by Life Stages, the LHIs examine the interrelationships between biological, social, economic, and environmental factors that affect individuals' abilities to achieve these indicators using a life stages perspective. The LHIs—such as physical activity, obesity, tobacco use, substance abuse, and infant deaths—are monitored and tracked over time (USDHHS, 2014).

The European region of the WHO created a similar initiative, *Health 2020,* as a policy for health and well-being for the WHO European region (WHO Regional Office for Europe, 2013). Adopted in 2012 by 53 member states of the region, *Health 2020* provides a vision, a strategic goal, priorities, and actions that can adapt to the many cultures of the European region (Jakab & Tsouros, 2015), much like *Healthy People, Health 2020* also provides an implementation package for policymakers, health ministries, and associated agencies and sectors. For example, a questionnaire asks if a country's policy documents address how the state will reduce the burden of disease and risk factors, enhance health and well-being, and improve governance and systems for health (WHO Regional Office for Europe, 2014). It asks specifically about such issues as integrated health policy, equity and universal coverage, health as a major societal resource and asset, and the social determinants of health. In addition, the document also examines equity, human rights and gender, health and intersectoral action, health systems and capacity, emergency response and preparedness, creation of resilient communities, and monitoring and evaluating public health research.

BASIC PUBLIC HEALTH PRINCIPLES OF DISEASE PREVENTION AND HEALTH PROMOTION

Consumer Health Education

An expert panel convened by the USDHHS describes high-quality health information as "accurate, current, valid, appropriate, intelligible, and free of bias" (Eng &

Gustafson, 1999, p. 630). Consumer health education can be quite complex, with multiple paths to achieving the desired information and behavior change. One individual may be very comfortable using Internet sources, while another may have difficulty reading printed information and have neither the ability nor the interest in searching the web for health information. Indeed, those with limited access to sources of health information may still have very profound needs. This is particularly true in the case of those individuals who have multiple (or co-occurring) health issues or chronic health issues (Gazmararian, Williams, Peel, & Baker, 2003). Groups with lower income levels and lower levels of education also present challenges to those seeking to provide health education. Nevertheless, to be sure, the need for health education includes all socioeconomic levels.

Health Literacy
Health literacy is defined as "the degree to which individuals have the capacity to obtain, process, and understand basic health information and services needed to make appropriate health decisions" by an Institute of Medicine report (Nielsen-Bohlman, Panxer, Kindig, & Institute of Medicine Committee on Health Literary, 2004). The WHO endorses a broader definition that encompasses an individual's ability to "gain access to, understand and use information in ways which promote and maintain good health" (Nutbeam & WHO Collaborating Centre for Health Promotion, 1998). Whichever definition is used, health literacy incorporates comprehension skills, literacy skills, and numeracy skills to be able to make health decisions and to decode health messages. For example, consider a patient who receives a message from a health care provider to limit salt intake to less than 1500 mg daily. To incorporate this health behavior, a patient must be able to read a nutrition label to locate the sodium content, calculate an adjustment based on a serving size, and total all of the food items eaten throughout a day to compare to the daily goal. Health literacy includes both the ability to access needed health information and the capability of using that information. Millions of people in the United States are affected by low health literacy, which increases the risk of preventable adverse drug reactions and increases costs to the health care delivery systems, running into the billions of dollars (Nielsen-Bohlman et al., 2004).

Screening tools to identify patients at-risk for low health literacy have been studied (e.g., the Test of Functional Health Literacy in Adults and the Rapid Estimate of Adult Literacy in Medicine), and shortened tools have been adapted for ease of use (e.g., Newest Vital Sign; Dumenci, Matsuyama, Kuhn, Perera, & Siminoff, 2013; Wali & Grindrod, 2016; Yeung et al., 2017). Many health care professionals utilize a "Universal Precautions Method" and strive to improve communication and education overall instead of a targeted approach to patients identified as having low health literacy (Weiss et al., 2016). This includes using simple, easy-to-read educational handouts, encouraging questions, and using teach-back counseling techniques

(Callahan et al., 2013). From a pharmacy perspective, a health-literate individual would be able to understand a prescription label (including dosing and administration), be aware of alternate treatments that might also be considered, evaluate the effects of the medication (efficacy and adverse effects), understand the purpose for each medication, and negotiate health care systems for follow-up and further treatment.

Sender, Audience, Message, and Medium

Another issue in consumer health education is the design of the message and the mode of delivery. Usually, using only a single message or a single medium is less effective than a multidimensional approach. The message is more effective when considering the various parts of the communications process, including the sender, the audience, the message, and the medium to be used to deliver the message. Health communications often use famous or well-known individuals as senders to relay messages that would appeal to a certain audience, but care must be used to carefully match the appeal of the communicator with the needs of the audience. In addition to celebrities, peers, and individuals representing a trusted source, such as the health care provider, can also be effective.

Different audiences often require different communicators, messages, and mediums. In a pharmacy chain serving multiple ethnic backgrounds, translations into other languages may be essential in an effective communication program. Older individuals may need larger print, while younger individuals may prefer social media as their source of health information.

Usually messages with a simple point told in a straightforward format work best. For many audiences, a message that includes a human-interest story is more powerful than statistics and facts, even though these might also be included. The medium includes television, radio, email, regular mail, planned events, newspapers, and social media. When using multiple media, a coordinated effort should consider how different "channels" may augment or work against each other. For example, something that identifies each message as part of a common program usually works well; however, sending the same message over numerous channels may waste valuable resources that could be used to convey different components of the health information. In this process, interference or noise can disrupt the process with too much information, conflicting messages, inappropriate cultural differences, and undesired emotional responses to the message. Having a logo or identifiable background can also help tie various messages together. Of course, we want to have a clear idea of why we are using social media and determine what we want to accomplish and what we want to persist, keeping things active, interesting, and engaging. To determine the effectiveness of the communication effort, feedback or assessment is important and should be an essential part of the program. Although feedback should document the effectiveness of the project, the lessons learned—whether the lessons are from successful programs or from mistakes—can make the next effort more effective.

The American Public Health Association has helpful information about using social media on its website (https://www.apha.org/news-and-media/social-media) as does the Centers for Disease Control and Prevention (https://www.cdc.gov/socialmedia/), reminding others that they can use many tools including Facebook, Twitter, Google, blogs, podcasts, Instagram, and LinkedIn, among many others.

Social Marketing

Social marketing, often used to increase the effectiveness of disease prevention and health promotion interventions, is defined as the "application of commercial marketing technologies to the analysis, planning, execution, and evaluation of programs designed to influence the voluntary behavior of target audiences in order to improve their personal welfare and that of their society" (Andreasen, 1995, p. 7). Social marketing uses audience research to segment the target audience into groups with common risk behaviors, similar motivations, and channel preferences. Intervention strategies are developed using the "Four Ps": (a) *product* (what behavior the consumer is asked to "buy into"), (b) *price* (what the consumer must give up in order to obtain the product), (c) *place* (how and where the product reaches the consumer), and (d) *promotion* (how information about the product is disseminated). The "marketing mix" of message and medium is continually refined based upon consumer feedback.

Using the social marketing model, the Centers for Disease Control and Prevention (CDC) developed "prevention marketing" that involves community representatives and stakeholders in the entire process, using principles from behavioral science, marketing, and community intervention (Kennedy & Crosby, 2002). Originally developed to address HIV transmission among youth (Ogden, Shepherd, & Smith, 1996), this model has applications in numerous settings. Tan et al. (2010) used a social marketing framework in the Baltimore Experience Corps Trial (BECT), a randomized controlled trial to recruit older adult volunteers for the purpose of health promotion and improving academic behaviors of children in public schools. Tan et al. suggest the BECT is an excellent model for the development of other volunteer programs designed to serve as public health interventions. The project discusses the Four P application, making useful refinements of the different types of product (core, actual, and augmented), price (replacing a sedentary or inactive lifestyle with high-intensity volunteering), place (school settings), and promotion (message and recruitment strategies). Thrasher et al. (2011) evaluated a high-exposure social marketing campaign in Mexico City that showed the effects of the implementation of Mexico City's comprehensive smoke-free law. The evaluation of the media campaign to support this legislation showed the campaign successfully promoted the law and positively reinforced knowledge and attitudes related to second-hand smoke and smoke-free laws.

Each of these four "p" words—product, price, place, promotion—can introduce a number of complex marketing topics. For example, one of the components of a product would be the life cycle of the product, and this applies well to social marketing efforts. Those planning such efforts need to be sensitive to the fact that their efforts may lose their appeal over time or after the initial excitement or curiosity has diminished. A new smoking-cessation program at a retail pharmacy may generate considerable initial interest but may lose the initial appeal if the pharmacy tends to see the same people from month to month. Products designed for a male audience will often use different phrases and branding than those targeted for women. This often presents a unique challenge. For example, if women are the target population of a public health program to reduce male violence against women but a change in both the men's and women's behaviors is the program goal, then the communicator has to consider how all of the messages will work together.

Similarly, with price, one must determine if one is more concerned with the cost of the materials and program production, the cost to the buyer who might be indigent, or the competitive costs when compared to other things the individual might do or purchase. What about the price to others, when the cook's diet leads to the entire family's weight loss? While pharmacists give free information about medications, they also charge for personal counseling sessions and sell paperbacks that contain drug information. Price is a consideration for each of these initiatives.

Placement raises questions such as whether to market directly to the consumer of the product. Does one use an intermediary to distribute the product? If so, where would the product be placed to receive optimum exposure? For example, if we are promoting calcium supplements, we may want to place a small display by athletic equipment or a sports injuries section to reach exercising individuals who may not think about walking over to the antacids section to find a cheap calcium source.

Promotion includes a consideration of what approach will best meet the targeted market. We will reach a variety of individuals who prefer receiving messages over certain media, whether the media is radio, television, phone, or computer. The important point is not to assume that everyone has access to technology, has a college education, or is a member of a more affluent socioeconomic group. There is a significant amount of literature on the differences among individuals and social groups in accessing and using information on health.

Differentiating between marketing and communication helps emphasize program goals. If the goal of a program is to change behavior, then marketing will play an important role. Our intention is to encourage a large number of people to buy into the program that we are developing. We want them to change their behavior from what they have done in the past to something new: initially that would be starting our program. If we are more interested in communicating important information, then we might assess our program by the level of public awareness or the change in base-level knowledge in a community. Monitoring the media coverage of our program might be a good measure of the effectiveness of our communication efforts in the community. Public awareness, however, is not necessarily a sign the program has led to desirable behavior change.

Whether our goal is behavior change or communication of information, successful programs include a good deal of front-end planning for a successful program launch to result. This would include preparing for a surge of requests once a program starts or after a media event has promoted the program. Ideally, this preparedness should take place before the program starts or the interview airs on the television. Do the staff people who handle the phone calls have answers to the most common questions? Are there enough people and phone lines? Are copies of program materials ready to go into the mail when requested? Do we have adequate capacity on our web pages? Are the web pages updated and working as we wish? Each program has a unique set of challenges, and identifying these in the planning stages is a key part of the process. While this kind of planning can be elaborate, it can also be as simple as logging onto a web page from home or having a friend call the 800 number for information.

PREVENTION PROGRAMMING

Community-centered prevention efforts have a public health focus of working at the community organizational level to implement change. One example of prevention programming was the CDC's federal HIV prevention activities (Ogden et al., 1996). Since the mid-1980s, the CDC had been responding to the HIV threat via the school systems and youth-serving organizations; however, high-risk and out-of-school youth remained underserved. Rural areas have also presented special challenges in HIV programming. The Prevention Marketing Initiative (PMI) funded demonstration projects with the goal of reducing sexually risky behavior among young people (Kennedy & Crosby, 2002). PMI sites and their community volunteers received marketing training, which included health departments, youth organization, AIDS organizations, religious groups, and schools. The programs used public service announcements, community workshops, telephone information, and unique branding for the programs. Today, the term "prevention programming" is used in many ways, including the prevention of sexual violence and as part of training programs on college campuses. In a 2006 review article on the literature in prevention programming, community-based prevention programs that were successful included a community ready for a prevention program, community coalitions, programming that fits the community, fidelity assessments, adequate resources, and appropriate training. Program evaluation is also an important component (Stith et al., 2006).

STAGE-BASED MODELS

Although there are many models to guide health communication, stage-based models are a useful approach to understanding human behavior. In the Transtheoretical

Model (also called "Stages of Change"), often used in smoking cessation counseling, there are five stages individuals undergo in the adoption of a new behavior or idea (Prochaska, DiClemente, & Norcross, 1992): (a) precontemplation (no knowledge or intent of new behavior), (b) contemplation (learns or is thinking about the new behavior), (c) preparation (intends to action, usually within the next 30 days), (d) action (the behavior is performed consistently), and (e) maintenance (the person consistently performs the behavior change long enough to change existing behavior; Prochaska et al., 1992).

Another stage-based measure, the Patient Activation Measure® (PAM®), identifies patients based on the level of activation (Hibbard, Stockard, Mahoney, & Tusler, 2004). The four stages are: Level 1, the patient believes his or her role is important; Level 2, the patient has the confidence and knowledge to take an action; Level 3, the patient takes the action; Level 4, the patient maintains the action even during times of stress. Strategies and information are then tailored to support patients at different levels of activation to be implemented in different clinical settings, situations, and approaches (Hibbard, 2017). The PAM® is also available as a commercial product that has been found useful in determining future emergency department visits, hospital admissions, and medication adherence.

Stage-based models appear to be linear, but human behavior is often nonlinear, with people moving back and forth or skipping stages as they make decisions. In prevention programming, individuals may fall back into old habits or find better ways of doing something. Stage-based models highlight the need for intervention programs that are appropriate for groups at various levels of willingness to adopt changes in their behaviors. Interventions are more likely to succeed when they incorporate the patient's understanding of health behaviors and readiness for change. Hence, understanding consumer motivation and choice/decision-making attributes may well drive the "next generation" of interventions.

Precede-Proceed Model

The Precede-Proceed model has been used in many health promotion and disease prevention research projects, education programs, and community applications for over 40 years and builds on the work of Lawrence W. Green and others (Green, 1974; Green & Kreuter, 1992). The Precede-Proceed framework is founded on disciplines that include epidemiology; the social, behavioral, and educational sciences; and health administration. The approach includes a focus on the desired outcomes and a plan to achieve them. The model moves from planning to evaluation, emphasizing the numerous forces that will affect a successful health program. The Precede component of the model includes predisposing, reinforcing, and enabling constructs. The Proceed component of the model includes policy, regulations, resources, and organization. The model can be very useful in providing a structure to apply various theories of health behavior. Working with the Precede-Proceed model, one can think of both a planning stage and an implementation stage. Part of the participation can involve an extensive data collection and analysis, not just laying the foundation but throughout the project and the evaluations. The data collection does require a strong community involvement in the project. The process can be broken down into stages, beginning with an initial assessment and concluding with an evaluation of the achievement of outcome (Gielen, McDonald, Gary, & Bone, 2008).

Intervention Programs

Effective intervention programs can be designed for individuals at very different age levels while sharing the goal of health promotion or disease prevention. For interventions that focus on those individuals who are too young to have graduated from high school, efforts would include the adolescents' social environments and would address multiple sources of influence within these environments. For prevention programs like smoking and drug abuse, these efforts are often most effective when applied early (e.g., in primary school years) and continued through adolescence. This kind of program usually would include teacher training, programming for students, and parent classes. Similarly, interventions for older adults should focus on the individual's knowledge and motivation, social settings and support systems, and even changes in laws and public policy. A successful flu immunization campaign at the public health level might address each of these areas (where and how much, community groups for the locations, and who receives first priority).

BASIC TASKS IN PROGRAM DESIGN

In disease prevention/health promotion campaigns, such as those already described, there are a number of basic tasks: (a) choosing a target audience(s) and setting objectives that are measurable in some way; (b) selecting a message and means of delivery, including the mix of media and messages; and (c) creating some form of evaluation to provide evidence of the successful of the program. It is critical to effective evaluation that programs are consistent in design and well integrated into the day-to-day management of programs.

Immunization

The CDC's Racial and Ethnic Adult Disparities Immunization Initiative program was a multiyear demonstration project conducted in five sites (Chicago, IL; Rochester, NY; San Antonio, TX; Milwaukee, WI; and the Mississippi Delta region) to increase flu and pneumonia vaccination rates for African Americans and Hispanics 65 years of age and older (Kicera, Douglas, & Guerra, 2005; Morita, 2006). The Mississippi program focused on both rural and urban African Americans, while the San Antonio program focused on Hispanics (Kicera et al., 2005). This research has explored the reasons why people chose to have a flu shot (family and health) or to avoid immunization (fear of becoming ill) and has looked at the realities of providing programming with similar goals to dissimilar target groups (Winston, Wortley, & Lees, 2006).

Tobacco

Successful programs designed to decrease the use of tobacco have included both individual and group foci, multiple approaches, and a continued effort to elicit target behaviors. A great deal of social and behavioral research has focused on smoking prevention (usually focused on young people in school) and smoking cessation (focused on tobacco users). Programs that have targeted both the community and the school system seem to be effective, perhaps because they address the issue of changing messages that experimental smokers may obtain from school programs, peers who are important to them, and family members. However, as of now, there are no common standards across all schools in all states (Bruckner et al., 2014).

Smoking cessation initiatives can be described as primary (those targeting the smoker) or secondary (those that have a secondary aim to increase smoking cessation rates but have a different primary aim). Successful primary initiatives include use of medications for smoking cessation, quitlines, smoking cessation services, and employer incentives for quitting. Secondary initiatives include government and business polices that limit exposure to second-hand smoke by prohibiting smoking in certain areas or limit access to or experimentation with smoking by increasing taxes on tobacco products. Quitlines offer free access to smoking cessation resources and counselors by telephone and provide an example of a successful program design. This novel approach was first implemented in in the 1980s by the U.S. National Cancer Institute and has expanded to state-based organizations and through a national platform (1-800-QUIT NOW). Awareness of quitlines has reached the public through national education campaigns, with 65% of smokers aware of these services (Kaufman, Augustson, Davis, & Finney Rutten, 2010). Quitlines have adapted, and many now offer Internet-based platforms and text messaging. Success of these programs is measured in 30-day smoking abstinence rates, and the use of dual technology increased the odds of being successful 1.51 times (Puckett et al., 2015).

PUBLIC POLICY AND CHANGES IN THE LAW

Health promotion and disease prevention strategies, as described in the discussion on tobacco, can include laws and regulations. Effective strategies in the area of smoking have included age restrictions for the sale of tobacco products, taxes that increase the price of cigarettes, and smoke-free businesses. In a similar vein, laws that have changed the design of automobiles, fostered safer road construction, and tightened seatbelt and infant car seat laws have reduced motor vehicle deaths. Altering human behavior is complicated, and these positive changes have come with a sustained long-term effort, using multiple approaches in a population that generally supports these social changes.

Implications for Public Health and Pharmacy Practice

One of the most significant challenges for health policy today is to understand and improve health behavior. Disease prevention and health promotion initiatives require coordinated and focused efforts from behavioral science, public health, health education, and translational research or the translation of science into practice. For pharmacists, the ability to integrate the best available knowledge from theory and research in pharmacy practice can help advance that agenda in the next decade. One of the challenges for pharmacists in public health is to move beyond simply doing what other health professionals are doing and develop programs and interventions that are grounded in the unique strengths of the pharmacist. Some pharmacy programs are adding particular areas or institutes with an explicit focus on public health (Dindial, Fung, & Arya, 2016). In 2014, the CDC provided a Public Health Grand Rounds titled "How Pharmacists Can Improve our Nation's Health" (Lee, Burns, Rodriguez de Bittner, & Hall, 2014). As part of that program, the pharmacist was identified as a key player in addressing the health outcomes of those with chronic disease, including the elderly (e.g., 9 of 10 older adults have taken at least one prescription drug in the last month usually for chronic disease). The potential for pharmacy and public health will continue to grow as the US population continues to age.

The potential of global health will also provide great opportunities for the practice of pharmacy and pharmacy education. Crawford (2005) described a pharmacy course that included an emphasis on health promotion and disease prevention as part of a general introduction to pharmacy and the health care system. This required course for first-year pharmacy students included a lecture on health promotion and disease prevention, with additional content in discussion topics and related areas (e.g., cholesterol screening, immunizations, and bioterrorism). The course had a public health focus, including population-focused care and some potential international issues such as responding to bioterrorism (Crawford, 2005). A few years later, Bailey and DiPietro Mager (2016) published a review of the pharmacy programs offering a global health education component (e.g., required course, a minor or certificate, dual degrees). Of the 133 pharmacy schools in the review, more than 50 offered an elective or required course related to global health and more than 50 had global health experiential education experiences. Their findings document the growing role of global health in pharmacy. While distinctions made between public health (especially focused on prevention), international health (focused on underdeveloped countries), and global health (as a broader category, including an integration of both population and individual patient concerns) may be helpful (Koplan et al., 2009), clearly public health responses in the community are responses to both local and international health issues.

Another issue surrounding health behavior is the increased opportunity for health professionals and patients to engage in interactive health communication through such innovations as online networks, personal digital assistants (including drug information), and text messaging. The potential for health interventions using these types of communication options are just starting to be used to change health behavior. The potential goes far beyond using the phone for a refill at the pharmacy and checking the web pages for information about the drug and the disease being treated. The evaluation of both drug information and pharmacy websites in terms of their public health contributions might be of both vital human interest and economic importance.

Payers for services, such as Medicare/Medicaid and pharmacy benefits management companies, also have significant potential influences in encouraging widespread improvements in disease prevention and health promotion through the structure of their programs. Benefit design decisions and reimbursement systems can encourage individuals to take advantage of cost-effective preventive services and can encourage providers to offer preventive and/or treatment services that promote effective health behavior. Reimbursements for pharmacy services that promote better use of medications or higher levels of compliance have the potential to foster population-based programs that would increase the health of the public.

The value of evaluation and assessment of programs will continue to be an important part of the future of public health pharmacy. While implementing a program with good intentions is laudatory, demonstrating that the efforts actually worked (and, hopefully, did no harm) should be a central component for public health pharmacy practice. In evidence-based health care systems, providing the documentation of one's successes is of immense value. Indeed, many of the behavior change strategies would also work for those seeking to expand the awareness of pharmacy's important role in public health.

Health promotion and disease prevention programs have a long history of successes, but those individuals working in public health have also learned from programs that have been less than successful. Changing human behavior is challenging. It usually requires a longitudinal effort, a variety of approaches, individual support, and population (or social group) acceptance. As challenging as this may be, the potential to have a life-long impact on the health of entire communities, populations, and even international regions is a compelling reason for an increased public health commitment by those in pharmacy. The alignment of individual responsibility, population norms, and international health offers great opportunities for the participation of pharmacists in public health pharmacy.

References

Ali, M., Nelson, A. R., Lopez, A. L., & Sack, D. A. (2015). Updated global burden of cholera in endemic countries. *PLoS Neglected Tropical Diseases, 9*(6), e0003832. doi:10.1371/journal. pntd.0003832

Andreasen, A. (1995). *Marketing social change: Changing behavior to promote health, social develop-ment and the environment.* San Francisco, CA: Jossey Bass.

Bailey, L. C., & DiPietro Mager, N. A. (2016). Global health education in doctor of pharmacy programs. *American Journal of Pharmaceutical Education, 80*(4), Article 71. doi:10.5688/ajpe80471

Bouvé College of Health Sciences. (2017). Doctor of pharmacy (PharmD). Retrieved from http://www.northeastern.edu/bouve/pharmacy/programs/pharmd/

Bruckner, T. A., Domina, T., Hwang, J. K., Gerlinger, J., Carpenter, C., & Wakefield, S. (2014). State-level education standards for substance use prevention programs in schools: A sys-tematic content analysis. *Journal of Adolescent Health, 54*(4), 467–473. doi:10.1016/j.jadohealth.2013.07.020

Callahan, L. F., Hawk, V., Rudd, R., Hackney, B., Bhandari, S., Prizer, L. P., . . . DeWalt, D. (2013). Adaptation of the health literacy universal precautions toolkit for rheumatology and cardiology—applications for pharmacy professionals to improve self-management and out-comes in patients with chronic disease. *Research in Social & Administrative Pharmacy, 9*(5), 597–608. doi:10.1016/j.sapharm.2013.04.016

Campbell University College of Pharmacy & Health Sciences. (2017). Wellness Institute. Retrieved from http://ww2.campbell.edu/cphs/centers-and-programs/wellness-institute/

Center for Pharmacy Care. (2017). Duquesne University Pharmacy and Center for Pharmacy Care. Retrieved from http://duq.edu/academics/schools/pharmacy/centers-and-programs/duquesne-university-pharmacy-and-center-for-pharmacy-care

Cockerham, W. C. (2004). *Medical sociology* (9th ed.). Upper Saddle River, NJ: Pearson Prentice Hall.

Commission on Social Determinants of Health. (2008). *Closing the gap in a generation: Health equity through action on the social determinants of health.* Geneva, Switzerland: World Health Organi-zation. Retrieved from http://apps.who.int/iris/bitstream/10665/43943/1/9789241563703_eng.pdf

Corelli, R. L., Fenlon, C. M., Kroon, L. A., Prokhorov, A. V., & Hudmon, K. S. (2007). Evaluation of a train-the-trainer program for tobacco cessation. *American Journal of Pharmaceutical Education, 71*(6), 109.

Crawford, S. Y. (2005). Pharmacists' roles in health promotion and disease prevention. *American Journal of Pharmaceutical Education, 69*(4), Article 73. doi:10.5688/aj690473

Desai, S. N., Pezzoli, L., Martin, S., Costa, A., Rodriguez, C., Legros, D., & Perea, W. (2016). A second affordable oral cholera vaccine: Implications for the global vaccine stockpile. *The Lancet: Global Health, 4*(4), e223–e224. doi:10.1016/s2214-109x(16)00037-1

Dumenci, L., Matsuyama, R. K., Kuhn, L., Perera, R. A., & Siminoff, L. A. (2013). On the validity of the Rapid Estimate of Adult Literacy in Medicine (REALM) scale as a meas-ure of health literacy. *Communication Methods & Measures, 7*(2), 134–143. doi:10.1080/19312458.2013.789839

Dindial, S., Fung, C., & Arya, V. (2016). A call for greater policy emphasis and public health applica-tions in pharmacy education. American Journal of Pharmaceutical Education, 76(8), Article 142. Retrieved from https://www.ncbi.nlm.nih.gov/pmc/articles/PMC3475771/

Eng, T. R., & Gustafson, D. H. (1999). *Wired for health and well-being: The emergence of interac-tive health communication.* Washington, DC: U.S. Department of Health and Human Services, Science Panel on Interactive Communication and Health. Retrieved from https://pdfs.seman-ticscholar.org/e6e1/402eccdfa6a1d63459c465a5f7e81a45c33e.pdf

Ferreira, S. (2016). Cholera threatens Haiti after Hurricane Matthew. *BMJ, 355,* i5516. doi:10.1136/bmj.i5516

Gazmararian, J. A., Williams, M. V., Peel, J., & Baker, D. W. (2003). Health literacy and knowledge of chronic disease. *Patient Education & Counseling, 51*(3), 267–275.

Gielen, A. C., McDonald, E., Gary, T. L., & Bone, L. R. (2008). Using the precede-proceed model to apply health behavior theories. In R. B. Glanz & V. K.(Eds.), *Health behavior and health educa-tion: Theory, research, and practice* (pp. 407–433). San Francisco, CA: Jossey-Bass.

Globe, D. R., Johnson, K., Conant, L., & Frausto, S. (2004). Implementing a community-based health promotion program into the pharmacy curriculum: The USC FUENTE initiative. *American Journal of Pharmaceutical Education, 68*(2), 32. doi:10.5688/aj680232

Gochman, D. S. (1982). Labels, systems and motives: Some perspectives for future research and programs. *Health Education Quarterly, 9*(2–3), 263–270.

Green, L. W. (1974). Toward cost-benefit evaluations of health education: Some concepts, methods, and examples. *Health Education & Behavior, 2*(1 Suppl.), 34–64. doi:10.1177/109019817400020S106

Green, L. W., & Kreuter, M. W. (1992). CDC's Planned Approach to Community Health as an application of PRECEDE and an inspiration for PROCEED. *Journal of Health Education, 23*(3), 140–147. doi:10.1080/10556699.1992.10616277

Grice, G. R., Tiemeier, A., Hurd, P., Berry, T. M., Voorhees, M., Prosser, T. R., ... Duncan, W. (2014). Student use of health literacy tools to improve patient understanding and medication adherence. *The Consultant Pharmacist, 29*(4), 240–253. doi:10.4140/TCP.n.2014.240

Hibbard, J. H. (2017). Patient activation and the use of information to support informed health decisions. *Patient Education & Counseling, 100*(1), 5–7. doi:10.1016/j.pec.2016.07.006

Hibbard, J. H., Stockard, J., Mahoney, E. R., & Tusler, M. (2004). Development of the Patient Activation Measure (PAM): Conceptualizing and measuring activation in patients and consumers. *Health Services Research, 39*(4 Part 1), 1005–1026. doi:10.1111/j.1475-6773.2004.00269.x

Hogue, M. D. (2005, February). *Successful models: Public health initiatives.* Paper presented at the interim meeting of the American Association of Colleges of Pharmacy, Washington, DC. Retrieved from http://www.aacp.org/InterimMeeting/hogue.html.

Jakab, Z., & Tsouros, A. D. (2015). Health 2020—achieving health and development in today's Europe. *Przeglad epidemiologiczny, 69*(1), 1–7, 105–112.

Kasl, S. V., & Cobb, S. (1966a). Health behavior, illness behavior, and sick role behavior. I. Health and illness behavior. *Archives of Environmental Health, 12*(2), 246–266.

Kasl, S. V., & Cobb, S. (1966b). Health behavior, illness behavior, and sick-role behavior. II. Sick-role behavior. *Archives of Environmental Health, 12*(4), 531–541.

Kaufman, A., Augustson, E., Davis, K., & Finney Rutten, L. J. (2010). Awareness and use of tobacco quitlines: Evidence from the Health Information National Trends Survey. *Journal of Health Communication, 15*(Suppl. 3), 264–278. doi:10.1080/10810730.2010.526172

Kennedy, M. G., & Crosby, R. A. (2002). Prevention marketing: An emerging integrated framework. In R. J. DiClemente, R. A. Crosby, & M. C. Kegler (Eds.), *Emerging theories in health promotion practice and research* (pp. 255–284). San Francisco, CA: Jossey-Bass.

Kicera, T. J., Douglas, M., & Guerra, F. A. (2005). Best-practice models that work: The CDC's Racial and Ethnic Adult Disparities Immunization Initiative (READII) Programs. *Ethnicity & Disease, 15*(2 Suppl. 3), S3-17-S3-3-20

Koplan, J. P., Bond, T. C., Merson, M. H., Reddy, K. S., Rodriguez, M. H., Sewankambo, N. K., & Wasserheit, J. N. (2009). Towards a common definition of global health. *The Lancet, 373*(9679), 1993–1995. doi:10.1016/s0140-6736(09)60332-9

Lee, M., Burns, A., Rodriguez de Bittner, M., & Hall, L. E. (2014). How pharmacists can improve our nation's health. *Grand Rounds.* [Webinar].

Marmot, M., Allen, J., Bell, R., Bloomer, E., & Goldblatt, P. (2012). WHO European review of social determinants of health and the health divide. *The Lancet, 380*(9846), 1011–1029. doi:10.1016/s0140-6736(12)61228-8

McBane, S. E., Corelli, R. L., Albano, C. B., Conry, J. M., Della Paolera, M. A., Kennedy, A. K., ... Hudmon, K. S. (2013). The role of academic pharmacy in tobacco cessation and control. *American Journal of Pharmaceutical Education, 77*(5), 93. doi:10.5688/ajpe77593

McWhorter School of Pharmacy. (2017). Samford University McWhorter School of Pharmacy: Program description. Retrieved from http://schoolpages.pharmcas.org/publishedsurvey/447#3

Morita, J. (2006). Addressing racial and ethnic disparities in adult immunization, Chicago. *Journal of Public Health Management & Practice, 12*(4), 321–329.

Mylan School of Pharmacy. (2017). Academic Partners Program. Retrieved from http://duq.edu/
    academics/schools/pharmacy/centers-and-programs/academic-partners-program
National Center for Health Statistics. (2001). *Healthy People 2000 final review*. Hyattsville, MD: U.S.
    Public Health Service. Retrieved from https://www.cdc.gov/nchs/data/hp2000/hp2k01.pdf
Nielsen-Bohlman, L., Panxer, A. M., Kindig, D. A., & Institute of Medicine Committee on Health
    Literary. (2004). *Health literacy: A prescription to end confusion*. Washington, DC: National
    Academy Press. Retrieved from http://iom.nationalacademies.org/Reports/2004/Health-
    Literacy-A-Prescription-to-End-Confusion.aspx
Nutbeam, D., & WHO Collaborating Centre for Health Promotion. (1998). *Health promotion
    glossary*. Geneva, Switzerland: World Health Organization, Division of Health Promotion,
    Education and Communications. Retrieved from http://www.who.int/healthpromotion/
    about/HPR%20Glossary%201998.pdf?ua=1
O'Donnell, M. P. (2009). Definition of health promotion 2.0: Embracing passion, enhancing moti-
    vation, recognizing dynamic balance, and creating opportunities. *American Journal of Health
    Promotion, 24*(1), iv. doi:10.4278/ajhp.24.1.iv
Ogden, L., Shepherd, m., & Smith, W. A. (1996). *The Prevention Marketing Initiative: Applying pre-
    vention marketing*. Atlanta, GA: Centers for Disease Control and Prevention. Retrieved from
    https://stacks.cdc.gov/view/cdc/6320
Prochaska, J. O., DiClemente, C. C., & Norcross, J. C. (1992). In search of how people change.
    Applications to addictive behaviors. *American Psychologist, 47*(9), 1102–1114.
Puckett, M., Neri, A., Thompson, T., Underwood, J. M., Momin, B., Kahende, J., . . . Stewart, S.
    L. (2015). Tobacco cessation among users of telephone and web-based interventions—four
    states, 2011–2012. *MMWR: Morbidity and Mortality Weekly Report, 63*(51), 1217–1221.
Rowlands, G., Shaw, A., Jaswal, S., Smith, S., & Harpham, T. (2015). Health literacy and the social
    determinants of health: A qualitative model from adult learners. *Health Promotion International.*
    doi:10.1093/heapro/dav093
[Staff]. (2016, October 12). World Health Organization to send 1 million doses of cholera vaccine
    to Haiti to avert new cases. *The Pharmaceutical Journal.* doi:10.1211/PJ.2016.20201829
St. Louis College of Pharmacy, & St. Louis County Department of Public Health. (2017). *PGY1
    pharmacy residency: St. Louis College of Pharmacy & St. Louis County Department of Public
    Health learning experiences*. St. Louis, MO: Author. Retrieved from https://stlcop.edu/resi-
    dencies/_files/pgy1-department-of-health-learning-experience.pdf
Stith, S., Pruitt, I., Dees, J. E., Fronce, M., Green, N., Som, A., & Linkh, D. (2006). Implementing
    community-based prevention programming: A review of the literature. *Journal of Primary
    Prevention, 27*(6), 599–617. doi:10.1007/s10935-006-0062-8
Tan, E. J., Tanner, E. K., Seeman, T. E., Xue, Q. L., Rebok, G. W., Frick, K. D., . . . Fried, L. P. (2010).
    Marketing public health through older adult volunteering: Experience Corps as a social
    marketing intervention. *American Journal of Public Health, 100*(4), 727–734. doi:10.2105/
    ajph.2009.169151
Thrasher, J. F., Huang, L., Perez-Hernandez, R., Niederdeppe, J., Grillo-Santillan, E., & Alday, J.
    (2011). Evaluation of a social marketing campaign to support Mexico City's comprehen-
    sive smoke-free law. *American Journal of Public Health, 101*(2), 328–335. doi:10.2105/
    ajph.2009.189704
U.S. Department of Health and Human Services. (1990). *Healthy People 2000: National health pro-
    motion and disease prevention objectives*. Rockville, MD: Author. Retrieved from http://files.
    eric.ed.gov/fulltext/ED332957.pdf
U.S. Department of Health and Human Services. (2000). *Healthy people 2010*. Washington,
    DC: Author. Retrieved from http://purl.access.gpo.gov/GPO/LPS8595
U.S. Department of Health and Human Services. (2010). *Healthy People 2020*. Washington,
    DC: Author. Retrieved from http://www.healthypeople.gov/2020/

U.S. Department of Health and Human Services. (2014, March). *Healthy People 2020 leading health indicators: Progress update.* Washington, DC: Author. Retrieved from https://www.healthy-people.gov/sites/default/files/LHI-ProgressReport-ExecSum_0.pdf

University of California at San Francisco School of Pharmacy. (2017). Clinician-assisted tobacco cessation. Retrieved from http://rxforchange.ucsf.edu/

University of Southern California School of Pharmacy. (2017, March 14). Dr. Jessica Núñez de Ybarra to speak at commencement [Press release]. Retrieved from https://pharmacyschool.usc.edu/dr-jessica-nunez-de-ybarra-to-speak-at-commencement/

Virginia Commonwealth University School of Pharmacy. (2017). MPH dual degree programs. Retrieved from http://familymedicine.vcu.edu/epidemiology/mph/dual-degrees/

Wali, H., & Grindrod, K. (2016). Don't assume the patient understands: Qualitative analysis of the challenges low health literate patients face in the pharmacy. *Research in Social & Administrative Pharmacy, 12*(6), 885–892. doi:10.1016/j.sapharm.2015.12.003

Weiss, B. D., Brega, A. G., LeBlanc, W. G., Mabachi, N. M., Barnard, J., Albright, K., . . . West, D. R. (2016). Improving the effectiveness of medication review: Guidance from the Health Literacy Universal Precautions Toolkit. *Journal of the American Board of Family Medicine, 29*(1), 18–23. doi:10.3122/jabfm.2016.01.150163

Winston, C. A., Wortley, P. M., & Lees, K. A. (2006). Factors associated with vaccination of Medicare beneficiaries in five U.S. communities: Results from the racial and ethnic adult disparities in immunization initiative survey, 2003. *Journal of the American Geriatrics Society, 54*(2), 303–310. doi:10.1111/j.1532-5415.2005.00585.x

World Health Organization. (2016). Social determinants of health. Retrieved from http://www.who.int/social_determinants/sdh_definition/en/

World Health Organization Regional Office for Europe. (2013). *Health 2020: A European policy framework and strategy for the 21st century.* Copenhagen, Denmark: Author. Retrieved from http://www.euro.who.int/__data/assets/pdf_file/0011/199532/Health2020-Long.pdf?ua=1

World Health Organization Regional Office for Europe. (2014). *Qualitative indicators for monitoring Health 2020 policy targets.* Copenhagen, Denmark: Author. Retrieved from http://www.euro.who.int/__data/assets/pdf_file/0004/259582/Qualitative-indicators-for-monitoring-Health-2020-policy-targets-Eng.pdf

Yeung, D. L., Alvarez, K. S., Quinones, M. E., Clark, C. A., Oliver, G. H., Alvarez, C. A., & Jaiyeola, A. O. (2017). Low-health literacy flashcards & mobile video reinforcement to improve medication adherence in patients on oral diabetes, heart failure, and hypertension medications. *Journal of the American Pharmacists Association, 57*(1), 30–37. doi:10.1016/j.japh.2016.08.012

6

Cultural Perspectives in Public Health

BARRY A. BLEIDT, CARMITA A. COLEMAN, AND PETER D. HURD

The World Health Organization (WHO; 1948, p. 1) defines health as "a state of complete physical, mental and social well-being and not merely the absence of disease or infirmity." Public health is "the science and art of preventing disease, prolonging life and promoting health through organized efforts and informed choices of society, organizations, public and private, communities and individuals" (Winslow, 1920, p. 30). In general, public health is concerned with issues that impact the health outcomes of a population in contrast to the health of an individual. The population in question can be as small as a handful of people within a community or as widespread as the people living in one or more countries. Today, the burden of preventable, chronic diseases and the existence of global communicable diseases significantly affect and challenge public health and health care.

In order to deliver effective health care and public health services, an awareness of and appreciation for culture's influence on the social determinants of health is fundamental. Figure 6-1 illustrates how and where culture has a significant influence on a patient's health beliefs and health. Health disparities among different groups is attributed to poorer overall health and decreased health outcomes. Culturally competent delivery of care is a primary contributor to reducing the more expansive concern of health disparities (U.S. Department of Health and Human Services [USDHHS], 2010).

There are many facets to understanding the concept of culture and its influences. First, each person is a member of multiple cultures. Second, some aspects of culture may be visibly obvious on an individual (such as ethnicity, gender, or religion), while other aspects may not be as readily apparent at all (such as sexual orientation). Third, another less discussed aspect of culture is there can be tremendous diversity within a defined culture. For example, the Hispanic or Latino culture is very diverse, representing customs, beliefs, and values from different hemispheres and many countries. Fourth, there are numerous cultures to which a patient could identify that may not be immediately recognizable as a distinct culture by a novice in his or her cultural-integration journey, such as

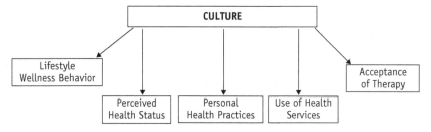

Figure 6-1. Culture's influence on a patient's health beliefs and health.

- Generational (to which generation does a patient belong);
- Disability (physical, psychological, emotional);
- Health professional (versus patient);
- Primary spoken language (e.g., French, Creole, Arabic, Spanish);
- Lifestyle (vegan, cross-fit); and
- Gender (transsexual, questioning).

In this chapter, we define culture, including its role and influence as a social determinant of health, and discuss the concepts of cultural awareness and cultural competency, which are the foundation of a patient-centered approach to better health outcomes and wellness. We also discuss the current status of cultural consideration in health care as a public health problem and present the need for culturally competent services delivery, along with an exploration of what is involved in the cultural integration journey.

When public health issues arise to affect health negatively, it becomes imperative to identify and prioritize these concerns using a pragmatic framework that leads to positive action. Silvia Rabionet, associate professor of public health at Nova Southeastern University College of Pharmacy, established eight criteria that must be met for an issue to be defined as a public health problem. Professionals involved in addressing the public's health can use the following framework to define, advocate, and articulate when to approach an issue from a public health perspective:

1. Does it affect the health and well-being of the population?
2. Is it widespread and increasing in scope and magnitude within a population or in a subgroup of a population?
3. Does it affect health-related and other societal resources (e.g., economic and social impacts)?
4. Does it challenge cultural norms and/or raise questions about values of life?
5. Does its solution rest in collective measures and interventions based in disease prevention, health promotion, and education?
6. Does it require interprofessional collaboration?

7. Does it call for organized government intervention?

8. Does it merit urgent action?

The complexity of delivering culturally competent care that is respectful of a heterogeneous patient population will multiply as the US and world populations become more diverse. Past failures to recognize the role of culture significantly affected the health and well-being of the populace; these failures also drastically influenced the utilization of resources and challenged how we value the individuality of a patient.

Actions undertaken to resolve the lack of culturally competent care include interprofessional collaboration and governmental action. Therefore, culturally competent care meets these criteria to be classified as a public health problem. Modern public health practice requires interprofessional and transdisciplinary teams of public health workers and health care professionals including pharmacists, physicians, dentists, psychologists, epidemiologists, biostatisticians, physical therapists, medical assistants, nurses, environmental scientists, dietitians and nutritionists, veterinarians, public health engineers, public health lawyers, sociologists, community development workers, communications experts, and bioethicists, among others.

The ethnic make-up of the population of the United States is continuously evolving and rapidly expanding. By 2060, the nation's population is expected to increase to under 417 million people, an average increase of 2.1 million people per year (Colby & Ortman, 2015). At that time, it is projected those that are now considered minorities will be a collective majority. Figure 6-2 shows a graphic representation and ethnic breakdown of the US population for the years 2014 and 2060. These

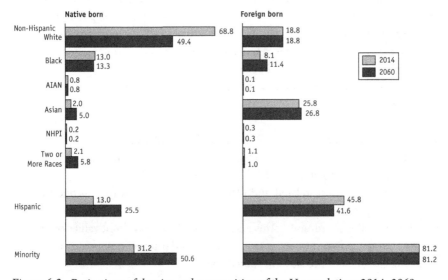

Figure 6-2. Projections of the size and composition of the U. population: 2014–2060.

substantial changes demonstrate clearly how and why culture has become a huge influence on health. Interestingly, 20% of that population will include new immigrants to the United States.

Purnell and Paulanka (2012, p. 2) define culture as "the totality of socially transmitted behavioral patterns, arts, beliefs, values, customs, life-ways, and all other products of human work and thought characteristics of a population of people that guide their worldview and decision-making." It is important to understand as ethnic diversity continues to expand within the United States, cultural considerations must be recognized as an integral factor in patient care to a greater extent than now. Cultural values and norms can determine health-seeking behaviors, self-management of a disease, and certainly cross-cultural communication with health care providers. Public health practitioners who do not recognize that culture is the background for many of the decisions made relating to health will most likely encounter mistrust from the patient but also professional frustration from the lack of impactful patient outcomes regardless of the intervention. Purnell and Paulanka (2012) further identified 12 domains of culture that could impact how a patient would approach an issue such as health care. The 12 domains encompass both personal and social practices, as well as cultural and family heritage, health attitudes and beliefs, and physiological/genetic aspects that affect health. Tying each cultural domain into a pertinent health care scenario helps practitioners understand elements that may need addressing from a culturally competent perspective. For example, in some cultures, obesity is a sign of affluence, not disease. Some cultures may not have a framework or construct for prenatal or postnatal care, which may affect pregnancy and childbirth health practices.

The Need for Cultural Competence in Healthcare Delivery

Findings reported in a 2016 Roundtable on Population Health Improvement workshop on health equity indicated that it is important to increase the racial and ethnic diversity among health care providers (National Academies of Sciences, Engineering, and Medicine, 2016). Although studies have found that racial and ethnic minority practitioners are significantly more willing to serve in minority and medically underserved areas than their majority counterparts (Smedley, Butler, & Bristow, 2004), there are a number of medically underserved populations and communities across the United States. Many reported health disparities and health inequities are found in medically underserved populations in medically underserved areas and in areas that are designated "health professional shortage areas" (Health Resources and Services Administration, 2016).

Box 6-1 **SNPhA Mission Statement**

SNPhA is an educational service association of pharmacy students who are concerned about pharmacy and health care–related issues and the poor minority representation in pharmacy and other health-related professions.

The purpose of SNPhA is to plan, organize, coordinate, and execute programs geared toward the improvement for the health, educational, and social environment of the community.

Medically underserved populations include groups of persons who face socioeconomic, cultural, or linguistic barriers to health care. *Medically underserved areas* range in size and designation from a whole county or a group of contiguous counties, a group of county or civil divisions, or a group of urban census tracts. *Health professional shortage areas* are defined as the shortage of primary medical care, dental, or mental health providers in urban or rural areas across a variety of population groups or across medical or other public facilities (Health Resources and Services Administration, 2016). However, the defining factor is that residents have a shortage of personal health services.

Greater diversity among health care professionals is associated with increased patient choices of clinicians, satisfaction, improved patient–practitioner communication, and better access to care for minorities (LaVeist & Pierre, 2014; Smedley et al., 2004; Williams, Walker, & Egede, 2016). The profession of pharmacy is fortunate to have at one professional student society whose primary mission is to improve the health of the medically underserved and increase the number of minority pharmacists: the Student National Pharmaceutical Association (SNPhA, 2016). In 1972, the SNPhA was formed in order to promote these interests among student pharmacists. As illustrated by its mission shown in Box 6-1, SNPhA develops and implements programming and clinical initiatives that target improving minority health outcomes.

SNPhA has at its core six patient outreach initiatives, including HIV/AIDS, chronic kidney disease, and diabetes (SNPhA, 2013). Annually, SNPhA measures the number of initiative events and patient interventions. There were more than 108,000 patient encounters. These astounding numbers show that student pharmacists can have significant impact on the public health of a nation.

Cultural Competence

Delivering efficient and effective health care and public health services requires an understanding of the differences among various cultures to which a patient identifies. There are five steps involved in the journey toward cultural integration (Bleidt, 1992). Starting with ethnocentricity and moving along to ethnic diversity,

a practitioner may find him- or herself working from cultural insensitivity to awareness, sensitivity, competency, and finally cultural integration.

An individual practitioner can be at many points along this continuum depending on which culture(s) he or she is encountering at the time. There is no set starting
point either, as proper attitudes and learned techniques and practices advance the
clinician along the continuum with each new cultural engagement. Although the
continuum applies to both individuals and organizations, the primary purpose of
this chapter is to discuss individual journeys.

With each new cultural experience, a person evolves toward cultural integration.
The four benchmarks on the continuum address *insensitivity, awareness, sensitivity,*
and *integration*. *Cultural insensitive* is defined as not being aware of or having knowledge of cultural differences or their impact and/or lacking the desire to learn about
various cultures. *Cultural awareness* is the stage that involves self-examination of
one's own cultural background, what makes it unique, and what bearing these dis-
coveries may have. In *cultural sensitivity*, public health professionals have an awareness and begin to develop a deeper cultural knowledge about others but have not
assimilated this knowledge into practice successfully. In the last step, *cultural integration*, cultural knowledge is placed into practice in order to communicate better
and serve the patient more effectively.

A culturally competent practitioner possesses the knowledge, skills, attitudes,
and abilities to provide optimal health care services to patients from a wide range of
cultural and ethnic backgrounds. In a culturally competent organization, clinicians
can move through the steps fairly rapidly and the patient feels comfortable as this
learning process occurs.

In the absence of cultural competency, miscommunication between clinician
and patient can occur leading to medical misadventures, misdiagnosing, and failure
to consider differing responses to medications. Skills in seeking, interpreting, and
understanding relevant person-specific nuances are valuable to serving patients or
those who seek services. Resources, especially time, must be given to those who
serve other so that they may obtain these needed abilities.

Cultural competence comprises the collective knowledge, abilities, attitudes,
and aptitudes of practitioners to provide optimal services to a broad variety of culturally and ethnically different patients. Competence begins with having skills to
assemble pertinent cultural information. It is a critical step in the patient's care to
determine if a cultural assessment is needed to be conducted. A culturally skilled
practitioner is able to collect pertinent cultural data and perform a culturally appropriate physical assessment from a patient.

Culturalkinetics

Culturalkinetics is a process (Bleidt, 1992); it is defined as the movement along
the cultural integration continuum as new patients or cultures are seen. It involves

understanding that other cultures may not share your views or values. Baseline assumptions are established and used with each new encounter until enough relevant data has been obtained from a cultural assessment. Then the more specific, pertinent information is used with the patient. With each meeting, more data is gathered until as complete of an understanding of who he or she is can be achieved.

Through culturalkinetics, culturally competent behavior is a continuous process of self-awareness and self-improvement as more detailed knowledge is gained about each culture or patient, learning about cultural nuances and how they affect attitudes and health behaviors. Through this process one becomes more sensitive, understanding, and empathetic about these variances. Finally, cultural integration is reached when a practitioner is truly skillful in adapting and responding to those differences within appropriate contexts and circumstances.

The process of culturalkinetics involves a utilizing a set of skills needed to culturally assess a patient. According to Bleidt (1992), these skills include

- identifying and appreciating ethnospecific problems (such as bigotry);
- respecting the person as a human being and his or her right to be treated as one;
- accepting those who may be different as equals;
- communicating in a cross-cultural fashion at the patient's (consumer's) literacy level without being condescending;
- being a good listener, empathetic, and polite;
- understanding, without prejudice, differing value systems and beliefs the patient may hold;
- connecting with the underserved;
- identifying with a patient's background and using this to link with him or her;
- using innovative approaches from other cultures to solve individual problems;
- learning constantly about other cultures; and
- appreciating the differences among cultures.

From this list of essential skills core, we can determine which values and behaviors are most relevant to create culturally competent organizational policies and processes that can be embodied within standards and guidelines. Such standards, by definition, would employ broader definitions of culture that go beyond traditional frames of race, ethnicity, health, and services provision and settings. This is reflected by the following recommendations of the National Center for Cultural Competence (2016, para. 3), For an organization to achieve cultural competence, it must

- have a defined set of values and principles and demonstrate behaviors, attitudes, policies, and structures that enable them to work effectively cross-culturally;
- have the capacity to (1) value diversity, (2) conduct self-assessment, (3) manage dynamics of difference, (4) acquire and institutionalize cultural knowledge,

and (5) adapt to diversity and the cultural contexts of the communities they serve; [and]

• incorporate the above in all aspects of policymaking, administration, practice, and service delivery and involve systematically consumers, key stakeholders, and communities.

The CLAS Standards

Since their release by the Office of Minority Health (OMH) in 1999, the National Standards for Culturally and Linguistically Appropriate Services in Health Care (CLAS Standards) have been the foundation of health and health care organizations' efforts to improve health equity, reduce health disparities, and improve quality of care (OMH, 1999, 2001). In the introduction to the CLAS Standards, the OMH emphasizes the relationship between health and the social determinants of health, that is, "those conditions in which individuals are born, grow, live, work and age" (WHO, 2016), such as socioeconomic status, education level, and the availability of health services.

Although the original 14 guidelines have been modified over time, the intent of the guidelines is still the same: to facilitate health care delivery for minority populations. They are aimed at health care organizations and the services that these organizations should provide. Specific services include

• education of staff in cultural and linguistic service delivery;
• provision of language assistance services and interpreters;
• promotion of a strategic plan outlining goals and policies in this area; and
• development of collaborative partnerships with the community.

In 2012, the OMH updated the CLAS Standards to clarify the meaning of the standards and broaden their scope. Standard 1 was made the Principal Standard. If all 14 standards are adopted, successfully implemented, and sustained with fidelity over time, then the Principal Standard is achieved: "Provide effective, equitable, understandable, respectful, and quality care and services that are responsive to diverse cultural health beliefs and practices, preferred languages, health literacy, and other communication needs" (OMH, 2013, p. 31). The remaining standards were regrouped under three categories: (a) governance, leadership, and workforce; (b) communication and language assistance; and (c) engagement, continuous improvement, and accountability. Table 6-1 shows the standards for each theme.

It is the primary goal of Western medicine to provide optimal care for *all* patients. In order to realize this goal, providers must acknowledge and understand the existence of cultural variations and beliefs. The ethos of pharmaceutical care

Table 6-1 **National Standards for Culturally and Linguistically Appropriate Services in Health and Healthcare**

Principal Standard: Provide effective, equitable, understandable, respectful, and quality care and services that are responsive to diverse cultural health beliefs and practices, preferred languages, health literacy, and other communication needs.

Theme 1: **Governance, Leadership, and Workforce**	2. Advance and sustain governance and leadership that promotes CLAS and health equity 3. Recruit, promote, and support a diverse governance, leadership, and workforce 4. Educate and train governance, leadership, and workforce in CLAS
Theme 2: **Communication and Language Assistance**	5. Offer communication and language assistance 6. Inform individuals of the availability of language assistance 7. Ensure the competence of individuals providing language assistance 8. Provide easy-to-understand materials and signage
Theme 3: **Engagement, Continuous Improvement, and Accountability**	9. Infuse CLAS goals, policies, and management accountability throughout the organization's planning and operations 10. Conduct organizational assessments 11. Collect and maintain demographic data 12. Conduct assessments of community health assets and needs 13. Partner with the community 14. Create conflict and grievance resolution processes 15. Communicate the organization's progress in implementing and sustaining CLAS

Note: CLAS = National Standards for Culturally and Linguistically Appropriate Services in Health Care.

(or pharmacy care, or patient care in pharmacy practice) is congruent with delivering the best possible individualized care, which requires taking into consideration the impact of a patient's culture on his or her illness, on the acceptance of therapy, and especially on your interaction and communication with them (Coleman & Bleidt, 2002).

In the late 1990s, the USDHHS prepared a report on national goals for a more healthy population titled *Healthy People 2000* (USDHHS, 1991). Since that initial document, *Healthy People 2010* and now *Healthy People 2020* have been developed and implemented federally (USDHHS 2000, 2010). One of primary goals of *Healthy*

People 2000 was to reduce health disparities among Americans. *Healthy People 2010* went further to set the goal of eliminating health disparities. Now, *Healthy People 2020* seeks to achieve health equity. This new concept of health equity is its loftiest undertaking in that it compels practitioners to assist patients in the "attainment of the highest level of health for all people" (National Partnership for Action to End Health Disparities, 2011, p. 9). Interestingly, these reports do not equate a patient's health to a singular rationale of the lack of a disease process but to broader determinants of health espoused by the United States (Secretary's Advisory Committee . . ., 2010) and the WHO (2016). Box 6-1 offers a brief review of these determinants from *Healthy People 2020*.

Implications for Public Health and Pharmacy Practice

As we end this chapter, we would like to present recommendations on how to facilitate and promote cultural competence in an organization. Adapted from Brown and Nichols-English (1999), these suggestions, if followed, would help to build a more culturally competent environment within a health care institution. They represent an excellent starting place to begin the continuous journey toward cultural integration:

- Create a supportive environment for practicing multicultural patient care;
- Allocate adequate resources to purchase culturally consistent patient-education materials, to attend workshops and courses, and to train staff and professional personnel;
- Accept diversity in the approaches and techniques used for different patient populations and be able to adapt and change one's practice in reference to the changing environment and differences in patient-population needs;
- Respect the differences in people; and
- Strengthen collaborative relationships with other health care providers.

By recognizing and understanding health disparities, pharmacists can effectively change practice and service delivery to ensure culturally competent care to all their patients. Simply by practicing culturalkinetics, changing the pharmacy environment to be more welcoming for different groups, and incorporating health promotion and disease prevention initiatives, pharmacists can improve the overall health of local communities. Minimizing or eliminating communication barriers contributes to quality of care (Vanderpool & Ad Hoc Committee on Ethnic Diversity and Cultural Competence, 2005). In Appendix A, the policies of the American Society of Health-System Pharmacists (ASHP) that directly relate to cultural competence are presented. See the American Pharmacists Association manual for its policies that directly relate to cultural competence (https://www.pharmacist.com/policy-manual).

In this chapter we have introduced the process of culturalkinetics and how to take the journey toward cultural integration. From an early age, most of us have learned the Golden Rule, which is "do unto others as you would have done unto you." However, in a fully culturally integrated scenario, the Platinum Rule would be followed, which is *do unto others as they want done unto them*. There is a very important distinction between these two guidelines. The Platinum Rule recognizes that the other individual has the right to be treated as he or she feels is appropriate.

The highest level of *cultural awareness*, cultural integration, is when one considers the individual difference in us all as worthy of recognition. This aspect of providing care becomes very important to patients we may see from other countries and to the lesbian, gay, bisexual, and transgender community that has been largely ignored by many health care practitioners for far too long. It is hoped that this chapter will provide a roadmap for greater understanding of how to provide better care for all.

Appendix A
ASHP Cultural Competence Policy
[Reprinted with permission of ASHP]

1613 CULTURAL COMPETENCY

Source: Council on Education and Workforce Development

To foster the ongoing development of cultural competency within the pharmacy workforce; further,

To educate health care providers on the importance of providing culturally congruent care to achieve quality care and patient engagement.

This policy supersedes ASHP policy 1414.

RATIONALE

The United States is rapidly becoming a more diverse nation. Culture influences a patient's belief and behavior toward health and illness. Cultural competence can significantly affect clinical outcomes. Research has shown that overlooking cultural beliefs may lead to negative health consequences.[1] According to the National Center for Cultural Competency, there are numerous examples of benefits derived from the impact of cultural competence on quality and effectiveness of care in relation to health outcomes and well-being.[2] Further, pharmacists can contribute to providing "culturally congruent care," which can be described as "a process of effective interaction between the provider and client levels" of health care that encourages provider cultural competence while recognizing that "[p]atients and families bring their own values, perceptions, and expectations to health care encounters which also influence the creation or destruction of cultural congruence."[3] The Report of the ASHP Ad Hoc Committee on Ethnic Diversity and Cultural Competence[4] and the ASHP Statement on Racial and Ethnic Disparities in Health Care[5] support ways to raise awareness of the importance of cultural competence in the provision of patient care so that optimal therapeutic outcomes are achieved in diverse populations.

1. Administration on Aging. *Achieving cultural competence. A guidebook for providers of services to older Americans and their families.* Available at: http://archive.org/details/achievingcultura00admi
2. Goode TD, Dunne MC, Bronheim SM. The evidence base for cultural and linguistic competency in health care. The Commonwealth Fund; 2006. Available http://www.commonwealthfund.org/usr_doc/Goode_evidencebasecultlinguisticcomp_962.pdf
3. Schim SM, Doorenbos AZ. A Three-dimensional Model of Cultural Congruence: Framework for Intervention. *J Soc Work End Life Palliat Care.* 2010; 6:256–70.
4. Report of the ASHP Ad Hoc Committee on Ethnic Diversity and Cultural Competence. *Am J Health-Syst Pharm.* 2005; 1924–30.
5. ASHP Statement on Racial and Ethnic Disparities in Health Care. *Am J Health-Syst Pharm.* 2008; 65:728–33.

Authors' Note

One of the coauthors, Dr. Bleidt, does not believe in race as a subdivision of mankind. When asked, he identifies himself as a member of the human race. Race is an artificial construct developed by British sociologists to justify slavery and treating others with less dignity than deserved. This chapter reflected these views.

References

Bleidt, B. (1992). Understanding multicultural pharmaceutical education. *Journal of Pharmacy Teaching,* 3(2), 141–151. doi:10.1300/J060v03n02_15

Brown, C. M., & Nichols-English, G. (1999). Dealing with patient diversity in pharmacy practice. *Drug Topics,* 143(17), 61–70.

Colby, S. L., & Ortman, J. M. (2015, March). *Projections of the size and composition of the U.S. population: 2014 to 2060.* Washington, DC: U.S. Census Bureau Retrieved from https://www.census.gov/content/dam/Census/library/publications/2015/demo/p25-1143.pdf

Coleman, C. A., & Bleidt, B. (2002). Considering the whole patient with hypertension: the ethos of pharmaceutical care. *Ethnicity & Disease, 12*(4), S3-72-75.

Health Resources and Services Administration. (2016). Lists of designated primary medical care, mental health, and dental health professional shortage areas. *Federal Register, 81*(127), 43214–43215.

LaVeist, T. A., & Pierre, G. (2014). Integrating the 3Ds—social determinants, health disparities, and health-care workforce diversity. *Public Health Reports, 129*(Suppl.) 2, 9–14.

National Academies of Sciences, Engineering, and Medicine. (2016). *Framing the dialogue on race and ethnicity to advance health equity: Proceedings of a workshop.* Washington, DC: National Academies Press.

National Center for Cultural Competence. (2016). Conceptual frameworks/models, guiding values and principles. Retrieved from http://nccc.georgetown.edu/foundations/framework.html

National Partnership for Action to End Health Disparities. (2011, April). National stakeholder strategy for achieving health equity. Retrieved from https://minorityhealth.hhs.gov/npa/templates/content.aspx?lvl=1&lvlid=33&ID=286

Office of Minority Health. (1999). *Assuring cultural competence in health care: Recommendations for national standards and an outcomes-focused research agenda.* Washington, DC: Author. Retrieved from http://minorityhealth.hhs.gov/Assets/pdf/checked/Assuring_Cultural_Competence_in_Health_Care-1999.pdf

Office of Minority Health. (2001). *National standards for culturally and linguistically appropriate services in health care: Final report.* Washington, DC: Author. Retrieved from http://www.omhrc.gov/assets/pdf/checked/executive.pdf

Office of Minority Health. (2013). *National standards for culturally and linguistically appropriate services in health and health care: A blueprint for advancing and sustaining CLAS policy and practice.* Washington, DC: Author. Retrieved from https://www.thinkculturalhealth.hhs.gov/pdfs/EnhancedCLASStandardsBlueprint.pdf

Purnell, L. D., & Paulanka, B. J. (2012). *Transcultural health care: A culturally competent approach* (4th ed.). Philadelphia, PA: F.A. Davis.

Secretary's Advisory Committee on National Health Promotion and Disease Prevention Objectives for 2020. (2010, July 6). *Healthy People 2020: An opportunity to address societal determinants of health in the U.S.* Washington, DC: U.S. Department of Health and Human Services.

Smedley, B. D., Butler, A. S., & Bristow, L. R. (2004). *In the nation's compelling interest: ensuring diversity in the health-care workforce.* Washington, DC: National Academies Press.

Student National Pharmaceutical Association. (2013, October). *Initiative protocols.* Retrieved from http://snpha.org/wp-content/uploads/2014/08/Initiative-Protocols-20141.pdf

Student National Pharmaceutical Association. (2016). Mission statement. Retrieved from http://snpha.org/about/

U.S. Department of Health and Human Services. (1991). *Healthy people 2000.* Washington, DC: Author.

U.S. Department of Health and Human Services. (2000). *Healthy people 2010.* Washington, DC: Author. Retrieved from http://purl.access.gpo.gov/GPO/LPS8595

U.S. Department of Health and Human Services. (2010). *Healthy People 2020.* Washington, DC: Author. Retrieved from http://www.healthypeople.gov/2020/

Vanderpool, H. K., & Ad Hoc Committee on Ethnic Diversity and Cultural Competence. (2005). Report of the ASHP Ad Hoc Committee on Ethnic Diversity and Cultural Competence. *American Journal of Health System Pharmacy, 62*(18), 1924–1930. doi:10.2146/ajhp050100

Williams, J. S., Walker, R. J., & Egede, L. E. (2016). Achieving equity in an evolving healthcare system: Opportunities and challenges. *The American Journal of the Medical Sciences, 351*(1), 33–43. doi:10.1016/j.amjms.2015.10.012

Winslow, C.-E. A. (1920). The untilled field of public health. *Modern Medicine, 2,* 183–191.

World Health Organization. (1948). *Preamble to the Constitution of the World Health Organization as adopted by the International Health Conference, New York, 19–22 June, 1946; signed on 22 July 1946 by the representatives of 61 States (Official Records of the World Health Organization, no. 2, p. 100) and entered into force on 7 April 1948.* Geneva, Switzerland: Author.

World Health Organization. (2016). Social determinants of health. Retrieved from http://www.who.int/social_determinants/sdh_definition/en/

7

Pharmacists' Roles in the Increase of Health Literacy Among Patients

BARRY A. BLEIDT, CARMITA A. COLEMAN,

SILVIA E. RABIONET, AND ARDIS HANSON

Introduction

Many of the challenges people face in today's society have their origins in the early years and experiences of life, including problems with words, numeracy, and problem-solving. It is not easy being a patient (inpatient or outpatient). Entering into the strange realm of the sick role is a significant change from everyday life for most people. When a person becomes a patient, many facets of his or her existence are different, for example:

- Language—words and phraseology are both foreign and can be very difficult to understand;
- Culture—in a health care setting, there are different rules, eccentric guidelines, and peculiar ways of doing things;
- Time—health facilities generally have specific times in which they operate (appointments are generally between 8:00 AM and 4:30 PM when most people work) or people are awakened at 6:00 AM to take their medications;
- Space—inpatient rooms generally have room for only one to two people when many cultures have much larger families/extended families;
- Dress—in many circumstances, patients must wear a gown or other strange garb that is unflattering, immodest, and makes one most vulnerable, at best; and
- Expectations—patients may not be sure what to expect. They have crossed into a situation, for example, that may be both paternalistic and mutualistic; they could be expected to participate in their own therapy while it also being assumed that they will follow the practitioner's recommendation(s).

As a person becomes a patient, he or she must enter into a world very different from his or her normal, practiced routine and remain there throughout the course of treatment (which may be for life, in the case of a chronic condition). Many times, this existence will run parallel with day-to-day living; thereby increasing its intricacy. Hence, being a patient is a complex situation. This complexity is exacerbated significantly in patients who have low health literacy and numeracy.

Health Literacy Defined

SOCIAL DETERMINANTS OF HEALTH

According to the World Health Organization (WHO, 2016b, para. 1), the social determinants of health

> are the conditions, in which people are born, grow, work, live, and age, and the wider set of forces and systems shaping the conditions of daily life. These forces and systems include economic policies and systems, development agendas, social norms, social policies and political systems.

A primary determinant of health and wellness is people's ability to process health information correctly in a timely manner, to balance the presented options, and to use sound judgement to make a decision regarding their health or improving their quality of life. These collective skills empower a patient to be a partner and more involved in his or her own health care: these skills are also known as health literacy (Sørensen et al., 2012).

The relationship between literacy and health is very intricate. A patient's literacy skills affect his or her health knowledge, health status, and how easily he or she can navigate health service systems. Literacy also affects a person's income level, occupation, education, living quarters, and access to health care. Adults who live below the US poverty level have lower health literacy on average than adults who live above the poverty threshold, with 42% of persons with chronic mental disorders and 33% of persons with chronic physical disorders reporting scores at the "Below Basic" level of literacy (National Network of Libraries of Medicine, n.d.).

DEFINITIONS

A person's ability to listen, read, analyze, and apply pharmacy directions or other health information requires specific analytical and conceptual skills. These proficiencies, which collectively are referred to as *health literacy*, are "defined as the understanding and application of words (prose), numbers (numeracy), and forms (documents)" (Pfizer, 2011, p. 4). The WHO defines *health literacy* as "the cognitive and social skills which determine the motivation and ability of individuals to gain access to, understand and use information in ways which promote and maintain good health" (Nutbeam & WHO Collaborating Centre for Health Promotion, 1998, p. 10). *Healthy People 2010* defined *health literacy* as "The degree to which individuals have the capacity to obtain, process and understand basic health information and services needed to make appropriate health decisions" (Office of Disease Prevention and Health Promotion, 2000).

Health literacy goes beyond knowledge and the mere skills of reading, writing, processing numbers, and communicating verbally. It also includes a complex set of aptitudes that translate into the ability to access, understand, process, and act upon health information. Being health literate means being able to interpret instructions on prescription drug bottles and deliver the correct amount of medication at the correct time for the correct duration. In some cases, a dose must be calculated (e.g., for a child's over-the-counter product) or the correct dose must be measured (for liquid medications); these tasks are complex. In addition, patients must decode appointment slips, health information brochures, doctor's directions, and consent forms, as well as navigate through and negotiate around complex health care systems (National Network of Libraries of Medicine, n.d.).

Furthermore, these capabilities should translate into the ability to advocate for personal health and the health of others in the community (Freedman et al., 2009). Health literacy has little relationship to a patient's education level or general reading ability. A person may function adequately at work or home and still have marginal or inadequate literacy in a health care environment. Several other definitions also exist; the fact there are a number of different health literacy definitions demonstrates the field is evolving.

HEALTH LITERACY AS A PUBLIC HEALTH PROBLEM

Patients who have low health literacy and numeracy encounter certain circumstances as they attempt to access health care systems. First, such patients are unable to clearly understand their treatment options, nor are they able to comprehend the therapy they have been prescribed. As the country's population increases, the number of patients affected by low health literacy grows. Also, by not recognizing health literacy as a problem, prescribed medicine and other therapeutic recommendations may be used inefficiently, used incorrectly, not taken, or not followed at all.

Low health literacy is a significant public health problem based on meeting the conditions set forth in the definition. Healthcare systems and health care are complex; they can be difficult to access, to navigate, to engage with as an equal partner, and to exit when appropriate in ideal situations. As the US population increases in number and diversity, problems will multiply. An understanding of how health literacy impacts an individual as he or she navigates a particular health care system and various therapeutic options is a critical piece to the larger puzzle of engaging in patient-centered care.

Low Health Literacy's Impact on Patient Care

AT-RISK POPULATIONS

Culture plays an integral role in communication. Recognition of this fact provides a base for understanding health literacy. Culture strongly influences a person's health literacy level. Different cultural backgrounds shape patients' health literacy through their health belief system, religious observances, familial hierarchy, gender roles, education, traditional healer inputs, and communication style. The National Network of Libraries of Medicine (n.d., para. 4) emphasizes, "even though culture is only one part of health literacy, it is a very important piece of the complicated topic of health literacy." The U.S. Department of Health and Human Services (USDHHS) Office of Disease Prevention and Health Promotion (2007, p. 2.1) recognizes that "culture affects how people communicate, understand and respond to health information."

In its publication, *National Action Plan to Improve Health Literacy*, the Office of Disease Prevention and Health Promotion identified particular groups that are most likely to experience low health literacy. Those populations include patients who are over 65 years of age. In these patients, there is a higher probability of diminished visual acuity, decline in cognition, and a loss of reading abilities (when people stop reading, they start losing their ability to read), all progressively deteriorating over time. Also included are people who have had a lack of educational opportunity (people with a high school education or lower). "Reading abilities are typically three to five grade levels below the last year of school completed. As a result, people with a high school diploma, typically read at a seventh or eighth grade reading level" (National Network of Libraries of Medicine, n.d.).

Other groups include ethnic and cultural minorities; people with incomes at or below the federal poverty level; non-native speakers of English; people with physical, cognitive, or learning disabilities; patients with a compromised health status; and people with a combination of these attributes (USDHHS, 2010). Other at-risk groups include recent immigrants, patients with low visual acuity, and others who may be strangers to US health care systems. These categories highlight the significance of the social determinants of health when attempting to increase health literacy in the population.

PREVALENCE

While the aforementioned populations are disproportionally affected, practitioners should not be deceived that low health literacy is an issue that is solely reserved to them. In the United States, the National Assessment of Adult Literacy (NAAL) measures health literacy of adults. Four performance levels are used to quantify health literacy: (a) Below Basic, (b) Basic, (c) Intermediate, and (d) Proficient. The last reported results from NAAL showed that around 36% have limited health literacy (14% at Below Basic level plus 22% at the Basic level). Approximately 5% were not literate in English. This same report cites that only 12% of English-speaking adults in the United States have proficient health literacy skills (Kutner, Greenburg, Jin, & Paulsen, 2006). Poor health literacy is much more prevalent than many practitioners realize.

IMPACT ON PATIENT OUTCOMES

It is widely recognized that people make health decisions as a response to information, environments, resources, and social support systems. Higher levels of health literacy contribute to the alignment of the patients' health decisions and positive health outcomes (Kickbusch, Pelikan, Apfel, & Tsouros, 2013). Conversely, low health literacy is associated with poorer health outcomes and higher costs and is also considered a primary determinant of health inequalities (Heijmans et al., 2015). The following summarizes a few of the research findings on the association between limited health literacy and health outcomes.

- Patients are significantly more likely to report their health as poor (Baker, Parker, Williams, & Clark, 1998; Baker et al., 1996; Kutner et al., 2006).
- Patients are more likely to avoid preventive services such as mammograms, pap smears, and flu immunizations (Scott, Gazmararian, Williams, & Baker, 2002).
- Patients tend to enter a health care system sicker than patients with higher health literacy levels (Bennett et al., 1998).
- Patients are more likely to suffer from chronic conditions and manage them less effectively (Batterham, Hawkins, Collins, Buchbinder, & Osborne, 2016; Beauchamp et al., 2015; Wernick et al., 2016).
- Patients have higher rates of hospitalization and use of emergency services (Griffey, Kennedy, D'Agostino McGowan, Goodman, & Kaphingst, 2014) and a higher rate of preventable hospital visits and admissions (Auerbach et al., 2016; McNaughton et al., 2015; McNaughton et al., 2013)
- Patients find their status to be a social barrier to access health care services (Palumbo, 2015).

In conclusion, low health literacy patients consume more health care services, have an increased risk for hospitalization, and utilize, to a greater extent, expensive services, such as emergency department and inpatient care (National Institutes of Health, 2016).

ECONOMIC IMPACT

Besides the aforementioned low health literacy's consequences on the patient, there are also major economic impacts on society (Rusa, Bawa, Suminski, Snella, & Warady, 2015). One report, *Low Health Literacy: Implications for National Health Policy*, approximated low health literacy's annual costs to the US economy to be between $106 billion and $238 billion. These 2007 figures equaled between 7% and 17% of the total amount of personal health care spending (Vernon, Trujillo, Rosenbaum, & DeBuono, 2007). More recent data places the societal economic costs in the United States at more than $360 billion per year (World Literacy Foundation, 2015).

Lack of medication compliance and adherence add to these costs and compound the problem. Nearly 30% of patients fail to fill new prescriptions, and new prescriptions for new chronic conditions are not filled between 20% and 34% of the time (Pharmaceutical Research and Manufacturers of America [PhRMA], 2011). In addition, chronically ill patients who regularly fill their prescriptions may actually take half of the doses incorrectly (PhRMA, 2011).

CHARACTERISTICS OF POOR READERS

Pharmacists should be proactively aware of the common characteristics of a poor reader. One pharmaceutical manufacturer, Pfizer, Inc., concerned with the issue of low health literacy, has funded research and helpful interventions targeting low health literacy as have a number of government agencies, such as the Centers for Disease Control and Prevention and the Agency for Healthcare Quality and Research. Attributes common to patients who are poor readers or are having trouble understanding what is being presented to them fall within three distinct areas: language knowledge and processing ability, cognitive ability, and metacognitive strategic competence. Box 7-1 lists a number of characteristics of poor readers,

---

Box 7-1 **Characteristics of Poor Readers**

- Read slowly, missing meaning
- Skip over hard words
- Miss the context
- Tire quickly
- Interpret visuals literally
- Have difficulty because their eyes wander without finding a central focus
- Mix languages to express simple ideas
- Skip principle features
- Get lost in the details rather than focus on the main features

which can help practitioners know when an intervention is necessary to address the particular needs of these patients.

HEALTH LITERACY BARRIERS

Patients often confront complicated information and complex treatment decisions. They need to have certain abilities in order to be health literate. The lack of any or all of these capacities would pose barriers for the low literate patient. The following seven skills are needed to be health literate Patients need to be able to

1. Access and navigate health care services (when, where, and how);
2. Weigh relative risks and benefits;
3. Determine dosages and dosage schedule (mathematical calculations);
4. Converse with and listen to clinicians;
5. Assess information for credibility and quality;
6. Decode test results; and
7. Discover needed health information. (National Network of Libraries of Medicine, n.d.)

Patients may also need to behave additional skills, such as visual, computer, information, and numeric literacy. These skills are critical to be able to understand graphs or other visual information, operate a computer, obtain and apply relevant information, and calculate or reason numerically (National Network of Libraries of Medicine, n.d.).

Oral language and communication skills are also critically important. Patients need to be able to convey their health concerns accurately and describe their symptoms precisely. There is also a significant need to be able to ask relevant questions and comprehend oral treatment directions or medical options. Additionally, patients need sound decision-making abilities in order to share responsibility as a partner with practitioners. As the Internet has become an important source of health information, health literacy may now include searching capabilities and website evaluation skills (National Network of Libraries of Medicine, n.d.).

There are also barriers preventing patients from being proficient in health literacy. These include low numeracy abilities and limited reading skills. A more detailed discussion of these obstacles is found later in this chapter in the "Pharmacists' Identification of Low Health Literacy Patients" section.

Programs to Improve Health Literacy

In its 2001 report, *Crossing the Quality Chasm*, the Institute of Medicine (IOM) indicated that health care systems must be restructured if the needs of low-literate patients are to be met. Three years later, the IOM issued a vanguard report on health literacy. A prominent quote from this document stated "efforts to improve quality, reduce costs, and reduce disparities cannot succeed without simultaneous improvements in health literacy" (Nielsen-Bohlman, Panxer, Kindig, & Institute of Medicine Committee on Health Literary, 2004, p. xiv). Early on, it was recognized that pharmacists and the profession of pharmacy are key partners in helping patients with their health literacy. The pharmacy related tasks include going to get a prescription filled, listening to the counseling, taking the drug accurately, assessing the printed health information accompanying the medicines, completing forms, and understanding the health insurance coverage, among other responsibilities (IOM, 2001).

The Joint Commission is the organization that accredits health care organizations and programs in the United States. As a key element of quality care, the Joint Commission emphasizes the importance of health literacy. In its 2007 report, *What Did the Doctor Say? Improving Health Literacy to Protect Patient Safety*, the Commission stated

> Health literacy issues and ineffective communications place patients at greater risk of preventable adverse events. If a patient does not understand the implications of her or his diagnosis and the importance of prevention and treatment plans, or cannot access health care services because of communications problems, an untoward event may occur. (Joint Commission, 2007, p. 6)

Also in 2007, the Agency for Healthcare Research and Quality developed a publication titled *Is Our Pharmacy Meeting Patients' Needs? A Pharmacy Health Literacy Assessment Tool User's Guide* (Jacobson et al., 2007). This volume is a guide for conducting a health literacy assessment in a pharmacy, which is an essential quality improvement tool for businesses and other groups serving low health literate patients. This first step in the quality-improvement process raises awareness of health literacy among pharmacy staff and pharmacists, identifies obstacles that patients may encounter, and reveals improvement areas. Performing this baseline assessment at the beginning also permits an evaluation of the pharmacy's impact by implementing a follow-up measure (Jacobson et al., 2007).

The puzzle of poor health literacy is not a static one. It is important to remember, as the system becomes more complex, the problem will continue to grow (Palumbo, 2015). The aforementioned landmark reports and others moved health literacy from an "under-recognized silent epidemic to an issue of health policy and reform" (National Network of Libraries of Medicine, n.d.).

FEDERAL-LEVEL INITIATIVES

Over the past decade, there have been several initiatives at the federal government level to address the issue of low health literacy. These laws and programs elevate the importance of health literacy as a key factor in improving the overall health of the US population, reduce costs, and decrease the incidence of medical errors.

The Patient Protection and Affordable Care Act of 2010 (ACA) contains several provisions that address the need for greater attention to health literacy. There are also requirements for health plans to communicate health information clearly, promote prevention, and be patient-centered. The ACA also codified the concept of medical or health homes to assure equity and cultural competency and deliver high-quality care. The *National Action Plan to Improve Health Literacy* (USDHHS, 2010), in collaboration with over 700 public and private-sector entities, provides a framework for future research and action. The *Plan* includes seven goals and strategies that researchers and practitioners can use to design studies and interventions. The Plain Writing Act of 2010 requires all new publications, forms, and publicly distributed documents from the federal government to be written in a "clear, concise, well-organized" manner. The law requires that federal agencies use "clear Government communication that the public can understand and use" (Plain Writing Act, p. 2861).

INTERNATIONAL-LEVEL INITIATIVES

All the regions of the world, through WHO regional offices, developed frameworks, action plans, and toolkits to engage health professionals alongside patients, communities, and stakeholders in increasing health literacy. WHO regional offices are also involved in building health literacy and patient empowerment in conjunction with mobile health and e-health initiatives (World Health Organization & International Telecommunication Union, 2012).

The WHO Regional Office for South-East Asia developed a comprehensive health literacy toolkit to inform health professionals, policymakers, communities, and patients in low- and middle-income countries. The toolkit offers resources and specific strategies on how to target specific populations by age, disability, and heath condition. It also provides guidelines to raise health literacy among ethnic and language minorities, refugees, and asylum seekers (Dodson, Good, & Osborne, 2015; IOM, 2013).

In 2013, WHO's Regional Office for Europe published the document *Health Literacy—The Solid Facts* as a practical guide to inform actions to strengthen people's health literacy in Europe (Kickbusch et al., 2013). Some examples in the European region include programs to prevent and manage chronic and other noncommunicable diseases, to improve mental health, and to heighten patients' rights. The document summarizes existing evidence of the role health literacy plays in promoting heath and preventing disease. The document also highlights the importance of health literacy initiatives within health care delivery systems. Specifically regarding adherence to medication, it calls for improving drug labeling, better clinical communication during patient–provider encounters, enhanced education and information distributed at pharmacies, and providing hospital discharge information in more effective ways (Kickbusch et al., 2013).

As part of the Healthy Europe 2020 initiative, the European Union commissioned an expert panel to deliberate on effective ways of investing in health. In May 2016, the panel released its recommendations. The report emphasizes the need for types of data collection, better monitoring to identify the magnitude of problems for access and utilization, and more effective evaluation and assessment "to measure changes over time and across groups of people and to enhance international comparability" (Expert Panel on Effective Ways of Investing in Health, 2016, p. 15). The report discusses the role and impact of health literacy within the context of delivering quality and safe health care services. The small amount of data available (from eight countries only) suggests that low health literacy is a prevalent problem affecting the entire continent. The results paint a picture very similar to what is happening in the United States in that low health literate patients have poorer health and higher health care use. The report calls for evidence-based strategies to improve health literacy because what is currently available is weak (Expert Panel on Effective Ways of Investing in Health, 2016).

Additionally, the International Pharmaceutical Federation (FIP) through its foundation embarked on an initiative to promote the use of pictograms to improve communications about medications to low literate patients and others. These efforts are described later in this chapter.

OTHER INITIATIVES

The National Patient Safety Foundation developed a patient education program designed to assist low health literate patients. The *Ask Me 3*™ product aims to foster communication among patients and health care providers in order to increase positive health outcomes. It encourages patients to ask three simple and basic but necessary questions at each health care encounter, including the pharmacy. They are also asked to be sure to understand the answer to these questions. These questions are

1. What is my main problem?
2. What do I need to do?
3. Why is it important for me to do this? (National Patient Safety Foundation, 2016)

Numerous health care providers and organizations have adopted these questions as part of their everyday practice. Among them, CVS Health's Minute Clinics™, the medical clinics located in CVS/Pharmacy, became the first retail clinic provider in the nation to implement the *Ask Me 3*™ program in 2014 (CVS Caremark, 2014). Other useful strategies and tactics are also available to address health literacy concerns for both patients and clinicians.

Health Literacy and Health Promotion

Health professionals in the 21st century are expected to practice in an environment that promotes measurable positive health outcomes, health equity, and effective and efficient health care delivery. They are increasingly responsible for engaging in patient-centered care, where patients are expected to participate actively in the decision-making process about their health and treatment options. Shared health decision-making poses various challenges to patients and providers, as both need to develop the skills and be ready to make collaborative decisions that result in positive outcomes. In today's environment of information explosion and technological advances, pharmacists can play a leading role in educating and empowering patients with recommendations on accurate sources of information, with the skills needed to be a good partner, and by assisting them in navigating complex health care systems.

We can expand the scope of practice of the pharmacist by showing them how to address the health literacy of their patients through the use of "health promotion" and public health frameworks. Some key components are necessary in order to embrace a population framework for health literacy. First, clear links need to be established between health literacy and health promotion. Literacy begins with the ability to stay healthy and recognizes the potential of the individual to impact the health and wellness of others. Second, pharmacists need to embrace their role as a patient educator, independently of their practice site. Third, the links between health equity and health literacy need to be clearly understood. At-risk populations are more vulnerable to misunderstanding health information and to the sequelae that follow.

Primacy should be given to the understanding of the societal-level factors that affect the acquisition and progression of diseases. By approaching health literacy from a public health framework, pharmacists can identify how they can become change agents in a wide variety of practice sites, in different disease stages, and with different population groups that are at risk or who might become at risk.

According to the WHO (1986, para. 3), "health promotion is the process of enabling people to increase control over, and to improve, their health." The WHO recognizes that, in aiming for healthier populations, health promotion strategies are an essential component in disease prevention and early clinical interventions. Health promotion activities, alongside medications and biomedical interventions, are critical in addressing chronic and communicable diseases and in avoiding unnecessary burden and facilitating recovery, particularly among poor and marginalized groups. The WHO (2016) encourages carrying out health promotion in "settings where people live, work, learn, and play" as an effective and creative method of health improvement and increasing the quality of life (World Health Organization, [2016a]). Further, from a social determinants of health perspective, more personal forms of communication and community-based educational outreach can incorporate basic (functional) interactive health literacy skills and critical health literacy skills to ensure that individuals can gather and understand information, evaluate the importance and relevance of information in context to make health decisions, and address negative external factors that might inhibit health promotion (Nutbeam, 2000; Rowlands, Shaw, Jaswal, Smith, & Harpham, 2015).

Pharmacists can help patients in community and institutional settings to promote their health and prevent disease. They can be proactive in developing skills in their patients, such as (a) reading and following physical activities guidelines, (b) interpreting food and product labels, (c) finding health information on the Internet and participating in online networks, and (d) analyzing risk factors in advertisements for prescription medicines, among others (Gazmararian, Curran, Parker, Bernhardt, & DeBuono, 2005). Skill-building activities in these areas can be integrated or combined with other interventions and strategies that are already in place and that are becoming the standard of practice, such as feedback techniques, handing out written information upon prescription retrieval, medication management sessions, and transition of care counseling. We discuss how to develop these skills later in the "Pharmacists' Interventions" section of this chapter.

Health literacy interventions, in addition to promoting the understanding of words and numbers, should create awareness of the social, political, environmental, and economic forces that impact health (Freedman et al., 2009). In order to do so, pharmacists need to develop their own critical social skills and strong civic orientation while assisting patients in achieving health literacy levels to overcome social and structural barriers. Pharmacists with critical social skills should be able to communicate information about health risks factors (e.g., smoking, obesity, violence, addictions) not only as an individual patient concern but also as a challenge affecting the larger community and its resources. Moreover, pharmacists should welcome civic engagement and promote a health literacy among their patients (Freedman et al., 2009).

The Roles of Pharmacists

PHARMACISTS' IDENTIFICATION OF LOW HEALTH LITERACY PATIENTS

Because of the unique access patients have to the pharmacist, they are uniquely positioned to identify patients with low health literacy and numeracy and have a positive impact upon them. When we encounter such a patient, it is important to understand that low literacy status or poor communication skills do not automatically translate into a lack of intelligence. Quite the opposite is true many times; it is highly likely that many of these patients have developed sophisticated coping skills to help them navigate increasingly complex health care systems. As an example, patients will bring family members, including their own children, to help complete forms and to interpret instructions. With these survival mechanisms already in place, it is often the case that the clinician will not realize the patient is not able to comprehend what is being said and is, therefore, unable to implement supposedly agreed-upon care plans. For these reasons, it is important for pharmacists to be able to identify patients that could be at risk, including those who may be poor readers. The characteristics of poor readers were discussed in an earlier section of this chapter.

Many factors are involved in low health literacy. However, within the context of health care delivery, patients need additional skills and knowledge to enable them to hear, process, understand, synthesize, and implement health information and instructions in their own care. The IOM, in its consensus report *Health Literacy: A Prescription to End Confusion*, describes health literacy as functional, in that it requires an individual to understand information and perform tasks that are outside his or her usual knowledge and activities (Nielsen-Bohlman et al., 2004). There are several skill sets that even the most literate person must have at a proficient level to be able to engage fully in his or her own care (DeWalt et al., 2010). The skill sets required for a proficient level of health literacy are presented in Box 7-2.

Box 7-2 **Skill Sets Required for a Proficient Level of Health Literacy**

- Basic anatomy and physiology (name and function of body parts and systems)
- Definition of health
- Healthy behaviors and choices
- Understanding of the etiology of disease
- Mathematical concepts (probability, measurements, frequency, timing/scheduling, ranges, and calculations)
- Numerical logic (what makes sense from a mathematical point of view)
- Information processing, problem-solving, and decision-making skills
- Ability to complete written forms
- Vocabulary to describe symptoms, needs, and preferences
- Ability to comprehend and follow directions
- Ability to use medical devices and tools such as thermometer, glucometer, bandage, tweezers, etc.
- Ability to notice and report changes in health status
- Ability to read and perform functions on a medication label
- Ability to negotiate treatment
- Ability to advocate for services

Pharmacists must be able to identify and remove barriers to patient understanding. The removal of these barriers can lead to improved patient outcomes and better communication within the pharmacy. Examples of these barriers to health literacy proficiency are shown in Table 7-1.

Table 7-1 **Barriers to Health Literacy With Examples**

Barriers	Potential Examples of Barriers
Determinants of health	• Economic policies (e.g., state Medicaid laws) • Social and cultural norms
Literacy	• Inability to read • Inability to complete forms • Inability to provide patient preferences
Numeracy	• Calculation skills • Statistical ranges • Measurements
Age	• Loss of visual acuity • Loss of independence • Decreased ambulation • Polypharmacy
Disability or illness	• Decreased cognition • Inability to concentrate • Decreased communication skills • Increased need for assistance
Language	• Need for interpretative services • Need for print media translation • Need for cultural congruence in provider interactions
Culture	• Differing definitions and value of health • Language used • Procedures and protocols of health care settings
Emotion	• Decreased cognition • Inability to concentrate • Need to revisit previous instructions or care plans
Access to care	• Limited public transportation • Limited child care options • Facility hours • Welcoming environment

(continued)

Table 7-1 **Continued**

Barriers	Potential Examples of Barriers
Complexity of the health care system	• Polypharmacy • Shorter hospital stays • Increased reliance on forms and written materials • Increase self-care • Managed care regulations
Rapidly advancing medical technologies	• Biotechnologies/biopharmaceuticals • Point-of care diagnostic tools • More complex medication regimens • More complex drug delivery systems and medications

PHARMACISTS' INTERVENTIONS

It would be beneficial to have techniques and tools that would specifically address the known needs of these populations. Pharmacists are uniquely positioned as health professionals to have a positive impact on the health care needs of low-literacy patients. Because community pharmacies enable the delivery of health-related services in close proximity to patients, they develop a natural trust of community pharmacists and may be more willing to share their needs or perceived inadequacies with their neighborhood pharmacist. When working with patients, it is important for pharmacists to remember that reading, writing, and comprehension are skills that must be developed over time.

In an individual patient encounter, there are two evidence-based techniques to assist low health literacy and numeracy patients with comprehending and being able to use health information better. The first strategy is to prepare for and engage in an effective oral counseling session. The second method is to use appropriately written health care materials. These two practices should be used collaboratively and synergistically. The low health literacy patient can be positively impacted by receiving consistent, simple oral directions that can be easily understood with the addition of written materials at an accessible grade level would supplement the instructions during the session and after the encounter.

THE COUNSELING SESSION

In Box 7-2, eight approaches are listed that should be utilized when counseling a patient with low health literacy. By utilizing these suggestions, pharmacists can increase the effectiveness of their communication with limited health literacy patients. Each approach is discussed in more detail next (Jacobson et al., 2007).

Limit Number of Objectives

Most patients have difficulty remembering everything a pharmacist would like to impart to them regarding their medications or their disease state(s). Moreover, with an additional layer of potential environmental distractions that could be present due to an illness or presence of a disease, attention span and focus could be at a minimum. It is important in the preparation of a counseling session the pharmacist provides the most essential information in the initial encounter. Giving too much information, too rapidly, could confuse the patient, particularly one that is primarily reliant on verbal communications.

The American Society of Health-System Pharmacists developed a website, Safe Medication (www.safemedication.com), which provides a framework of five questions that patients could ask their pharmacists to initiate the exchange of information. These queries are presented in Box 7-3. Conversely, pharmacists could also use these questions as a starting point for their consultation with the patient (National Patient Safety Foundation, 2016).

Once again, it is critical to provide the patient with the basic necessities to help him or her successfully start their medications during initial contact. It is important to realize there are additional opportunities to provide information by extending the encounter through scheduled consultation sessions, follow-up telephone conversations, providing appropriate written materials, or using technological prompts and contacts.

Cluster Information

In preparation for the counseling session, pharmacists need to determine how to present information in a format that is easily palatable for the patient. It is helpful to group information in analogous clusters instead of just presenting random

---

Box 7-3 Counseling Approaches for Patients with Low Health Literacy and Numeracy

- Limit number of objectives
- Cluster information
- Use common words
- Start sentences with a verb
- Consider the environment and distractions
- Use metaphors and analogies to make information more relatable
- Use pictographs, objects, models, and/or demonstrations
- Ensure understanding using repetition and teach back

facts. As we try to understand information, our brains arrange it in a logical manner. Pharmacists can help that process along by presenting the needed medication information in way that makes sense to the patient. For example, if there is a need to discuss dietary changes required as part of a patient's therapy, the pharmacist could provide all of the dietary information together before moving on to discuss another aspect of his or her treatment.

Use Common Words

Medical professionals, including pharmacists, have a plethora of jargon and phrases to explain bodily functions, disease processes, medication activities, and treatment plans. The key to a successful interaction is not to impress patients with complex medical language but to build the therapeutic relationship by being open and willing to speak with patients in a manner and with words they understand. Patients need to be able to use the information provided by their health care professional to deal with their illness. A patient can only use the information effectively if it is understood.

The Institute for Healthcare Improvement (2016) defines four categories of words that are commonly used that have a high likelihood of causing confusion or providing misinformation: medical words, concept words, category words, and value judgment words. In Table 7-2, examples of problem words used in a counseling session that can cause confusion are presented along with suggestions for replacing them. We highly recommend that pharmacists interested in providing better patient-centered care to those with low health literacy review this reference to learn more about these words.

Start Sentences with a Verb

During the counseling sessions, pharmacists should start their sentences with a verb. This tactic helps the patient put recommendations into action. While using this technique, pharmacists must take special care not to be overly demanding while providing instruction. However, "Apply this medication to the wound five times per day" is more effective than "This medication should be applied to the wound five times per day." Action words upfront remind patients they must do their part in caring for the wound.

Consider Environment and Distractions

During the counseling session, care must be taken to ensure that counseling is performed in a place that lends itself to privacy, comfort, and minimal disruptions. Seldom do patients want their issues made known to those around them. Pharmacists and the pharmacy staff need to be cognizant of the potential of "listening ears" especially in smaller community settings where there may be more

Table 7-2 **Words Used in Counseling Sessions That Can Cause Confusion**

Word Type	Problem Word Examples	Consider Using Instead
Medical Words • Words frequently used by medical professionals in care instructions	Ailment	Sickness, problem
	Dysfunction	Problem
	Inhibitor	Drug that stops something that is bad for you
	Oral	By mouth
	Intermittent	Off and on
Concept Words • Words used to describe an idea, metaphor, or notion	Active role	Take part in, participate
	Avoid	Stay away from
	Gauge	Measure, get a better idea of
	Intake	What you eat or drink
	Referral	See another doctor
Category Words • Words that describe a group or subset and may be unfamiliar	Adverse	Something that is bad
	Hazardous	Not safe, dangerous
	Generic	Not brand name
	Poultry	Chicken, turkey, etc.
	Prosthesis	Replacement for body part
Value Judgment Words • Words that may need an example or visual to convey their meaning with clarity	Adequate	Be specific, such as five servings of vegetables per day
	Cautiously	Carefully, such as making sure to get up slowly when rising
	Excessive	Too much, such as if going to the bathroom multiple times at night
	Moderately	Not too much, such as limit the amount of salt you are using in your food
	Progressive	Slowly becoming better or worse; such as "you should be feeling better in about two or three days with your medication"

Note: Words to Watch is a component of the Ask Me 3 program, which is a registered trademark licensed to the Institute for Healthcare Improvement.

Reprinted with permission by Institute for Healthcare Improvement (2016).

customer camaraderie. Ensuring a private environment removes at least one worry from the pharmacist–patient encounter. Patients can feel free to express their concerns and hear the instructions from the pharmacist more clearly.

Oftentimes there can be other distractions that can impede the pharmacist–patient interaction. Care must also be taken to ensure that counseling is performed at a time when the patient is able to focus on the health information. This strategy is more important for low health literacy patients. If a person has just been given a difficult or complex diagnosis, it may not be the opportune time to provide medication information. When the pharmacist perceives this situation, scheduling a discussion after the patient has had an opportunity to process his or her news would be more effective. If the pharmacist proceeds when the patient is distracted by emotional news, it is more likely the patient will not hear much of is said during the conversation. In these circumstances, patients are s usually processing the perceived changes that will have to occur in their life and how it will affect their families. Additionally, facing anxiety of the unknown and the perception of loss of personal control are factors that are present when facing such diagnoses.

Pharmacists also have to be considerate when the patient is accompanied by a crying, febrile child or when a caregiver needs to get the patient home quickly to begin convalescing. Obviously, in these cases, the patient or caregiver has more pressing priorities than listening to a counseling session. It is difficult enough to listen, understand, remember, and eventually act on the counseling provided by the pharmacist under good conditions. Once again, the pharmacist should consider extending the counseling session by either scheduling a later time to provide more information than just the basics or by using technology to be in contact with the patient.

Use Metaphors and Analogies to Make Information More Relatable

Certainly, pharmacists want the patient to get the most out of his or her counseling session. If a patient can relate the provided information, it is more likely the patient can make it useable in his or her care. The use of metaphors and analogies helps patients to compare their new knowledge with more familiar topics and concepts. For example, comparing human vasculature to a common garden hose can assist the patient in understanding blood flow and how it can be impacted.

Use Pictographs, Objects, Models, and/or Demonstrations

Employing the use of pictographs, objects, models, and patient demonstration can assist the patient in understanding and processing health information. A pictogram (or "pictograph") is a symbol that is a picture that represents an object or concept (e.g., a triangular road sign meaning "yield to oncoming traffic"; Merriam-Webster, 2016). They are common in everyday life.

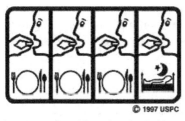 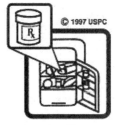

Take 4 times a day, with meals and at bedtime.   Store in refrigerator.

Figure 7-1. Two examples of USP pictograms.

In 1997, the United States Pharmacopeial Convention (USP) released a comprehensive library of 81 different pictograms that were developed as standardize graphic images to "help convey medication instructions, precautions, and/or warnings to patients and consumers" (USP, 2016). In Figure 7-1, two examples of USP pictograms are shown.

Pharmacists and patients are able to download these symbols to graphically communicate medication instructions, particularly for patients with low health literacy and numeracy, patients with limited visual acuity, and patients for whom English is a second language. After accepting the USP licensing agreement, these pictorial tools can be downloaded for use.

Nearly 20 years later, the FIP engaged in a project to improve upon the use of pictograms that can give pharmacists "a means of communicating medication instructions" to patients with low health literacy, with no common language, who have slight cognitive impairments and/or have seeing difficulties. These symbols are larger, simpler, and more informative than their predecessors (FIP Foundation for Education and Research, n.d.). They can be downloaded from the FIP website and can be used as a medication label, a medication storyboard, a medication instruction sheet, and/or a medication calendar. In Figure 7-2, four examples of FIP pictograms are shown. After accepting the contact information request web page, the software needed to create these symbols also can be downloaded from the site.

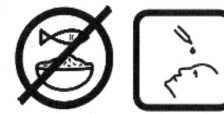 

Figure 7-2. Three examples of FIP pictograms.

If there is an especially active requirement for the use of a medication besides simply taking a common solid dosage form, it will be important to have patients demonstrate how they will use the medication after they leave the pharmacy. For example, a patient that has been prescribed an inhaler can be shown to use it and then demonstrate the proper administration technique to ensure not only the patient's understanding but also his or her ability to use it properly. By witnessing the patient's demonstration in this way, the pharmacist can determine if he or she needs additional assistance, could use a spacer, or requires reteaching of the method. Having the patient demonstrate the technique onsite also provides an opportunity for other questions to be asked about the medication. Demonstrations help with a variety of other dosage forms as well such as ophthalmic and aural drops, nasal sprays, and others. Moreover, asking patients to demonstrate their self-dosing technique can help to correct old methods that may be ineffective.

Ensure Patient Understanding Using Repetition and Teach Back

One of the most effective methods that can be used to ensure that patients are able to process health information provided is to simply ask them questions to test their understanding. Pharmacists can help to make the patient more comfortable by taking on the onus of using such a counseling technique. The use of a phrase such as "Just to be sure I have provided the correct information to you, would you please show me how you are going to take this medication?" helps patients share responsibility of their treatment regimen with their pharmacist. The pharmacist can verify understanding while helping the patient to avoid the feeling of being "tested."

APPROPRIATELY WRITTEN HEALTHCARE MATERIALS

There is an obvious and unfortunate gap between prescription drug and medical literature and most patients' reading levels. Generally, health care materials are written at a tenth-grade level, but most patients read at an eighth-grade level. Moreover, about 18% of the adult US population reads at a fifth-grade level (Rampey et al., 2016).

In order to overcome the chasm that exists between patient needs and the available health care literature, there are several techniques that can be used by pharmacists. While this chapter does not cover readability formulas to assess the literature that pharmacists are using, those with a particular interest in health literacy can use these formulas to prepare materials that are helpful for a variety of patients. Instead, this chapter explores easy-to-apply techniques that can be performed in a matter of minutes. In general, health information should be organized as a typical counseling session. Some of the same methods that were used to make a counseling session more meaningful will be employed in this area as well.

Written materials should be easy to read. There should not be an information overload, and written materials should emphasize by priority the desired actions of the patient. Because written materials should be culturally and linguistically appropriate, they should engage readers with a conversational style, using common words, and they should use an active voice. Just as was suggested in the counseling session guidelines previously discussed, written materials should cover similar topics at one time to assist the patient in focusing on one issue at a time.

Written materials should be visually pleasing to the patient, avoiding glossy paper or hard-to-read, fancy fonts. Glossy paper and ornate fonts cause particular difficulty for those with low visual acuity. The document should be arranged with plenty of white space. A large amount of dense, prose text can be disconcerting for a patient who feels overwhelmed while reading. The use of bold lettering, bullet points, and strategic indentations can focus the patient's eyes on important points. Because visual acuity can decrease with age, having patient literature in clear, matte, appropriately contrasting colorization, and spatial arrangements with nonelaborate fonts are particularly accommodating for geriatric patients.

Written materials should use captions, pictograms, or other visuals that have meaning related to the subject matter rather than distracting or entertaining cartoons or photos. It is more important to show visuals that motivate, clarify, or demonstrate the desired outcomes. Fortunately, many community pharmacy retailers are now developing easy-to-access written materials for use with low health literacy patients. Pharmacists are able quickly to individualize the materials depending on the situation and provide the materials in multiple languages.

Prescription drugs are quite byzantine and have intricate nuances to their use; this is why they are regulated as Rx only by the U.S. Food and Drug Administration. Taking a prescription medication at the right time, in the right manner, in the right amount, for the right duration, can be easily misunderstood and then misused. For example, what is the correct timing for "TID" (three times a day) directions? Is it every eight hours around the clock, or is it at times better suited for real life? Most patients' therapies involve multiple prescription medications, plus over-the-counter drugs, and possibly nutritional supplements. How are these balanced? Does the patient consider drug-drug interactions (chemical or physiological)? What about more complicated dosage forms such as inhalers, injectables, or eye drops? Are they being used correctly?

The pursuit of low health literacy solutions has been ongoing. Intervention research has been investigating ways to improve patient outcomes. In 2013, the National Council for Prescription Drug Programs introduced the concept of a

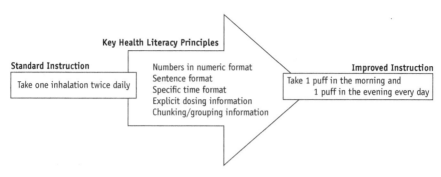

Figure 7-3. Universal Medication Schedule.

Universal Medication Schedule (UMS). UMS simplifies medication administration instructions for patients and/or their caregivers, increases patient understanding and adherence to their medication instructions, and results in improved health outcomes. The consistent and widespread use of these standards will assist patients in understanding and adhering to their medication regimen. As an example, instructions that indicate "take one pill in the morning and take one pill in the evening" are clearer than "take twice a day" (National Council for Prescription Drug Programs, 2013). Figure 7-3 shows the adaptation of standard inhaler instructions to the National Council for Prescription Drug Programs (2013) recommended language.

At Northwestern University, Wolf et al. (2016) studied the impact of the UMS. They found that over 90% of the patients interpreted UMS directions correctly, the benefit was greater in more complex regimens, and UMS directions showed a greater comprehension versus standard instructions on a prescription label. Patients with low health literacy showed the most significant results. Table 7-3 shows the timing for common dosage regimens according to the UMS guidelines drafted by the National Council for Prescription Drug Programs (2013). The guidelines emphasize using full sentences and explicit dosing information, grouping information in a more understandable format, using numeric format (using numerals, not spelling out the number), and using specific time information with a graphic format.

Table 7-3 **Universal Medication Schedule**

Do not drink alcoholic beverages while taking this medicine.	Take	1 pill in the morning 1 pill in the evening		
	Morning	Afternoon	Evening	Bedtime
	7–9 AM	11–1 PM	4–8 PM	9–11 PM
	1		1	

Implications for Public Health and Pharmacy Practice

Until recently, health literacy was defined and measured as an individual aptitude. Currently, health literacy is a multifaceted concept incorporating basic functional numeracy, prose literacy, communicative/interactive literacy, and problem-solving literacy. In other words, other characteristics such as the capacity, readiness, and preparedness to manage one's own health actively are also germane (Sørensen et al., 2012). In the past, low health literacy was perceived as an individual patient's deficit; that is, a patient had a lack of skills to be able to process health information leading to a lack of knowledge regarding health issues. Now, health literacy is recognized as a health care system issue. It is system-wide, reflecting the complexity of both the presentation of health information and navigation of health care systems. Current research is paying more attention to a patient's social support system (e.g., partner, family, community, and workplace) and to health care systems' role in remedying low health literacy problems.

Poor health literacy is more common than many practitioners realize. Therefore, for pharmacists, the approach to practice should be to ensure all patients receive the individualized tools to manage their care positively. There are also negative psychological effects of low health literacy, with one study reporting patients having a sense of shame about their limited health literacy skills (Parikh, Parker, Nurss, Baker, & Williams, 1996). In order to maintain their dignity, many of them may hide their reading or vocabulary difficulties (Baker et al., 1996).

In general, communication among people is a complex process. It involves many factors that impact the transmission and/or receipt of the message. These influences are called barriers. Examples include proxemics, kinesics, culture, generation, paralanguage, environmental, and distracting factors among others. As part of everyday life, communication transpires simultaneously at many parallel levels.

When suddenly, out of nowhere, a person is stricken with a health problem that forces him or her to exit the wellness role and adopt the sick role, the transition of roles is very difficult, at best. If healing (getting better) is to follow, then this change-over must occur; thus the patient enters into a dissimilar dominion from everyday life. Add to this complex situation the following inputs (interferences):

- New places must be found in a complicated facility with strange-sounding names;
- Unfamiliar documents, with too many lines, asking a voluminous number of questions must be completed;
- A new partnership must be established with one or more health professionals, some of whom may be unfamiliar;
- A new language is spoken, using many acronyms, at a faster pace than is reasonably listenable;

- Tests are performed, sometimes using weird, cold probes, with minimal explanation as to why;
- Numbers and measurements are presented that have little to no meaning;
- Questions are asked that seemingly have no answers;
- Decisions must be made in a far-to-fast timeframe that could have potentially serious ramifications; and
- The patient's everyday life has to continue.

Patients experience any or all of these scenarios as they travel through the various US health care systems. A patient's health literacy level determines how many of these interferences apply and how harshly they may affect the situation. Now, add to these situations disease-induced interference with cognition, multiple comorbidities, and/or a low health literacy level, and the potential for nonadherence, lack of understanding, and negative outcomes becomes very high.

Low health literacy is a health care system problem and requires system-wide solutions. It is not the patient's fault for failing to comprehend health information that has been given to him or her. All of us, no matter how literate, are at risk for interpreting health information incorrectly or not understanding it at all. This situation is especially true if the therapy is very complicated or the diagnosis is an emotionally charged one that involves a loved one or oneself (National Institutes of Health, 2016). It is possible that patients think they have the correct directions but may be too ashamed or embarrassed to seek further clarifying information to confirm their understanding.

Communicating the concepts of risks and benefits in a balanced, clear manner is challenging under optimal circumstances. In low health literate patients, the complexity of this situation is significantly exacerbated. The massive volume of health information now available on the Internet has made it much harder to determine what is evidenced based versus what is pseudo-science, false and misleading advertisements, quackery, or gimmickry. These added complexities only increase the vulnerability of all patients for receiving misinformation and, in actuality, decreases their literacy level.

Choosing to be healthy, realizing when and knowing how to seek health care, and engaging in preventive measures to stay well require that a patient comprehends and uses health information correctly. This "ability to obtain, process, and understand health information needed to make informed health decisions is known as health literacy" (Office of Disease Prevention and Health Promotion, 2007, p. 2.5).

When pharmacists are "clinicianing" (the process of being a clinician rather than practicing), they must think and engage in finding solutions to how best to serve their patents most effectively. Then they can put these strategies and tactics into practice. Improving communication between the patient and pharmacist regarding health information reduces health care costs and increases the quality of health care.

Health literacy is a complicated, crazy conundrum. In the words of the National Institutes of Health (2016), solving the problem of low health literacy "saves lives, saves time, saves money."

References

Auerbach, A. D., Kripalani, S., Vasilevskis, E. E., Sehgal, N., Lindenauer, P. K., Metlay, J. P., . . . Schnipper, J. L. (2016). Preventability and causes of readmissions in a national cohort of general medicine patients. *JAMA Internal Medicine, 176*(4), 484–493. doi:10.1001/jamainternmed.2015.7863

Baker, D. W., Parker, R. M., Williams, M. V., & Clark, W. S. (1998). Health literacy and the risk of hospital admission. *Journal of General Internal Medicine, 13*(12), 791–798.

Baker, D. W., Parker, R. M., Williams, M. V., Pitkin, K., Parikh, N. S., Coates, W., & Imara, M. (1996). The health care experience of patients with low literacy. *Archives of Family Medicine, 5*(6), 329–334.

Batterham, R. W., Hawkins, M., Collins, P. A., Buchbinder, R., & Osborne, R. H. (2016). Health literacy: Applying current concepts to improve health services and reduce health inequalities. *Public Health, 132*, 3–12. doi:10.1016/j.puhe.2016.01.001

Beauchamp, A., Buchbinder, R., Dodson, S., Batterham, R. W., Elsworth, G. R., McPhee, C., . . . Osborne, R. H. (2015). Distribution of health literacy strengths and weaknesses across socio-demographic groups: A cross-sectional survey using the Health Literacy Questionnaire (HLQ). *BMC Public Health, 15*, 678. doi:10.1186/s12889-015-2056-z

Bennett, C. L., Ferreira, M. R., Davis, T. C., Kaplan, J., Weinberger, M., Kuzel, T., . . . Sartor, O. (1998). Relation between literacy, race, and stage of presentation among low-income patients with prostate cancer. *Journal of Clinical Oncology, 16*(9), 3101–3104.

CVS Caremark. (2014, February 14). Low health literacy compromises health, increases costs. WP BrandStudio. Retrieved from http://www.washingtonpost.com/sf/brand-connect/wp/2014/02/14/low-health-literacy-compromises-health-increases-costs/

DeWalt, D. A., Callahan, L. F., Hawk, V. H., Broucksou, K. A., Hink, A., Rudd, R., & Brach, C. (2010). *Health literacy universal precautions toolkit* (AHRQ Publication, no. 10-0046-EF). Rockville, MD: Agency for Healthcare Research and Quality. Retrieved from http://www.ahrq.gov/sites/default/files/wysiwyg/professionals/quality-patient-safety/quality-resources/tools/literacy-toolkit/healthliteracytoolkit.pdf

Dodson, S., Good, S., & Osborne, R. H. (2015). *Health literacy toolkit for low and middle-income countries: A series of information sheets to empower communities and strengthen health systems.* New Delhi, India: World Health Organization, Regional Office for South-East Asia. Retrieved from http://www.searo.who.int/entity/healthpromotion/documents/hl_tookit/en/

Expert Panel on Effective Ways of Investing in Health. (2016). *Access to health services in the European Union.* Brussels, Belgium: European Commission. Retrieved from http://ec.europa.eu/health/expert_panel/sites/expertpanel/files/015_access_healthservices_en.pdf

FIP Foundation for Education and Research. (n.d.). Pictograms support. The Hague, The Netherlands: Author. Retrieved from http://www.fip.org/fipfoundation/Our-work/2239/Pictograms_support/

Freedman, D. A., Bess, K. D., Tucker, H. A., Boyd, D. L., Tuchman, A. M., & Wallston, K. A. (2009). Public health literacy defined. *American Journal of Preventive Medicine, 36*(5), 446–451. doi:10.1016/j.amepre.2009.02.001

Gazmararian, J. A., Curran, J. W., Parker, R. M., Bernhardt, J. M., & DeBuono, B. A. (2005). Public health literacy in America: An ethical imperative. *American Journal of Preventive Medicine, 28*(3), 317–322. doi:10.1016/j.amepre.2004.11.004

Griffey, R. T., Kennedy, S. K., D'Agostino McGowan, L., Goodman, M., & Kaphingst, K. A. (2014). Is low health literacy associated with increased emergency department utilization and recidivism? *Academic Emergency Medicine, 21*(10), 1109–1115. doi:10.1111/acem.12476

Heijmans, M., Uiters, E., Rose, T., Hofstede, J., Devillé, W., van der Heide, I., . . . Rademakers, J. (2015, June). *Study on sound evidence for a better understanding of health literacy in the European Union: Final report.* Brussels, Belgium: European Commission. Retrieved from http://ec.europa.eu/health/health_policies/docs/2015_health_literacy_en.pdf

Institute for Healthcare Improvement. (2016). *Words to watch: Fact sheet.* Boston, MA: Author. Retrieved from https://c.ymcdn.com/sites/npsf.site-ym.com/resource/resmgr/AskMe3/Words-to-Watch_dwnld.pdf

Institute of Medicine. (2001). *Crossing the quality chasm: A new health system for the 21st century.* Washington, DC: National Academy Press.

Institute of Medicine. (2013). *Health literacy: Improving health, health systems, and health policy around the world: Workshop summary.* Washington, DC: National Academies Press. Retrieved from https://www.nap.edu/download/18325

Jacobson, K. L., Gazmararian, J. A., Kripalani, S., McMorris, K. J., Blake, S. C., & Brach, C. (2007, October). *Is our pharmacy meeting patients' needs? A pharmacy health literacy assessment tool user's guide* (AHRQ Publication No. 07-0051). Rockville, MD: Agency for Healthcare Research and Quality. Retrieved from http://www.ahrq.gov/sites/default/files/publications/files/pharmlit.pdf

Kickbusch, I., Pelikan, J. M., Apfel, F., & Tsouros, A. D. (2013). *Health literacy: The solid facts.* Copenhagen, Denmark: World Health Organization Regional Office for Europe. Retrieved from http://www.euro.who.int/__data/assets/pdf_file/0008/190655/e96854.pdf

Kutner, M., Greenburg, E., Jin, Y., & Paulsen, C. (2006). *The health literacy of America's adults: Results from the 2003 National Assessment of Adult Literacy.* Washington, DC: U.S. Department of Education, National Center for Education Statistics.

McNaughton, C. D., Cawthon, C., Kripalani, S., Liu, D., Storrow, A. B., & Roumie, C. L. (2015). Health literacy and mortality: A cohort study of patients hospitalized for acute heart failure. *Journal of the American Heart Association, 4*(5). doi:10.1161/jaha.115.001799

McNaughton, C. D., Collins, S. P., Kripalani, S., Rothman, R., Self, W. H., Jenkins, C., . . . Storrow, A. B. (2013). Low numeracy is associated with increased odds of 30-day emergency department or hospital recidivism for patients with acute heart failure. *Circulation: Heart Failure, 6*(1), 40–46. doi:10.1161/circheartfailure.112.969477

Merriam-Webster. (2016). Pictogram. Retrieved from http://www.merriam-webster.com/dictionary/pictogram?utm_campaign=sd&utm_medium=serp&utm_source=jsonld

National Council for Prescription Drug Programs. (2013, March). *Universal Medication Schedule White Paper, Version 1.0.* Scottsdale, AZ: Author. Retrieved from http://ncpdp.org/NCPDP/media/pdf/wp/NCPDP-UMS-WhitePaper201304.pdf

National Institutes of Health. (2016). Clear communication: Health literacy. Rockville, MD: Author. Retrieved from https://www.nih.gov/institutes-nih/nih-office-director/office-communications-public-liaison/clear-communication/health-literacy

National Network of Libraries of Medicine. (n.d.). Health literacy. Rockville, MD: Author. Retrieved from https://nnlm.gov/outreach/consumer/hlthlit.html

National Patient Safety Foundation. (2016). Ask me 3: Good questions for your good health. Boston, MA: Author. Retrieved from https://npsf.site-ym.com/default.asp?page=askme3

Nielsen-Bohlman, L., Panxer, A. M., Kindig, D. A., & Institute of Medicine Committee on Health Literacy. (2004). *Health literacy: A prescription to end confusion.* Washington, DC: National Academy Press. Retrieved from http://iom.nationalacademies.org/Reports/2004/Health-Literacy-A-Prescription-to-End-Confusion.aspx

Nutbeam, D. (2000). Health literacy as a public health goal: A challenge for contemporary health education and communication strategies into the 21st century. *Health Promotion International, 15*(3), 259–267. doi:10.1093/heapro/15.3.259

Nutbeam, D., & World Health Organization Collaborating Centre for Health Promotion. (1998). *Health promotion glossary* (WHO/HPR/HEP/98.1). Geneva, Switzerland: World Health Organization Division of Health Promotion, Education and Communications. Retrieved from http://www.who.int/healthpromotion/about/HPR%20Glossary%201998.pdf?ua=1

Office of Disease Prevention and Health Promotion. (2000). Health communication. In U.S. Department of Health and Human Services (Ed.), *Healthy People 2010:* Vol. 1. *Objectives for improving health.* Washington, DC: Author. Retrieved from http://www.healthypeople.gov/2010/document/pdf/Volume1/11HealthCom.pdf.

Office of Disease Prevention and Health Promotion. (2007). *Quick guide to health literacy.* Washington, DC: U.S. Department of Health and Human Services. Retrieved from https://health.gov/communication/literacy/quickguide/Quickguide.pdf

Palumbo, R. (2015). Discussing the effects of poor health literacy on patients facing HIV: A narrative literature review. *International Journal of Health Policy and Management, 4*(7), 417–430. doi:10.15171/ijhpm.2015.95

Parikh, N. S., Parker, R. M., Nurss, J. R., Baker, D. W., & Williams, M. V. (1996). Shame and health literacy: The unspoken connection. *Patient Education and Counseling, 27*(1), 33–39.

Patient Protection and Affordable Care Act, 42 U.S.C. § 18001 et seq., Pub. L. No. 111–148 (2010). Retrieved from https://www.gpo.gov/fdsys/pkg/PLAW-111publ148/pdf/PLAW-111publ148.pdf

Pfizer. (2011, February). *The newest vital sign: A health literacy assessment tool.* New York, NY: Author. Retrieved from https://www.pfizer.com/files/health/nvs_flipbook_english_final.pdf

Pharmaceutical Research and Manufacturers of America. (2011, January). *Improving prescription medicine adherence is key to better health care: Taking medicines as prescribed can lower costs and improve health outcomes* Washington, DC: Author. Retrieved from http://phrma-docs.phrma.org/sites/default/files/pdf/PhRMA_Improving%20Medication%20Adherence_Issue%20Brief.pdf

Plain Writing Act, 5 U.S.C. § 301 et seq., Pub. L. No. 111–274 (2010). Retrieved from https://www.gpo.gov/fdsys/pkg/PLAW-111publ274/pdf/PLAW-111publ274.pdf

Rampey, B. D., Finnegan, R., Goodman, M., Mohadjer, L., Krenzke, T., Hogan, J., & Provasnik, S. (2016). *Skills of U.S. unemployed, young, and older adults in sharper focus: Results from the Program for the International Assessment of Adult Competencies (PIAAC) 2012/2014: First look* (NCES 2016-039rev). Washington, DC: U.S. Department of Education. Retrieved from http://nces.ed.gov/pubs2016/2016039rev.pdf

Rasu, R. S., Bawa, W. A., Suminski, R., Snella, K., & Warady, B. (2015). Health literacy impact on national healthcare utilization and expenditure. *International Journal of Health Policy and Management, 4*(11), 747–755. doi:10.15171/ijhpm.2015.151

Rowlands, G., Shaw, A., Jaswal, S., Smith, S., & Harpham, T. (2015). Health literacy and the social determinants of health: A qualitative model from adult learners. *Health Promotion International.* doi:10.1093/heapro/dav093

Scott, T. L., Gazmararian, J. A., Williams, M. V., & Baker, D. W. (2002). Health literacy and preventive health care use among Medicare enrollees in a managed care organization. *Medical Care, 40*(5), 395–404.

Sørensen, K., Van den Broucke, S., Fullam, J., Doyle, G., Pelikan, J., Slonska, Z., & Brand, H. (2012). Health literacy and public health: A systematic review and integration of definitions and models. *BMC Public Health, 12*, 80. doi:10.1186/1471-2458-12-80

The Joint Commission. (2007). *What did the doctor say? Improving health literacy to protect patient safety.* Oakbrook Terrace, IL: Author. Retrieved from https://www.jointcommission.org/assets/1/18/improving_health_literacy.pdf

U.S. Department of Health and Human Services, Office of Disease Prevention and Health Promotion. (2010). *National action plan to improve health literacy.* Washington, DC: Author. Retrieved from http://www.health.gov/communication/hlactionplan/pdf/Health_Literacy_Action_Plan.pdf

U.S. Pharmacopeial Convention. (2016). USP pictograms. Rockville, MD: Author. Retrieved from http://www.usp.org/usp-healthcare-professionals/related-topics-resources/usp-pictograms

Vernon, J. A., Trujillo, A., Rosenbaum, S., & DeBuono, B. (2007). *Low health literacy: Implications for national health policy*. Washington, DC: George Washington University, Center for Health Policy Research. Retrieved from http://publichealth.gwu.edu/departments/healthpolicy/CHPR/downloads/LowHealthLiteracyReport10_4_07.pdf

Wernick, M., Hale, P., Anticich, N., Busch, S., Merriman, L., King, B., & Pegg, T. (2016). A randomised crossover trial of minimising medical terminology in secondary care correspondence in patients with chronic health conditions: Impact on understanding and patient reported outcomes. *Internal Medical Journal, 46*(5), 596–601. doi:10.1111/imj.13062

Wolf, M. S., Davis, T. C., Curtis, L. M., Bailey, S. C., Knox, J. P., Bergeron, A., . . . Wood, A. J. (2016). A patient-centered prescription drug label to promote appropriate medication use and adherence. *Journal of General Internal Medicine.* doi:10.1007/s11606-016-3816-x

World Health Organization. (1986). *The Ottawa Charter for Health Promotion.* Geneva, Switzerland: Author. Retrieved from http://www.who.int/healthpromotion/conferences/previous/ottawa/en/index.html

World Health Organization. (2016a). Health promotion: About us. Geneva, Switzerland: Author. Retrieved from http://www.who.int/healthpromotion/about/en/

World Health Organization. (2016b). Social determinants of health. Geneva, Switzerland: Author. Retrieved from http://www.who.int/social_determinants/sdh_definition/en/

World Health Organization, & International Telecommunication Union. (2012). *National eHealth strategy toolkit.* Geneva, Switzerland: Author. Retrieved from http://www.who.int/ehealth/publications/overview.pdf

World Literacy Foundation. (2015, August 24). *The economic & social cost of illiteracy: A snapshot of illiteracy in a global context.* London: Author. Retrieved from https://worldliteracyfoundation.org/wp-content/uploads/2015/02/WLF-FINAL-ECONOMIC-REPORT.pdf

8

Behavioral Health

ARDIS HANSON, CAROL A. OTT, AND BRUCE LUBOTSKY LEVIN

How is behavioral health defined? The World Health Organization (WHO, 2003, p. 7) defines mental health as more than a lack of mental disorders, it is "a state of well-being whereby individuals recognize their abilities, are able to cope with the normal stresses of life, work productively and fruitfully, and make a contribution to their communities." Behavioral health, defined by the U.S. Substance Abuse and Mental Health Services Administration, is similar to that of the WHO, "a state of mental/emotional being and/or choices and actions that affect wellness." (Substance Abuse and Mental Health Services Administration, 2011, p. 1).

Both definitions focus on well-being and can be influenced by national or cultural expectations of what wellness comprises at a personal and at a community-level. This chapter defines behavioral health as the study of alcohol, drug abuse, and mental disorders from a population or public health perspective.

If behavioral health is grounded in wellness, then what are behavioral disorders? Behavioral disorders generally include substance abuse or misuse, alcohol and drug addiction, mental disorders, and co-occurring mental and substance use disorders. However, defining behavioral disorders is a complex undertaking. Unlike earlier definitions of mental disorders as clusters of behaviors, the National Institute of Mental Health's (NIMH, 2008) *Strategic Plan* framed mental illnesses as brain disorders, specifically disorders of brain circuits affected by genetic, neurobiological, environmental, experiential, and behavioral factors. In 2011, behavioral disorders were named as mental, neurological, and substance-use (MNS) disorders in the NIMH's Grand Challenges in Global Mental Health Initiative (Collins et al., 2011). MNSs include all conditions that affect the nervous system and are leading causes of disease burden, estimated on the basis of disability adjusted life years (DALYs).

How behavioral disorders are defined also may change across populations. In the United States, for example, adults have serious mental illnesses (SMI), while children have serious emotional disabilities (SED). The definitions for SMI and SED, developed in the 1990s are still in use today. The definitions limit diagnosis of SMI or SED to specific age groups, the current time period or within the past year, meeting specific *Diagnostic and Statistical Manual of Mental Disorders* (DSM) criteria, and resulting in one or more functional impairment(s) that substantially limits or constrains one or more major life activities (U.S. Department of Health and Human Services, 1997, 1999,).

Epidemiology

When we talk about the burden of disease, it is critical to understand major health problems often drive policy, which then drives legislation, which finally drives practice. Taking a public health perspective is useful for determining the burden of diseases, injuries, and leading risk factors. We start with the prevalence and incidence of a disease. Based on a national sampling of adults in the United States in 2012, SAMHSA estimated that 43.7 million adults aged 18 or older (18.6%) experienced having a mental illness in the past year (Substance Abuse and Mental Health Services Administration, 2013).

However, the number of people with a disease is not enough to determine burden of disease or the importance of a health condition as a national or global priority. To do that, we also examine the data on behavioral disorders and the effect these disorders have on the morbidity (years lived with disability [YLDs]) and mortality (years of life lost [YLLs]).

MEASURING BURDEN OF DISEASE

The first global measure of morbidity, the DALY is the sum of years of potential life lost due to premature mortality and the years of productive life lost due to disability (Murray & López, 1996). Whiteford and colleagues (2013) estimate mental and substance use disorders accounted for 183.9 million (7.4%) DALYs globally. It is estimated that 13.6% of DALYs in the United States are caused by behavioral disorders and seven of the top 20 disorders affecting morbidity are mental illnesses: (a) major depressive disorders, (b) drug use disorders, (c) anxiety disorders, (d) alcohol use disorders, (e) schizophrenia, (f) bipolar disorder, and (g) dysthymia (U.S. Burden of Disease Collaborators, 2013). Breaking it down into YLDs and YLLs, Whiteford and colleagues (2013) estimate mental and substance use disorders across the globe accounted for 175.3 million YLDs and 8.6 million YLLs, with mental and substance use disorders as the leading cause of YLDs worldwide.

COMORBIDITY

Most serious behavioral disorders are chronic, long-term conditions that frequently co-occur with, and may exacerbate, other somatic or behavioral health conditions.

The majority of individuals who have the most serious mental illnesses and co-occurring disorders die, on average, at age 53 from treatable medical conditions or lifestyle changes, such as poor diets, tobacco smoking, obesity, high blood pressure, lack of exercise, and alcohol abuse (Parks, Svendsen, Singer, & Foti, 2006).

Diagnosing Behavioral Disorders

In the fourth edition of the DSM, there is a significant passage that notes that "although this manual provides a classification of mental disorders, it must be admitted that no definition adequately specifies precise boundaries for the concept of 'mental disorder'" (American Psychiatric Association, 1994, pp. xxi–xxii). So although we can classify symptoms into clusters of behaviors that define or frame behavioral disorders, there is no concrete or consistent operational definition of "mental disorder." Just as physical disorders are defined by symptom presentation, pathology, physiological norms, and etiology, mental disorders are defined by behavioral and emotional responses that are observable. Further, the DSM also notes that, to be a disorder, the response to a particular event must not be an expected and/or culturally sanctioned response, such as grief for the death of a loved one.

We would argue that diagnosis is much more than just identifying the set of symptoms presented to the clinician and addressing those symptoms. Diagnosis of a disorder should provide a prediction of supportive services that an individual may need or the level(s) of care that is currently or may become necessary in the future. Diagnosis alone is not enough data for health planning or disease management, especially for behavioral disorders. Diagnosis should also address the functional limitations faced by persons with specific or co-occurring disorders that affect an individual's ability to perform daily activities of living (ADLs).

ADLs are basic self-care tasks, such as feeding, toileting, selecting proper attire, grooming, maintaining continence, putting on clothes, bathing, walking, and being able to get around (mobility). In addition to ADLs, there are also instrumental activities of daily living (IADLs), which are the complex skills needed to successfully live independently in the community. IADLs include managing finances, driving or navigating public transit to work, shopping, preparing meals, using communication devices (telephone, Skype, etc.), performing housework and basic home maintenance, and managing medications.

Assessing symptomatology, ADLs, and IADLs can determine what kind of medications and assistance an individual may need on a day-to-day basis. However, to diagnose and evaluate across disorder and functional limitations (ADLs/IADLs) requires a number of diagnostic tools and may change depending upon a country's use of diagnostic tools as well as societal/cultural constructs of behavioral health.

INTERNATIONAL STANDARDS

At a global level, the WHO provides a family of international classifications to assist in the diagnosis of disorders. The first is the International Statistical Classification of Diseases and Related Health Problems (ICD). Now in its 10th revision, the ICD is used by more than 110 countries, including the United States, for epidemiology (surveillance, vital statistics, morbidity, and mortality), health management (reimbursement and resource allocation decision-making), and clinical purposes. Translated into 43 languages, 117 member states of the WHO use the ICD-10 to report mortality data. The ICD-10 contains more than 14,000 codes for diseases, signs and symptoms, abnormal findings, and external causes of injury or diseases. The basic structure of the ICD-10 code is as follows: Characters 1–3 (the category of disease), 4 (etiology of disease), 5 (body part affected), 6 (severity of illness), and 7 (placeholder for extension of the code to increase specificity). Not surprisingly, due to the cultural, social, and religious heterogeneity of the member states of the WHO, there is an overarching "ICD-10 rule" for diagnostic criteria of not using interference with social role performance as a criterion.

The ICD has been adapted for specialty areas, including two adaptations for mental and behavioral disorders: one for *Diagnostic Criteria for Research* and one for *Clinical Descriptions and Diagnostic Guidelines*. The *ICD-10 Classification of Mental and Behavioral Disorders: Diagnostic Criteria for Research* (DCR-10; WHO, 1993), referred to as the "Green Book," has the diagnostic classification schema and ICD-10 coding but does not have the descriptions of the clinical concepts. That is found in the *Clinical Descriptions and Diagnostic Guidelines* (WHO, 1992), commonly referred to as the "Blue Book." Each disorder is described with its main clinical features and other important but less specific associated features. The guidelines also provide the number and balance of symptoms that must be present before a diagnosis can be made with confidence. The DRC-10 follows the ICD-10 structure on social role performance with the exception of certain diagnoses for adults (e.g., dementia, simple schizophrenia, and dissocial personality disorder) and certain childhood disorders due to the complicated role relationships within or among families, peers, or communities. These "culture specific" disorders are found in Appendix 2 of the DRC-10.

In addition to the ICD, there are two other important diagnostic tools: International Classification of Functioning, Disability and Health (ICF) and the International Classification of Health Interventions (ICHI). The ICF is a classification of health and health-related domains in relationship to functioning and disability and measures functioning at both the individual and the population levels. Still in development, the ICHI is meant to provide a standard measure for the reporting and analysis of health interventions to allow comparison of behavioral, medical, surgical, and other health-related interventions across countries and populations.

NATIONAL STANDARDS

The National Center for Health Statistics is the federal agency responsible for use of the ICD-10 in the United States (Pickett, Berglund, Blum, & Wing, 1999). The U. S. ICD-10-CM has more than 68,000 codes, many of them new, that are and mapped to address measures of quality of care as well as outcomes of care. The ICD-10-CM includes the level of detail needed for morbidity classification and diagnostic specificity and uses code titles and language commonly used in accepted clinical practice. The Centers for Medicare and Medicaid Services in the United States also developed a new Procedure Coding (ICD-10-PCS) for inpatient procedures that harmonizes with the ICD-10. When the United States implemented the ICD-10 in 2016, a number of strategies made the implementation go smoothly (Goldstein, 2015).

In the United States, the fifth edition of the DSM (DSM-5; American Psychiatric Association, 2013) is the standard diagnostic tool for determining mental disorders. The DSM-V underwent a significant structural reorganization to correspond with the reorganized arrangement of disorders in the newest version of the ICD (the ICD-11). It was also harmonized to the United States ICD-CM to allow for easier integration for diagnostic and medical coding.

Diagnostic standards are important from a public health perspective since they can provide important data when planning for an individual or community level of care and services, as well as for broader statewide or nationwide services. Since persons with behavioral disorders often require a number of supportive services, having knowledge of diagnoses, ADLs, and IADLs can inform what services or supports are necessary (e.g., rehabilitation, employment, housing, transportation, medication management, etc.).

This also informs our ability to develop behavioral, medical, pharmacological, and technological interventions that will allow individuals to perform the tasks they need to do to be successful in living at home, to work in the community, or to engage socially with others outside of a residence. For example, if we know what changes occur in an individual's body functions and systems, an individual's level of capacity in a standard environment, and what an individual is able to do in his or her usual environment (level of performance), then we can design options to optimize their functional capacity and performance. It can also inform how we develop and implement interventions to improve the quality of lives of persons with behavioral disorders and how we can assess their effectiveness and efficacy in improving patient outcomes.

Service Delivery Challenges

Based upon the challenges identified by NIMH (Collins et al., 2011), we define global mental health services research as collaborative, interdisciplinary approaches to examining transnational problems that have relevance to many nations or that may have determinants or solutions that work across national borders to reduce disease burden and increase health equity. Within the framework of "how mental health services research findings can be used most effectively to influence the delivery of services," we can begin to examine challenges for both public behavioral health and public health pharmacy.

FORMULARIES

As managed care has continued to evolve and with the passage of the Patient Protection and Affordable Care Act in the United States, medication coverage remains a major focus in the provision of behavioral health and in public health pharmacy services. Strategies include pharmaceutical benefit managers (PBMs) and tiered formularies. PBMs negotiate pricing with pharmacies or establish which drugs will be included in formularies. Tiered formularies, increasingly used by private insurers, prefer to use generic and nonpreferred brand names. Nonpreferred brand names require special authorization for use and are used only when a patient fails to improve on a less costly medication before a more expensive medication will be approved. With the results of the Clinical Antipsychotic Trials of Intervention Effectiveness study comparing typical and atypical antipsychotic medication (Covell, Finnerty, & Essock, 2008) and Medicare D medication coverage (Centers for Medicare & Medicaid Services, 2015), newer managed care strategies create formularies that review prescribing practices that do not meet current best practices or algorithms (Moore et al., 2007).

The Mental Health Medicaid Pharmacy Partnership program in Missouri, for example, chose practice guidelines of the American Psychiatric Association, the Expert Consensus Guidelines Series, and the Texas Medication Algorithm Project and sent informational mailings to prescribers in the system about problematic prescribing patterns (Parks, 2006).

Medications used for behavioral disorders have traditionally been costly and subject to formulary restrictions within insurance programs, both private and public payer sources. Formularies are developed using clinical trial information for efficacy in the affected patient population; generally, if the data does not show significant clinical difference in effect, cost becomes the most important factor. In the case of psychoactive drugs, the effectiveness of individual agents within a class of drugs is largely similar, leading to cost as the driving force for formulary inclusion decisions.

Formulary systems often initially include a very limited number of preferred medications that must be ineffective for a patient before consideration can be given to the use of more expensive, nonpreferred drugs. It is often not clear what the insurer defines as an adequate trial in terms of dose and duration, so patients and providers must navigate a confusing and inconsistent system to obtain nonpreferred drugs.

While formulary systems are created with the goal of providing appropriate treatment of medical and psychiatric conditions in the most cost-effective manner possible, research has suggested that, as drug costs are decreased, the expenditures to the insurer are shifted to increased money spent in nonmedication areas. A study by Goldman, Dirani, Fastenau, and Conrad (2014) evaluated the impact of strict formularies for antipsychotic drugs to treat schizophrenia and revealed that restrictions on atypical antipsychotics resulted in increased total medical expenditures for schizophrenia and bipolar disorder, estimating a total annual increased cost of approximately $1 billion for state Medicaid systems. In addition, strict formularies caused patients to return to previously failed antipsychotic therapies or to discontinue treatment, increasing the use of other acute care medical services while decreasing drug costs (Seabury et al., 2014).

Quantity limits per prescription and prior authorization (PA) requirements are other methods that are used in an attempt to ensure appropriate use of medications and decrease costs. A quantity limit is defined as limiting the number of dose units (tablets or capsules) dispensed to the patient for each prescription based on the usual recommended dosing of the individual drug for a 30-day supply. For example, the usual recommended maximum dose of risperidone is 8 mg total dose daily. Risperidone is available as a 4 mg tablet, so the maximum quantity limit for risperidone 4 mg tablets for a 30-day supply would be 60 tablets. Commonly, recommended maximum doses for a drug are obtained from initial clinical registration trials that may include a less ill patient population as the study sample, and the results of the trials may not translate to the more extremely ill patient population. Higher doses are occasionally required for some patients, which leads to the need for PA before a prescription can be paid for by the payer and dispensed to the patient.

Prior authorizations are required for prescriptions when the drug, dose, or quantity exceeds those allowed by the insurance program or when a patient is also receiving another drug in the same class. Prior authorization criteria vary based upon the drug in question and can also differ relative to the place of the drug as preferred or nonpreferred; in some states, open access to behavioral health medications means that all medications used for psychiatric indications are covered by the Medicaid program, but access may be restricted based on clinical appropriateness and previously tried therapies.

Step therapy is another means used to control medication use in an insurance system. Step therapy requires a patient to try preferred medications for a given condition in the order of use required by the insurer. For example, a patient who needs an antidepressant medication may be required to try fluoxetine first, then sertraline, then venlafaxine in that order and in adequate doses and durations before moving on to a nonpreferred agent. A PA would then be required to obtain the nonpreferred agent.

Several studies have evaluated the impact of PAs on medication access and use of other medical care services. The results of this research suggests that PA restrictions

are associated with an increased risk of incarceration, increased discontinuation of medications prematurely, decreased number of psychiatric provider visits
after discontinuation of medications, increased emergency department visits, and
decreased initiation of nonpreferred medications without an offsetting increase in
preferred drugs (Goldman, Fastenau, et al., 2014; Lu et al., 2011; Lu, Soumerai,
Ross-Degnan, Zhang, & Adams, 2010).

MEDICATION ADHERENCE

The issue of medication adherence and its role in chronic disease management and
reduced use of acute care medical services is well-documented. It is assumed by
most healthcare professionals that those with mental disorders are more nonadherent to treatment, including medications, than those with other chronic disorders. The reality is that mental disorders lead to treatment nonadherence similarly
to chronic medical disorders, but often for different reasons. Several causes of nonadherence to medications have been identified, including the stigma associated
with having a mental illness, insight of the patient into his or her illness, the illness
symptoms, social isolation, the drug class and formulation, substance use, access to
healthcare, employment and insurance status, and lack of social and/or family support (Haddad, Brain, & Scott, 2014; Shuler, 2014). The risks to the patient and the
health system are great when a patient does not take medications as prescribed or
at all. There is increased risk of relapse of illness symptoms and hospitalization for
any cause, greater length of stay when hospitalized, increased self-harm by patients
experiencing symptoms, increased cost of care to the patient, and decreased quality of life (Haddad et al., 2014; Offord, Lin, Wong, Mirski, & Baker, 2013).

Overall, studies show that approximately 64% of patients with a mental illness
have partial adherence or nonadherence to medication therapy (Offord et al.,
2013). In one study of patients with depression, those studied had a 1.76 times
risk of being nonadherent to medications for chronic medical diseases if they were
depressed and undertreated (Grenard et al., 2011). A study by Markowitz, Karve,
Panish, Candrilli, and Alphs (2013) of the rates of rehospitalization for patients
with schizophrenia were greatest during the first 60 days after hospital discharge
with the greatest financial cost in rehospitalization and pharmacy costs.

Many strategies have been studied and employed as interventions for medication nonadherence. Of these, psychoeducation, psychosocial interventions, long-
acting antipsychotic injections, electronic reminders, simplification of medication
regimens, shared decision-making, financial incentives for adherence, and good
communication with the patient regarding drug therapy had the greatest impact
(Haddad et al., 2014). Medication education alone did not improve the rate of
nonadherence for most patients. In a study by Chong, Aslani, and Chen (2011),
interventions to improve adherence to antidepressants were evaluated. Medication
support, patient educational strategies, and telephone follow-up to monitor progress

were most effective. Overall, these strategies required a multidisciplinary approach, which provides an opportunity for pharmacist interaction.

Patients with mental illnesses often feel uncomfortable in the community pharmacy setting, and pharmacists have been shown in some studies to be uncomfortable counseling patients with mental illness. Good communication with patients receiving psychoactive medications is paramount to improving medication adherence. Pharmacists should counsel patients about the expected outcomes of their drug therapy, the most common (and sometimes debilitating) side effects that can be encountered, and ways to manage these side effects.

The use of long-acting injection (LAI) dosage forms of antipsychotics is a common way to ensure adherence to medications in the patient population with a psychotic disorder. Unfortunately, most patients believe that if a LAI dosage form is recommended, it is a punishment for nonadherence to oral medications. Promoting the idea of convenience to this patient population is an advantageous way to make LAIs a positive consideration for these patients.

Das, Malik, and Haddad (2014) performed and evaluated a survey of 11 patients with early psychosis and schizophrenia and their attitudes regarding LAI antipsychotic medications. The average age of these patients was 24 years; these were young patients in the beginning of their illness and their understanding of schizophrenia. Three areas were studied: (a) treatment alliance and the psychiatrist recommendation for LAI therapy, (b) patient knowledge and beliefs regarding LAIs, and (c) patient views about the appropriateness of LAI treatment.

The researchers suggest that the recommendation of the psychiatrist has value, validating the need for a strong therapeutic alliance. The knowledge and beliefs about LAI therapy were generally more positive for those who were already receiving LAI treatment, with convenience of dosing and not having to remember daily antipsychotic doses being the most common positive response. Among those not receiving LAIs, lack of awareness, stigma, and misperceptions of treatment were most often cited as reasons for the lack of acceptance of LAI treatment. Overall, this study reveals that a positive therapeutic alliance with the patient and the provision of clear information about the treatment allows for an informed discussion and greater positive response to treatment by the patient (Das et al., 2014).

BARRIERS TO TREATMENT

Behavioral health services are provided by a diverse number of systems, facilities, and providers, in primary care, specialty care, community-based, and public care settings (Hanson, Levin, Ott, & Meldrum, 2012). Within primary care, behavioral health services are delivered in medical care settings (general hospital emergency rooms and psychiatric units in general hospitals), long-term care facilities, the Veterans Administration medical care systems, and managed healthcare settings. Within the specialty behavioral health care sector, behavioral health services are available through many systems and settings, including (but not limited to) state/county mental hospitals, private psychiatric hospitals, community mental health centers, ambulatory mental health facilities, substance abuse centers, and an assortment of behavioral health practitioners. Within the community-based care settings, behavioral health is provided at public health centers, places of employment (employee assistance programs), places of worship, peer counseling centers, support groups, recreation facilities, and schools. Within public sector behavioral health care sector, behavioral health services are available through child welfare, foster care, corrections, juvenile justice, schools, court diversion programs, and integrated care. This is by no means an exhaustive list on trajectories into behavioral health services and treatment.

However, with all the different trajectories into care, there are also a number of barriers, particularly since successful treatment often requires an individual to have regular access to behavioral health care professionals and a number of support services. In addition to the persistent stigma surrounding behavioral disorders, there are issues of reimbursement; costs of care, availability of care based on provider, geographic availability, policy limitations, formulary restrictions, transportation, provider knowledge, patient knowledge, attitudinal/evaluative barriers, medication compliance, family support (or lack of it), inconvenience or inability to obtain an appointment, and refusal of treatment.

United States

Mojtabai et al. (2011) examined barriers to treatment identified by adults using findings from the U.S. National Comorbidity Survey-Replication. The most common reasons were attitudinal or evaluative barriers (97.4%), low perceived need (44.8%), and structural barriers (22.2%). Of the attitudinal/evaluative barriers, wanting to handle the problem by oneself ranked first (72.6%), followed by perceived severity of problem (16.9%), perceived ineffectiveness (16.4%), thought that things would get better (11.5%), and stigma (9.1%). Structural barriers were identified as financial (15.3%), availability (12.8%), transportation (5.7%), and inconvenience (9.8%). Mojtabai et al. also found that, across levels of severity, low perceived need was the most commonly reported barrier to treatment. These findings are significant and consistent with findings from numerous other studies conducted regarding access/utilization (Alonso et al., 2004a; Codony et al., 2009; Sareen et al., 2007). From a cross-national perspective, structural barriers, specifically financial barriers, are reported as another major barrier to care (Alonso et al., 2004b; Codony et al., 2009; Sareen et al., 2007).

Europe

The European Study of the Epidemiology of Mental Disorders (ESEMeD) project, funded by the European Union, examined access and patterns of use of behavioral health services in Belgium, France, Germany, Italy, the Netherlands, and Spain. ESEMeD showed that less than 30% of those with a behavioral disorder accesses or utilizes services (Alonso et al., 2007). Alonso et al. (2004b) found that approximately one-third of persons who reported having a behavioral disorder did not seek treatment. In addition, 21% of individuals who had contacted a behavioral health professional had not started a specific treatment for their disorder. Codony et al. (2009) found that 50% of the respondents identified there was a perceived need for treatment. Across countries, the prevalence of perceived need was 5% in Italy, 7.9% in Germany, 9% in Spain, 12.1% in the Netherlands, 12.3% in Belgium, and 13.5% in France. For individuals in certain countries, the lack of insurance coverage for treatment of behavioral disorders restricted access (Alonso et al., 2004b) as does certain personal characteristics (such as age and gender; Codony et al., 2009). Behavioral disorders were also determined to be more important determinants of work role disability and quality of life than physical disorders, and behavioral disorders had generally stronger "cross-domain" effects (Alonso et al., 2004a).

UNDERDETECTED ILLNESSES

For people with severe mental illnesses, public mental health systems offer rehabilitative, recovery-focused care. However, persons with other insurance plans or adults with less severe mental health conditions who are uninsured may face significant gaps in coverage and in access to services. Further, since in the United States behavioral health is "carved out" from the larger public health care system, persons with mental illnesses must navigate two separate and distinct systems of care.

Underdetected or underdiagnosed illnesses in persons with behavioral disorders is a growing concern. Numerous conditions are underdiagnosed because they have vague or even negligible symptoms, such as type 2 diabetes, hypertension, hyperlipidemia, osteoporosis, chronic kidney disease, and hypothyroidism or other thyroid disorders. Other conditions that are underdiagnosed due to lack of awareness on the part of the physician include depression, attention deficit hyperactivity disorder and hyperactivity in adults, sleep disorders (McWhirter, Bae, & Budur, 2007) bipolar disorders (Kim et al., 2013), and asthma (Gibson, McDonald, & Marks, 2010; van Huisstede et al., 2013).

Adults who report nonspecific psychological distress, major depressive disorder, or posttraumatic stress symptoms (post-traumatic stress disorder and posttraumatic stress syndrome) have more problems with their physical health than persons who do not report such symptoms. In addition, primary care providers routinely miss the connection between somatic illnesses and symptoms of mental illnesses. This may be due to lack of time spent with patients, deficits in a physician's own knowledge and skills, or the limited availability of specific treatment guidelines and psychosocial treatment alternatives (Satter et al., 2012).

Not only are persons with behavioral disorders more likely to have poorer dietary habits, live more sedentary lifestyles, and smoke, but they are more prone to hypertension, hyperlipidemia, obesity, asthma, and diabetes, leading to more serious medical conditions. The more serious the medical condition, the more likely the patient will experience a mental illness. For persons with asthma, for example, when a patient's depressive symptoms and anxiety increase, there is a corresponding increase in the frequency and severity of the attacks. Depression is also a major factor in pain management and immune functioning. Underdetected diseases also extend to treatments. Some of the novel antipsychotic medications are associated with complications, such as obesity, high blood glucose levels, and diabetes. Mental and somatic disorders routinely coexist, and the presence of a mental disorder impairs patient functioning and his or her ability to sustain effective disease management.

National and State Policy for Pharmacy Practice and Behavioral Health

The Paul Wellstone and Pete Domenici Mental Health Parity and Addiction Equity Act of 2008 (MHPAEA) was enacted to prevent group health plans and health insurers that provide mental or substance use disorder benefits from establishing limitations to treatment that were less than those given for medical or surgical benefits (MHPAEA 2008). The goal of this act was to provide similar coverage for mental health or addictions treatment as was provided for medical conditions. This generally applied to large group health plans and disallowed the imposition of annual or lifetime dollar limits on mental health benefits and substance use disorder treatment.

This act was amended by the Patient Protection and Affordable Care Act and the Health Care and Education Reconciliation Act of 2010 (referred to collectively as the Affordable Care Act). The Insurance Exchange Provisions within the Affordable Care Act require that all individual and group plans through the exchanges comply with federal mental health parity regulations and provide essential benefits. As of January 2014, the essential benefits included prescription drugs, mental health and addictions treatment, and rehabilitation treatments. The cost-sharing by plan type varies in payment level from 60% to 90%. The expansion of Medicaid coverage by states is another requirement of the Affordable Care Act. States must provide Medicaid coverage to people who are living at up to 133% of the federal poverty level. One caveat of this expansion is that, while mental health and addictions treatment services will be provided, new Medicaid enrollees in states may have more limited benefits than those previously enrolled in Medicaid under prior benefits (Paradise, 2015).

States may employ three strategies to meet the requirements for Medicaid expansion under the Affordable Care Act. The first is through a State Medicaid Amendment Plan that ensures coverage for mental health and substance use disorders and meets the MHPAEA requirements for parity. Mandatory patient enrollment into Medicaid Managed Care Organizations (MCOs) may also be considered; this requires that mental health and substance use disorder coverage be provided based on the determination of the managed care organization. States may also require patients to enroll voluntarily into Alternative Benefit Plans (ABPs). ABPs have existed for several years as a mechanism for enhancing coverage for Medicaid beneficiaries; these are now required to provide mental health and substance use disorder treatment as a part of the plan benefit.

Generally, state Medicaid programs are divided into fee-for-service (most seriously ill and disabled) and MCOs (healthier patients). The fee-for-service programs are more costly for the state Medicaid program but provide the most comprehensive benefits for the disabled patient population. Many state Medicaid programs will scale back their fee-for-service plan structure in favor of the MCO plans, which require the managed care organization to provide care for patients for a set fee per patient. There is a concern that those patients with disabilities who are transitioned to an MCO plan will not receive the same level of payment for care that was previously provided by the fee-for-service structure. These vulnerable patients often do not have the money to pay for services that are not covered by the MCOs (Burns, 2015). The expansion of Medicaid services will continue in most states for the next few years. It remains to be seen how many individuals in need of healthcare insurance will be covered by Medicaid expansion and how this treatment will be delivered.

Evidence-Based Practice in Mental Health: The Schizophrenia Example

The translation of clinical trial information and evidence-based practice in chronic medical disorders, such as hyperlipidemia, diabetes, and hypertension, is generally achieved in a rapid manner. New treatment guidelines or supplements to existing guidelines are generally published within several months of new evidence becoming available for these disease states. This is not often the case in the treatment of mental disorders. Here we use the example of the use of antipsychotics in the treatment of schizophrenia. The evidence base for the use of antipsychotics in schizophrenia leans heavily toward monotherapy, with little to no evidence of efficacy for polypharmacy (use of two or more routine antipsychotic medications) in most patients.

In 2005, Faries, Ascher-Svanum, Zhu, Correll, and Kane evaluated data regarding the use of monotherapy and polypharmacy treatment with atypical antipsychotics.

Thirty-six percent of patients in the study received monotherapy, while 27% were taking two or more antipsychotics. More than 30% of patients were receiving a mix of monotherapy and polypharmacy over the course of the study (Faries et al., 2005). A 2012 study evaluating the use of antipsychotic monotherapy versus polypharmacy noted that the trend from 2005 continues and the use of polypharmacy may be increasing (Novick et al., 2012). It is instructional to consider the fact that treatment guidelines for the management of schizophrenia do exist from several sources and are consistent in noting that monotherapy with an antipsychotic is the treatment of choice and continues to be so through several steps of each of the treatment guidelines (Dixon, Perkins, & Calmes, 2009; International Psychopharmacology Algorithm Project, 2015; Lehman et al., 2004; National Institute for Clinical Excellence, 2014). Unfortunately, while the American Psychiatric Association provided an updated guideline in 2009 and the National Institute for Clinical Excellence offered a revised guideline in 2014, the use of antipsychotic polypharmacy remains constant and is, in many cases, increasing.

Evidence suggests that not only is antipsychotic polypharmacy ineffective overall in the treatment of schizophrenia, but patients who are receiving multiple drugs have a lower rate of adherence to treatment and a greater risk of significant adverse drug events and side effects related to their treatment (Barnes & Paton, 2011). Several justifications are cited for the use of antipsychotic combinations. Healthcare providers may desire to target a specific symptom complex not covered by the current antipsychotic or may be concerned that an increase in the dose of the monotherapy antipsychotic may lead to greater side effect risk and add another antipsychotic in order to continue at lower overall daily doses.

Another common reason for antipsychotic polypharmacy is a patient who is being transitioned from one antipsychotic to another using a cross-tapering approach and the patient's symptoms of schizophrenia improve while in the middle of the transition. In this case, the provider may not want to continue to cross-taper or discontinue either drug because the patient is doing well on both medications (Barnes & Paton, 2011). Clozapine is an antipsychotic that is considered to have the best evidence for efficacy over other antipsychotics. Some treatment guidelines suggest that a trial of clozapine as monotherapy should be implemented prior to initiating antipsychotic polypharmacy. Wheeler, Humberstone, & Robinson (2009) studied the impact of prolonged clozapine treatment on outcomes for schizophrenia patients and describe improved occupational activities and lower hospitalization rates while lowering the overall cost of treatment.

While several studies have come to the same conclusion in recent years, there has been a paucity of prescribing of clozapine by healthcare providers. Healthcare providers often perceive that clozapine is difficult for both the patient and provider to use due to significant side effects and required white blood cell monitoring, which offers an opportunity for the pharmacist to provide drug information and support to both patients and providers.

It is clear that a gap exists between guideline recommendations and clinical practice. Simply providing information to healthcare providers has been unsuccessful in transitioning the evidence base to clinical practice. Several ways to modify practice have been suggested, including the use of treatment algorithms, educational outreach visits to providers, electronic reminders, and standardized assessments. Hirano et al. (2013) evaluated the use of algorithm-based treatment versus treatment-as-usual in schizophrenia patients. Forty-two patients with severe symptoms of schizophrenia were enrolled and randomized to one of the two treatment conditions; algorithm-based treatment compared favorably with the treatment-as-usual. Updated algorithms for the treatment of schizophrenia are being published. The Harvard South Shore Program recently provided an update for their Psychopharmacology Algorithm Project for Schizophrenia that mirrors available treatment guidelines and may be a good source of information for health care providers (Osser, Roudsari, & Manschreck, 2013).

The PA process within Medicaid programs has been described previously. In one state, the Medicaid program has open access to behavioral health drugs and uses the clinical evidence base to implement PA criteria for psychiatric medications. In early 2014, the state implemented a PA for antipsychotic polypharmacy that requires that the healthcare provider consider the use of clozapine monotherapy prior to receiving a PA for antipsychotic polypharmacy for a Medicaid patient. The Medicaid program recognized that some patients will not be eligible for clozapine due to psychosocial issues such as problematic clinic attendance or for clinical reasons like needle phobia or chronic medical conditions that could be worsened by the use of clozapine. The PA does not require that the patient try clozapine if these conditions exist but also does not allow the provider to disregard the use of clozapine because the provider is uncomfortable with its use. This is an example of a payer program attempting to modulate prescribing practices by forcing the provider to consider evidence-based treatment guidelines.

Implications for Public Health and Pharmacy Practice

There continues to be an increasingly important move toward the integration of primary health and behavioral health services in America. This increasing services delivery collaboration will impact education not only for primary care health providers and behavioral health providers but also pharmacy education.

Skills needed for working on an integrated team are not generally part of the academic preparation for health and behavioral health care professionals. For pharmacy education, this may require a retooling of curriculum and internships to provide more in-depth knowledge and practice for pharmacy students as well as for the continuing education of practicing community pharmacists. It also may require added emphasis on community-centered approaches to clinical psychiatric pharmacy practice. These include increased awareness of current epidemiologic and disease surveillance information as well as an increased emphasis on health information technologies, such as electronic health record systems and use of additional behavioral health information systems.

Federal and state policies are not structured to promote collaborative practice. State regulations for collaborative practice, including the definition of collaborative practice, differ significantly across states. For example, in one Midwest state, a clinical psychiatric pharmacist provides medication management services, including drug initiation and discontinuation, dose changes, refill authorizations, laboratory monitoring, and assessment for an outpatient mental health practice that includes more than 50 patients with early psychosis. The clinical psychiatric pharmacist practices under a scope of practice that is approved by the institution and signed by the clinic psychiatrists, which allows patients to be scheduled for individual clinic appointments with the pharmacist for medication management.

Pharmacists should take advantage of opportunities to engage in behavioral health policy work groups. This allows them to keep abreast of critical behavioral health issues and to bring their concerns regarding quality of care, care coordination, and patient-centered outcomes to policymakers and legislators.

Education of primary care medical providers about the training and ability of pharmacists to manage and monitor complex drug therapy regimens is paramount in gaining strong advocates for the expanded role of pharmacists in patient care and community practice. These are important considerations as community pharmacists and psychiatric clinical pharmacists continue to become a more integral part of behavioral health services delivery.

References

Alonso, J., Angermeyer, M. C., Bernert, S., Bruffaerts, R., Brugha, T. S., Bryson, H., Vollebergh, W. A. (2004a). Disability and quality of life impact of mental disorders in Europe: Results from the European Study of the Epidemiology of Mental Disorders (ESEMeD) project. *Acta Psychiatrica Scandinavica Supplementum, 420*, 38–46. doi:10.1111/j.1600-0047.2004.00329.x

Alonso, J., Angermeyer, M. C., Bernert, S., Bruffaerts, R., Brugha, T. S., Bryson, H., . . . Vollebergh, W. A. (2004b). Use of mental health services in Europe: results from the European Study of the Epidemiology of Mental Disorders (ESEMeD) project. *Acta Psychiatrica Scandinavica Supplementum* (420), 47–54. doi:10.1111/j.1600-0047.2004.00330.x

Alonso, J., Angermeyer, M. C., Bernert, S., Bruffaerts, R., Brugha, T. S., Bryson, H., . . . Vollebergh, W. A. (2004b). Use of mental health services in Europe: Results from the European Study of the Epidemiology of Mental Disorders (ESEMeD) project. *Acta Psychiatrica Scandinavica Supplementum, 420*, 47–54. doi:10.1111/j.1600-0047.2004.00330.x

Alonso, J., Codony, M., Kovess, V., Angermeyer, M. C., Katz, S. J., Haro, J. M., . . . Brugha, T. S. (2007). Population level of unmet need for mental healthcare in Europe. *The British Journal of Psychiatry, 190*, 299–306. doi:10.1192/bjp.bp.106.022004

American Psychiatric Association. (1994). *Diagnostic and statistical manual of mental disorders* (4th ed.). Washington, DC: Author.

American Psychiatric Association. (2013). *Diagnostic and statistical manual of mental disorders* (5th ed.). Washington, DC: Author.

Barnes, T. R., & Paton, C. (2011). Antipsychotic polypharmacy in schizophrenia: benefits and risks. *CNS Drugs, 25*(5), 383–399. doi:10.2165/11587810-000000000-00000

Burns, M. E. (2015). State discretion over Medicaid coverage for mental health and addiction serv ices. *Psychiatric Services, 66*(3), 221–223. doi:10.1176/appi.ps.201400440

Centers for Medicare & Medicaid Services. (2015). Medicare program; changes to the require-ments for Part D prescribers. Interim final rule with comment period. *Federal Register, 80*(87), 25958–25966.

Chong, W. W., Aslani, P., & Chen, T. F. (2011). Effectiveness of interventions to improve antide-pressant medication adherence: A systematic review. *International Journal of Clinical Practice, 65*(9), 954–975. doi:10.1111/j.1742-1241.2011.02746.x

Codony, M., Alonso, J., Almansa, J., Bernert, S., de Girolamo, G., de Graaf, R., . . . Kessler, R. C. (2009). Perceived need for mental health care and service use among adults in Western Europe: Results of the ESEMeD project. *Psychiatric Services, 60*(8), 1051–1058. doi:10.1176/appi.ps.60.8.1051

Collins, P. Y., Patel, V., Joestl, S. S., March, D., Insel, T. R., Daar, A. S., . . . Executive Committee of the Grand Challenges on Global Mental Health. (2011). Grand challenges in global mental health. *Nature, 475*(7354), 27–30. doi:10.1038/475027a

Covell, N. H., Finnerty, M. T., & Essock, S. M. (2008). Implications of CATIE for mental health services researchers. *Psychiatric Services, 59*(5), 526–529. doi:10.1176/appi.ps.59.5.526 10.1176/ps.2008.59.5.526

Das, A. K., Malik, A., & Haddad, P. M. (2014). A qualitative study of the attitudes of patients in an early intervention service towards antipsychotic long-acting injections. *Therapeutic Advances in Psychopharmacology, 4*(5), 179–185. doi:10.1177/2045125314542098

Dixon, L., Perkins, D., & Calmes, C. (2009). *Guideline watch (September 2009): Practice guideline for the treatment of patients with schizophrenia*. Retrieved from http://psychiatryonline.org/pb/assets/raw/sitewide/practice_guidelines/guidelines/schizophrenia-watch.pdf

Faries, D., Ascher-Svanum, H., Zhu, B., Correll, C., & Kane, J. (2005). Antipsychotic monotherapy and polypharmacy in the naturalistic treatment of schizophrenia with atypical antipsychotics. *BMC Psychiatry, 5*, 26. doi:10.1186/1471-244x-5-26

Gibson, P. G., McDonald, V. M., & Marks, G. B. (2010). Asthma in older adults. *The Lancet, 376*(9743), 803–813. doi:10.1016/s0140-6736(10)61087-2

Goldman, D. P., Dirani, R., Fastenau, J., & Conrad, R. M. (2014). Do strict formularies replicate failure for patients with schizophrenia? *American Journal of Managed Care, 20*(3), 219–228.

Goldman, D. P., Fastenau, J., Dirani, R., Helland, E., Joyce, G., Conrad, R., & Lakdawalla, D. (2014). Medicaid prior authorization policies and imprisonment among patients with schizophrenia. *American Journal of Managed Care, 20*(7), 577–586.

Goldstein, J. (2015). Strategies for successful ICD-10 implementation. *Health Management Technology, 36*(9), 12–13.

Grenard, J. L., Munjas, B. A., Adams, J. L., Suttorp, M., Maglione, M., McGlynn, E. A., & Gellad, W. F. (2011). Depression and medication adherence in the treatment of chronic diseases in the United States: A meta-analysis. *Journal of General Internal Medicine, 26*(10), 1175–1182. doi:10.1007/s11606-011-1704-y

Haddad, P. M., Brain, C., & Scott, J. (2014). Nonadherence with antipsychotic medication in schizophrenia: Challenges and management strategies. *Patient Related Outcome Measures, 5*, 43–62. doi:10.2147/prom.s42735

Hanson, A., Levin, B. L., Ott, C. A., & Meldrum, H. (2012). Mental health services. In R. L. McCarthy, K. W. Schafermeyer, & K. S. Plack (Eds.), *Introduction to health care delivery: A primer for pharmacists* (5th ed., pp. 273–294). Sudbury, MA: Jones & Bartlett.

Hirano, J., Watanabe, K., Suzuki, T., Uchida, H., Den, R., Kishimoto, T., . . . Kato, M. (2013). An open-label study of algorithm-based treatment versus treatment-as-usual for patients with schizophrenia. *Neuropsychiatric Disease and Treatment, 9*, 1553–1564. doi:10.2147/ndt. s46108

International Psychopharmacology Algorithm Project. (2015). The IPAP schizophrenia algorithm. Retrieved from http://www.ipap.org/algorithms.php

Kim, K. R., Cho, H. S., Kim, S. J., Seok, J. H., Lee, E., & Jon, D. I. (2013). Reevaluation of patients with bipolar disorder on manic episode: Improving the diagnosing of mixed episode. *Journal of Nervous and Mental Disease, 201*(8), 686–690. doi:10.1097/NMD.0b013e31829c505a

Lehman, A. F., Lieberman, J. A., Dixon, L. B., McGlashan, T. H., Miller, A. L., Perkins, D. O., & Kreyenbuhl, J. (2004). Practice guideline for the treatment of patients with schizophrenia, second edition. *American Journal of Psychiatry, 161*(2 Suppl.), 1–56. Retrieved from www.psychiatryonline.org/guidelines.

Lu, C. Y., Adams, A. S., Ross-Degnan, D., Zhang, F., Zhang, Y., Salzman, C., & Soumerai, S. B. (2011). Association between prior authorization for medications and health service use by Medicaid patients with bipolar disorder. *Psychiatric Services, 62*(2), 186–193. doi:10.1176/appi.ps.62.2.18610.1176/ps.62.2.pss6202_0186

Lu, C. Y., Soumerai, S. B., Ross-Degnan, D., Zhang, F., & Adams, A. S. (2010). Unintended impacts of a Medicaid prior authorization policy on access to medications for bipolar illness. *Medical Care, 48*(1), 4–9. doi:10.1097/MLR.0b013e3181bd4c10

Markowitz, M., Karve, S., Panish, J., Candrilli, S. D., & Alphs, L. (2013). Antipsychotic adherence patterns and health care utilization and costs among patients discharged after a schizophrenia-related hospitalization. *BMC Psychiatry, 13*, 246. doi:10.1186/1471-244x-13-246

McWhirter, D., Bae, C., & Budur, K. (2007). The assessment, diagnosis, and treatment of excessive sleepiness: Practical considerations for the psychiatrist. *Psychiatry, 4*(9), 26–35.

Mojtabai, R., Olfson, M., Sampson, N. A., Jin, R., Druss, B., Wang, P. S., . . . Kessler, R. C. (2011). Barriers to mental health treatment: Results from the National Comorbidity Survey Replication (NCS-R). *Psychological Medicine, 41*(8), 1751–1761. doi:10.1017/S0033291710002291

Moore, T. A., Buchanan, R. W., Buckley, P. F., Chiles, J. A., Conley, R. R., Crismon, M. L., . . . Miller, A. L. (2007). The Texas Medication Algorithm Project antipsychotic algorithm for schizophrenia: 2006 update. *Journal of Clinical Psychiatry, 68*(11), 1751–1762.

Murray, C. J., & López, A. D. (1996). *The global burden of disease: A comprehensive assessment of mortality and disability from diseases, injuries, and risk factors in 1990 and projected to 2020.* Cambridge, MA: Harvard School of Public Health.

National Institute for Clinical Excellence. (2014). *Psychosis and schizophrenia in adults: Treatment and management.* Retrieved from http://www.nice.org.uk/guidance/cg178

National Institute of Mental Health. (2008). *National Institute of Mental Health Strategic Plan.* Rockville, MD: Author.

Novick, D., Ascher-Svanum, H., Brugnoli, R., Bertsch, J., Hong, J., & Haro, J. M. (2012). Antipsychotic monotherapy and polypharmacy in the treatment of outpatients with schizophrenia in the European Schizophrenia Outpatient Health Outcomes Study. *The Journal of Nervous and Mental Disease, 200*(7), 637–643. doi:10.1097/NMD.0b013e31825bfd95

Offord, S., Lin, J., Wong, B., Mirski, D., & Baker, R. A. (2013). Impact of oral antipsychotic medication adherence on healthcare resource utilization among schizophrenia patients with Medicare coverage. *Community Mental Health Journal, 49*(6), 625–629. doi:10.1007/s10597-013-9638-y

Osser, D. N., Roudsari, M. J., & Manschreck, T. (2013). The psychopharmacology algorithm project at the Harvard South Shore Program: An update on schizophrenia. *Harvard Review of Psychiatry, 21*(1), 18–40. doi:10.1097/HRP.0b013e31827fd915

Paradise, J. (2015, March). Medicaid moving forward. *Issue Brief: The Kaiser Commission on Medicaid and the Uninsured,* 1–12.

Parks, J. J. (2006). A successful partnership to improve prescribing practices. *Psychiatric Services, 57*(10), 1528–1529.

Parks, J., Svendsen, D., Singer, P., & Foti, M. E. (2006). *Morbidity and mortality in people with serious mental illness.* Alexandria, VA: NASMHPD Medical Directors Council.

Paul Wellstone and Pete Domenici Mental Health Parity and Addiction Equity Act of 2008, Pub. L. 110–343, 42 USC 201 §511 et seq. (2008).

Pickett, D., Berglund, D., Blum, A., & Wing, L. (1999). A quick review of ICD-10-CM. *Journal of AHIMA: American Health Information Management Association, 70*(9), 99–100.

Sareen, J., Jagdeo, A., Cox, B. J., Clara, I., ten Have, M., Belik, S. L., . . . Stein, M. B. (2007). Perceived barriers to mental health service utilization in the United States, Ontario, and the Netherlands. *Psychiatric Services, 58*(3), 357–364. doi:10.1176/appi.ps.58.3.357

Satter, R. M., Cohen, T., Ortiz, P., Kahol, K., Mackenzie, J., Olson, C., . . . Patel, V. L. (2012). Avatar-based simulation in the evaluation of diagnosis and management of mental health disorders in primary care. *Journal of Biomedical Informatics, 45*(6), 1137–1150. doi:http://dx.doi.org/10.1016/j.jbi.2012.07.009

Seabury, S. A., Goldman, D. P., Kalsekar, I., Sheehan, J. J., Laubmeier, K., & Lakdawalla, D. N. (2014). Formulary restrictions on atypical antipsychotics: impact on costs for patients with schizophrenia and bipolar disorder in Medicaid. *American Journal of Managed Care, 20*(2), e52–e60.

Shuler, K. M. (2014). Approaches to improve adherence to pharmacotherapy in patients with schizophrenia. *Patient Preference and Adherence, 8*, 701–714. doi:10.2147/ppa.s59371

Substance Abuse and Mental Health Services Administration. (2011). *Leading change: A plan for SAMHSA's roles and actions 2011–2014.* Rockville, MD: Author.

Substance Abuse and Mental Health Services Administration. (2013). *National expenditures for mental health services and substance abuse treatment, 1986–2009.* Retrieved from https://store.samhsa.gov/shin/content/SMA13-4740/SMA13-4740.pdf

U.S. Burden of Disease Collaborators. (2013). The state of US health, 1990–2010: burden of diseases, injuries, and risk factors. *JAMA, 310*(6), 591–608. doi:10.1001/jama.2013.13805

U.S. Department of Health and Human Services. (1997). Estimation methodology for children with a serious emotional disturbance (SED). *Federal Register, 62*(193), 52139–52145.

U.S. Department of Health and Human Services. (1999). Estimation methodology for adults with serious mental illness (SMI). *Federal Register, 64*(121), 33890–33897.

van Huisstede, A., Castro Cabezas, M., van de Geijn, G. J., Mannaerts, G. H., Njo, T. L., Taube, C., . . . Braunstahl, G. J. (2013). Underdiagnosis and overdiagnosis of asthma in the morbidly obese. *Respiratory Medicine, 107*(9), 1356–1364. doi:10.1016/j.rmed.2013.05.007

Wheeler, A., Humberstone, V., & Robinson, G. (2009). Outcomes for schizophrenia patients with clozapine treatment: How good does it get? *Journal of Psychopharmacology, 23*(8), 957–965. doi:10.1177/0269881108093588

Whiteford, H. A., Degenhardt, L., Rehm, J., Baxter, A. J., Ferrari, A. J., Erskine, H. E., . . . Vos, T. (2013). Global burden of disease attributable to mental and substance use disorders: Findings from the Global Burden of Disease Study 2010. *The Lancet, 382*(9904), 1575–1586. doi:10.1016/S0140-6736(13)61611-6

World Health Organization. (1992). *The ICD-10 classification of mental and behavioural disorders: Clinical descriptions and diagnostic guidelines* Geneva: Author.

World Health Organization. (1993). *The ICD-10 classification of mental and behavioural disorders diagnostic criteria for research.* Geneva: Author.

World Health Organization. (2003). *Investing in mental health.* Geneva: Author.

9

Public Health Nutrition

LAURI WRIGHT AND MELODY CHAVEZ

Introduction

Nutrition is a vital component to life. It plays a dynamic role in all aspects of health including growth and development, health promotion, disease prevention, and acute and chronic disease management (Gilman, Chokshi, Bowen, Rugen & Cox, 2014). Obtaining and providing nutrition to our bodies allows essential nutrients such as carbohydrates, proteins, and lipids (fats) as well as minerals, vitamins, and water to promote overall health. Medical nutrition therapy, a therapeutic approach to treating medial conditions and their associated symptoms through a tailored diet, can help assist in the management of these chronic diseases. Nutrition is important to the practice of all health care professionals, especially community pharmacists.

Pharmacists are in a unique position to educate the public on nutrition in many areas of health care. They can make significant contributions in assuring adequate nutrition by advising patients about basic food needs, correcting improper food habits in children, advising special nutrition requirements, and suggesting special diet instructions for patients with diabetes and other illnesses throughout the life cycle. While many may associate a pharmacist's work in nutrition in the clinical setting, the Council for Pharmacy Education competencies indicate that students in a doctor of pharmacy program should "understand relevant diet, nutrition, and non-drug therapies" (Machen, Hammer & Odegard, 2007, p. 1). With the growing number of diet-related chronic diseases, there are many opportunities for pharmacists to educate patients about how behavior, nutrition, and physical activity can improve health in addition to medication. Therefore, the focus must be on recognizing the life cycle and how nutrition plays a role in the stages of life.

Planning a Healthy Diet

Good health starts with a balanced diet, which includes all six classes of nutrients and calories. Eating a balanced diet is oftentimes overlooked and should be the first thing considered for people of all ages. Pharmacists can be advocates for the community to assist in improving their nutrition, as millions of individuals have one or more preventable chronic diseases. About two-thirds of the US adults who are overweight can benefit from improvements in their dietary patterns. The U.S. Department of Agriculture (USDA) and Department of Health and Human Services (DHHS) have developed simple systems to help with the selection of healthy diets.

DIETARY GUIDELINES

The *Dietary Guidelines for Americans* are science-based advice to promote health and reduce the risk of chronic disease through diet and physical activity U.S. Dietary Guidelines Advisory Committee, 2015). A joint effort between the USDA and DHHS, the guidelines can assist community pharmacists in guiding the general public over two years of age to eat balanced daily meals. The guidelines include five basic activities:

1. Follow a healthy eating pattern across the lifespan;
2. Focus on variety, nutrient density, and amount;
3. Limit calories from added sugars and saturated fats and reduce sodium intake;
4. Shift to healthier food and beverages choices; and
5. Support healthy eating patterns for all.

In addition to the general guidelines, the document also addresses healthy eating patterns for US style, Mediterranean, and vegetarian diets and defines the core concepts of healthy eating and physical activity patterns.

MYPLATE

Another resource is *MyPlate*, the current nutrition guidelines published by the USDA. *MyPlate* is applicable to Americans over the age of two (Figure 9-1). The new *MyPlate* replaced the Food Guide Pyramid in 2011 and is designed to show Americans that nutrition does not have to be complicated. *MyPlate* is based on a 9-inch plate separated with divisions to encourage portion control. The colors

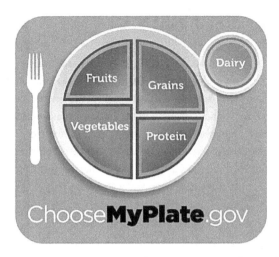

Figure 9-1. MyPlate guide for healthy eating (U.S. Department of Agriculture, 2016).

represent the types of foods that should be consumed. Pharmacists can utilize this tool to help the general public by personalizing their diet through access the *MyPlate* website (http://www.choosemyplate.gov). Encouraging individuals to follow the *MyPlate* method should assist in helping to main a healthy body weight and decrease the risk of nutrition-related chronic disease.

FOOD LABELS

Food labels are another tool that can assist a pharmacist with the general public in assessing the nutrient content of foods (Figure 9-2). Daily values on the label give the consumer the percentages per serving of each nutritional item listed based on a daily diet of 2,000 calories. Additional information on food labels can be found on the website (http://www.fda.gov/Food/default.htm). Figure 9-2 offers a quick review of the guidelines to assist the pharmacist in educating the public on how those nutrients affect an individual's health. The newly revised Food and Drug Administration label requirements address number of servings, caloric intake per serving, updated (%) daily values, changes in required nutrients, and a footnote explaining daily values.

Nutrition in the Lifecycle

NUTRITION DURING PREGNANCY AND LACTATION

Community pharmacists play a role in advising mothers-to-be about the nutritional requirements essential at each stage of pregnancy for both the short-term

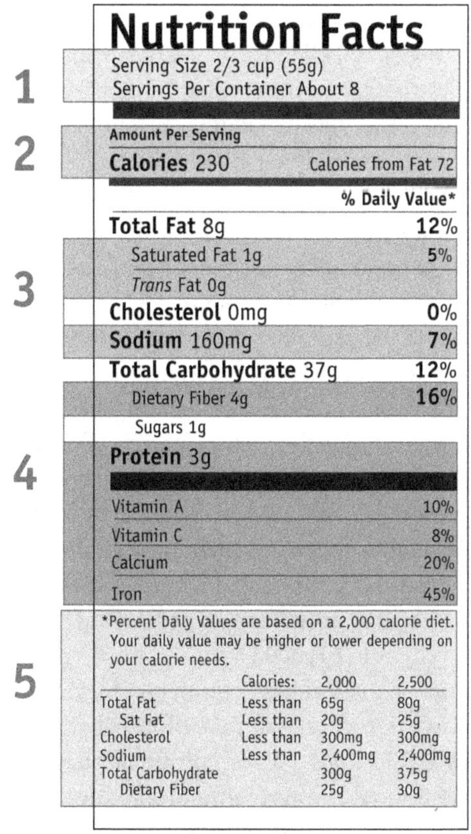

Nutrition Facts

1
Serving Size 2/3 cup (55g)
Servings Per Container About 8

2
Amount Per Serving
Calories 230   Calories from Fat 72

% Daily Value*

3
Total Fat 8g	**12%**
Saturated Fat 1g	5%
Trans Fat 0g	
Cholesterol 0mg	**0%**
Sodium 160mg	**7%**
Total Carbohydrate 37g	**12%**
Dietary Fiber 4g	**16%**
Sugars 1g	

4
Protein 3g

Vitamin A	10%
Vitamin C	8%
Calcium	20%
Iron	45%

5
*Percent Daily Values are based on a 2,000 calorie diet. Your daily value may be higher or lower depending on your calorie needs.

	Calories:	2,000	2,500
Total Fat	Less than	65g	80g
Sat Fat	Less than	20g	25g
Cholesterol	Less than	300mg	300mg
Sodium	Less than	2,400mg	2,400mg
Total Carbohydrate		300g	375g
Dietary Fiber		25g	30g

Figure 9-2. Nutrition fact label (U.S. Food and Drug Administration, 2016).

and long-term health of the baby. Many women may not be aware of the different nutritional requirements as well as planning food for these stages. Pharmacists can assist and focus on nutritional problems that may arise in pregnant women and suggest simple dietary changes for a safe pregnancy and good health of the child.

A woman's calorie and nutrient need increases significantly to support the growth of the developing fetus. The average weight gain during pregnancy is 25 to 35 pounds (Roth, 2014). Protein requirements increase to 60 grams of protein per day and are important for tissue building. The key nutrients foliate, iron, calcium, copper, zinc, and vitamin D are especially important considerations during pregnancy as well as for the long-term health of the baby. Teenage pregnancy is of concern, as these young women will need to know their own nutritional needs and the additional requirements for pregnancy. Pharmacists can assist in providing counseling on improvements in nutritional intake during pregnancy through such tools as *MyPlate*.

Community pharmacists can play a key role in breastfeeding promotion and support (Ronai, Taylor, Dugan, & Feller, E. 2009). Breast milk provides various hormones after delivery of the infant. It provides the right amount of lactose, water, essential fatty acids, and amino acids for brain development, growth, and digestion. It takes two to three weeks to fully establish a feeding routine, so no additional supplemental feedings should be given at this time (Roth, 2014). Breast milk is formulated to meet the infant's nutritional needs for the first six months of life. Some mothers may not want to or cannot breastfeed their infants. They may seek out their community pharmacist for a milk substitute (e.g. infant formula) and bottles and nipples, which are sold in the pharmacy. Pharmacists should be knowledgeable in the nutritional content of the breast milk substitutes and baby food.

The mother's calorie requirements increase during lactation and depend on the amount of milk produced. During the first six months of breastfeeding, an increase of 500 calories a day is required and then 400 calories a day for seven to nine months (Roth, 2014). If the mother's diet contains insufficient calories, the quantity of milk is reduced. This is often seen in women living in developing countries. It is important to educate women that they should not try to lose weight while breastfeeding. This is often seen in women living in developing countries (World Health Organization [WHO] & UNICEF, 2003).

Most chemicals a woman consumes enter the mother's milk, so it is important for women who breastfeed to check with their local pharmacist and/or physician regarding any current medications and/or nutritional supplements they might be taking. Alcohol in excess should be avoided, and if she does drink a mother should not breastfeed until the alcohol has completely cleared her system, which is generally two to three hours. Caffeine should be limited to the equivalent of two to three cups of coffee per day, as this may affect the baby's energy and sleep. Prescriptions such as methadone and oxycodone can make the baby drowsy and irritable. In a survey among pharmacists in Rhode Island, almost 50% reported receiving inquiries about breastfeeding and medication safety on a weekly or daily basis. Of those, 85% of responding pharmacists felt uncomfortable advising breastfeeding mothers on these concerns.

NUTRITION DURING INFANCY

The early stages of life are a period of rapid growth and development. During the first four to six months of a baby's life, his or her weight doubles; it triples by the end of the first year. The period of time from the first day of pregnancy until two years of age is called the "first 1,000 days." This period is recognized as a critical window of opportunity to shape long-term health. Nutrition plays a crucial role in this unique period. Nutritional needs are two to three times more than the adult requirements. Low birth rate infants and/or infants who have suffered from malnutrition may require more calories.

Infants' diets typically consist of breast milk or formula. Either type of feeding will provide the appropriate amount of nutrition; however, breastfeeding does provide additional benefits. Breast milk provides temporary immunity to many infectious diseases. It also provides bonding between the mother and child. Bottle-feeding can provide adequate nutrition as well. Pharmacists can provide information to mothers on commercial formulas and feeding instructions. They can also provide alternatives if the infant is extremely sensitive or allergic to infant formulas. Introduction of solid foods should occur after six months of age. Solid foods should be gradually introduced and, by the age of one year, most babies should be eating foods from all of the *MyPlate* groups.

NUTRITION FOR CHILDREN AND ADOLESCENTS

Children's nutritional needs vary as they grow and develop. Specific nutritional requirements affect physical, mental, and emotional growth and development (Roth, 2014). Studies have shown that children who fail to meet their nutritional needs can be affected intellectually as well as physically. Eating behaviors develop at this time, and it is important for parents to provide a positive feeding environment. However, many comorbid conditions begin during childhood and adolescence due to poor nutrition. These include cardiometabolic, pulmonary, and psychosocial complications for children that persist into adulthood, leading to poorer social and health outcomes as adults (Sahoo et al., 2015). Prevention and early intervention strategies are also critical to reversing the obesity epidemic (Gurnani, Birken, & Hamilton, 2015).

It is important for parents and/or caregivers to be patient and continue to encourage new foods. Children should be fed age-appropriate food that meets their nutritional needs. This is important as nutrient needs increase according to body size growth. Therefore, it is important that young children are given nutritious foods they will eat.

Adolescence is an important period of nutritional vulnerability due to increased dietary requirements for successful growth and development. Each stage of adolescence, from early adolescence (10–14 years of age), during late adolescence (15–19 years of age), to young adulthood (20–24 years of age) results in major nutritional changes for both females and males (Das et al., 2017). Requirements for energy-containing nutrients, vitamins, and minerals dramatically increase. During adolescence (ages 13 to 20), rapid growth occurs and can cause major changes for both females and males. Male requirements tend to be higher than females due to being bigger, more active, and increased muscle mass. Menstruation increases girls' need for iron as well as calcium for protein bone health.

Just as children imitate their parents' eating habits, adolescents imitate their peers' eating habits and consume large portions of low nutrient dense foods such as potato chips, sodas, and candy. Adolescent eating habits can be affected by busy schedules, part-time jobs, athletics, and social activities. Other social and environ-mental factors also affect eating patterns, such as food availability and preferences, cost, convenience, personal and cultural beliefs, the mass media, body image, and parental eating behaviors (Das et al., 2017). In the Identification and prevention of Dietary- and lifestyle-induced health EFfects In Children and infantS (IDEFICS) study, Iguacel and associates (2016) determined that socioeconomic inequalities, including social and accumulated vulnerability in childhood, may also determine long-term dietary patterns. The stressors during adolescence also increase the pos-sibility of at-risk behaviors, including being overweight or obese, prediabetes, eating disorders, alcohol abuse, and drug abuse. It is important to seek health care profes-sionals, such as pharmacists, if any of these is suspected.

NUTRITION DURING YOUNG, MIDDLE, AND LATE ADULTHOOD

Young adulthood, which overlaps the last stage of adolescence, is generally from 18 through 40 years of age. Growth is usually complete by the age of 25 years except if the individual is pregnant or lactating. Nutrient needs during this time change very little. Middle adulthood begins from age 40 through 60 years of age. The nutrition requirements begin to decrease as individuals reach middle age, as they are less active and may not be getting sufficient exercise. Weight control may become an issue if individuals are consuming more calories than needed. Chronic illnesses may begin during this time frame such as diabetes, metabolic syndrome, and hypertension.

Late adulthood begins at the age of 65 years. The fastest-growing population in the United States is people age 85 and older, also known as the frail elderly. Nutrient needs are affected by many physiological factors as the body function slows down. Poor nutrient intake and dentition problems can exacerbate a number of diseases, including cataracts, and osteoarthritis. Psychosocial changes such as no longer being fully independent or no longer feeling useful can also affect the individual's appetite. A decrease in income can also affect the quality of the individual's food intake, as he or she may not be able to afford healthy foods. According to the Centers for Disease Control and Prevention (CDC), older adults in the United States have one or more chronic diseases and at least 50% have two (CDC, 2016). The WHO (2016) sug-gests that 60% of all deaths are caused by chronic diseases, such as heart disease, stroke, cancer, chronic respiratory diseases, and diabetes. Further, of the 35 million individuals who died in 2005 from chronic disease worldwide, 50% were under the age of 70 and half of the deaths were women (WHO, 2016). Hence, proper nutri-tion continues to play a role in preventing, management, and stabilization of these disease states.

Because of these physiological, economic, and psychosocial changes, malnutri-tion is common among the elderly. Malnutrition rates vary by setting and are higher among those who are economically disadvantaged, socially isolated, or disabled. Kaiser and colleagues (2010) assessed the prevalence of malnutrition in older adults in various settings using the Mini Nutritional Assessment tool. In their dataset of 4,507 people from 12 different countries, the overall prevalence of malnutrition was 22.8%, with the prevalence in community-dwelling seniors being 5.8%. The overall prevalence of being "at risk for malnutrition" was 46.2%, with community dwelling seniors being most at risk for malnutrition at 31.9% prevalence (Kaiser et al., 2010).

Malnutrition is also associated with mortality and morbidity. The CDC estimates the rate of malnutrition mortality in the United States for all ages is 0.8 per 100,000 people. However, for the elderly, the mortality rate is much higher, 1.4 for 65- to 74-year-olds, 5.2 for 75- to 84-year-olds, and 20.9 for those 85 years of age and older (Lee & Berthelot, 2010). In fact, the CDC estimates that approximately 3,000 older adults die each year as a result of malnutrition (Xu, Murphy, Kochanek, & Bastian, 2016). Malnutrition among seniors also increases the risk for injury, illness, and premature institutionalization, all of which increase financial burdens (Gurvey et al., 2013; Wright, Vance, Sudduth, & Epps, 2015).

Pharmacists play a key role in delivering dietary advice throughout the stages of life. They are oftentimes the closest health professionals available in the community. Community pharmacists need to have a general knowledge about diet and disease states, as well as tools to provide the community with ways to improve their dietary habits. Nutrient needs during these phases of adulthood can be reviewed in the Dietary Guidelines for Americans (http://www.cnpp.usda.gov).

Medical Nutrition Therapy in Chronic Disease

The leading causes of death in the United States in descending order are heart disease, cancer, chronic lung disease, accidents, cerebrovascular diseases, Alzheimer's, diabetes, pneumonia, nephritis, and suicide. Heart disease has been consistently the leading cause of death for decades, with cancer the second leading cause of death. Diet has a great influence on mortality from these diseases. This section explores how pharmacists can assist in dietary interventions that can assist in the management of these disease states.

CARDIOVASCULAR DISEASE

The major causes of death around the world today are diseases of the heart and blood vessels; collectively known as cardiovascular disease. Atherosclerosis, hardening of the arteries, is considered to be the major cause of heart attacks and begins in childhood. Hyperlipidemia, hypertension, and smoking are major risk factors for the development of atherosclerosis. Dietary cholesterol and triglycerides also contribute to hyperlipidemia. Cerebrovascular accidents can also cause death due to blood flow blockage. Other risk factors have been identified and are known as the metabolic syndrome, which include

- Abdominal obesity;
- High blood lipids such a s high triglycerides, low HDL, and high LDL;
- High blood pressure;
- Insulin resistance; and
- Elevated highly sensitive C-reactive protein in the blood.

Medical nutrition therapy is the primary treatment for hyperlipidemia. The reduction of dietary fat typically corresponds to reduction in the amount of cholesterol and saturated fat ingested and a loss of weight. The American Heart Association developed guidelines with the American College of Cardiology, in which they recommend adults follow a diet that monitors fats and encourages an increase in fiber (Eckel et al., 2014). Community pharmacists can refer their patients to the American Heart Association website to learn more about heart healthy living (http://www.heart.org/HEARTORG/).

HYPERTENSION

Hypertension affects about one out of three adults in the United States. It contributes to heart attack, stroke, heart failure, and kidney failure and is often revered to as the "silent disease." In 90% of hypertension cases, the cause is unknown and is referred to as primary hypertension. The other 10% are caused by other conditions. Major risk factors for hypertension include aging, genetics, obesity, sodium sensitivity, and alcohol.

Lifestyle modifications and medications are both used to treat hypertension. Weight control is the primary dietary intervention if the individual is overweight. Regular physical aerobic activity can also reduce blood pressure directly. The Dietary Approaches to Stop Hypertension (DASH) diet is a lifelong approach to healthy eating that is designed to help treat or prevent high blood pressure (National Heart, Lung, and Blood Institute [NHLBI], 2003). The DASH diet encourages patients to reduce sodium intake and eat a variety of foods rich in nutrients, such as potassium, calcium, and magnesium, that help lower blood pressure. Emphasis is placed on fruits and vegetables for their potassium content, whole grains for their magnesium content, and low-fat calcium sources. Recommendations also include that individuals consume less red meat, sodium, sweets, and alcohol (NHLBI, 2003).

CANCER

Cancer is the second leading cause of death in the United States. The growth of malignant tissues that result from abnormal and uncontrolled cell division can develop slowly and continue for several decades. The etiology of cancer is not known; however, hereditary, viruses, environmental carcinogens, and possibly emotional stress contributes to its development. Food and cancer have not been proven to have an association; however, certain substances in food have been identified as carcinogenic. Nitrates from cured and smoked foods as well as high-fat foods have been associated with cancers. Individuals who drink alcohol and smoke are at greater risk of cancers. Finally, lifestyle factors such as lack of physical activity, obesity, and poor nutrition also serve as risk factors for certain cancers.

Nutritional care of the cancer patient is important. Energy demands are high because of the hypermetabolic states often caused by cancer. High-protein, high-calorie diets are typically recommended. Anorexia is a major problem and difficult to manage, as many patients with cancer tend to develop strong aversions to food. Chemotherapy can also lead to malnutrition due to nausea and the interruption of the absorption of nutrients. An individual's food habits may also change throughout the illness. Medications may be warranted to assist in nausea and pain. Enteral or parenteral nutrition may also become necessary if cachexia is extreme.

DIABETES

The prevalence of diabetes among children and adults has risen dramatically in the past decade. Diabetes is one of four priority noncommunicable diseases targeted by world leaders (WHO, 2016). In 2012, 29.1 million (9.3%) Americans had diabetes and another 86 million were prediabetes, with an estimated 1.4 million new cases each year (American Diabetes Association, 2016). In 2008–2009, there was an estimated 23,525 Americans under the age of 20 who were diagnosed with diabetes (CDC, 2014). In 2012, that figure rose to 208,000 (CDC, 2014). Blindness; heart and kidney disease; amputations of toes, feet, and legs; infections; and death are all conditions that can be attributed to diabetes. Diabetes remains the seventh leading cause of death in the United States (CDC, 2014).

Globally, an estimated 422 million adults were diagnosed with and/or living with diabetes in 2014 (WHO, 2016). Low- and middle income countries have seen a dramatic increase in the prevalence of diabetes, reflecting an increase in associated risk factors, such as being overweight or obese. In 2012, diabetes caused 1.5 million deaths and contributed to an additional 2.2 million deaths, due to increased risks for cardiovascular and other diseases (WHO, 2016). The economic impact of diabetes is estimated to be more than $827 billion, with families and individuals at risk for incurring catastrophic medical expenditures (WHO, 2016).

The etiology of diabetes is not known; however, genetics and environmental factors play a role in its occurrence. Types of diabetes include prediabetes, type 1, type 2, and gestational. Type 1 diabetes, also known as juvenile diabetes, develops when the body's immune system destroys the pancreatic beta cells. Individuals with type 1 diabetes must use exogenous insulin to survive. Type 2 diabetes is associated with obesity along with other factors such as aging, impaired glucose tolerance, lack of physical inactivity, race, and ethnicity. People with type 2 diabetes benefit most from a diet and physical activity program that controls glucose fluctuations and promotes weight loss. Gestational diabetes can occur in pregnancy between weeks 16 and 28. Typically it disappears after the infant is born; however, 35% to 60% of the women have a greater chance of diabetes in the next 10 to 20 years.

Diet is an important component of diabetes management. Controlling blood glucose levels provides optimal nourishment for the individual, prevents symptoms, and delays complications of the disease. Consuming carbohydrates consistently throughout the day can help maintain blood sugar. To maintain control of blood glucose levels, the diet should be designed to deliver consistent amounts of carbohydrates throughout the day. Because people with diabetes are considered at high risk for cardiovascular disease, their guidelines for dietary fat are similar. Increase in fiber appears to reduce the amount of insulin needed because it lowers blood glucose. Exercise has also helped the body use glucose; however, extra caution is needed as hypoglycemia can occur if insufficient calories and insulin are prescribed.

Food Insecurity and Hunger

Access to food has been an increasing issue for American families. Food insecurity is the inability to consistently access nutritious and adequate amounts of food necessary for a healthy life (Coleman-Jensen, Gregory, & Singh, 2014). The USDA estimates that 49 million people in the United States are living in food-insecure households, nearly 16 million of whom are children (Coleman-Jensen et al., 2014). Individuals at greatest risk for food insecurity include those individuals who are low income, are members of a minority, are elderly, and/or have children. Food-insecure adults have greater incidence of obesity and chronic diseases such as diabetes, less adherence to taking medications, and more mental health issues including anxiety and depression (Seligman, Laraia, & Kushel, 2010).

Food insecurity has proven to be somewhat difficult to measure. Early scales used household income levels to indirectly assess food insecurity. A national benchmark measure, the USDA Food Security Survey Module, was developed by the USDA Food and Nutrition Service in 1995 (Carlson, Andrews, & Bickel, 1999). The USDA Food Security Survey Module now has three forms in English and in Spanish: (a) a six-item short form, (b) a 10-item adult form, and (c) an 18-item household form, as well as a module for children 12 years of age and older.

With the growing numbers of food insecurity, multiple efforts are made to assist these individuals and families. Over $100 billion dollars is spent each year on federal food assistance programs. However, an increasing gap has been found between government food assistance programs and need (Feeding America, 2015; Roberts,

Povich, & Mather, 2012–2013). It has been nonprofit organizations that help fill the difference (Guo, 2010). Many of these nonprofits have created local food banks, food pantries, and meal programs.

Community pharmacists are in a unique position to identify patients who may be experiencing food insecurity. Several responses on the Food Security Survey Module are found to be most predictive of food insecurity (Hager et al., 2010). Two responses in the module, which pharmacists could ask, include (a) "Within the past 12 months, we worried whether our food would run out before we got money to buy more" and (b) "Within the past 12 months, the food we bought just didn't last and we didn't have money to get more."

In addition, pharmacists can learn about and direct their patients in need to their local food bank for more information on services available. National organizations, such as Feeding America and the Salvation Army, have created nationwide networks of local food banks, food pantries, and meal programs that serve communities across the country. In addition, there are many other local nonprofit organizations, such churches and schools, which offer food pantries and/or hot meals to those in need of food assistance. Pharmacists can also learn more about major federal assistance programs available in the United States for the food-insecure. Three programs of note include (a) the Supplemental Nutrition Assistance Program (SNAP), (b) the Women, Infants and Children (WIC), and (c) the Meals on Wheels program.

SNAP provides funds to purchase food for those demonstrating a financial need. Considered part of the national safety net for low-income households, there are national eligibility and benefits standards (USDA, 2012). Individuals can see if they qualify at their local health department. SNAP benefits are issued each month using an electronic benefit transfer card, similar to a debit card. SNAP recipients are only able to use their benefits at SNAP-approved stores and for SNAP-approved foods. Nonedible items, such as household goods, hot foods, medicine, alcohol, and cigarettes cannot be purchased with SNAP. SNAP is a supplemental program, meaning the amount of benefits does not provide all the food an individual needs (USDA, 2012.

WIC is a health care and nutrition program for low-income pregnant women, breastfeeding women, and infants and children under the age of five (Oliveira & Frazão, 2015). WIC eligibility, based on a financial need and a nutritional need (e.g., anemia or low body weight), allows WIC participants to buy nutritious food, including formula for infants, and services such as nutrition education breastfeeding support, and health care. Pharmacists may receive questions about what foods or formulas qualify for WIC benefits. The food items provided by WIC are juice, milk, breakfast cereal, cheese, eggs, fruits and vegetables, whole-wheat bread, whole-grain items (e.g., brown rice and tortillas), fish (canned), legumes, and peanut butter. The program also provides tofu, soymilk, and medical foods for children and women with various metabolic conditions or other diseases. Many studies have found the WIC program to be effective in decreasing health care costs (Oliveira & Frazão, 2015).

Home-delivered meals, or Meals on Wheels (MOW), are one of three Older Americans Act programs focused on improving the nutritional health of seniors. Hot, nutritious meals are delivered weekdays to homebound seniors. The meals must provide one-third of the nutrient needs of seniors. Eligibility is not based on financial need; rather, it is based on seniors being homebound and unable to prepare their own meals or shop for food. The MOW program has been shown to significantly improve nutrient intake, nutritional status, food security, loneliness, and social well-being (Wright, Vance, et al., 2015).

For community pharmacists who want to make a difference in their communities, being aware of the issues surrounding food insecurity for their patients is the first step to helping address this persistent national public health concern. NWS-13 in *Healthy People 2020* has as its objective to "reduce household food insecurity and in doing so reduce hunger" from 14.6% of households who were food insecure in 2008 to 6.0% (U.S. Department of Health and Human Services, 2010).

Global Perspective: Nutrition Transition

In this section, we discuss the rising prevalence of obesity and obesity-related disease experienced in developing countries with current thoughts on the etiology of the changes. Once considered a problem of high-income countries, obesity is quickly becoming a serious issue globally. Many low- and middle-income countries are facing a double burden of disease; these countries continue to struggle with problems of infectious diseases and undernutrition while experiencing a surge in obesity and noncommunicable diseases (WHO, 2013). The worldwide obesity prevalence has more than doubled since 1980 (Finucane et al., 2011). Obesity has clearly reached pandemic status, and it has debilitating repercussions.

The rise in worldwide obesity is thought to be due to the nutrition transition being experienced by developing countries. In the nutrition transition, there are significant changes in dietary and activity patterns. In country after country, a marked shift in the structure of the diet has been noted (Park, 2008; Popkin, Adair, & Ng, 2012; Wright, Corvin, Hoare, & Epps, 2015). Specifically, dietary changes include a large increase in the consumption of fat, added sugar, and animal products with a decrease in traditional foods, whole grains, and fiber (Popkin et al., 2012). Concurrently, there have been changes in activity patterns as well. Many countries are moving from agricultural economies to more industrialized economies. As a result, people are now working in less labor-intensive jobs. There has also been a change in leisure activities to more television viewing and computer browsing.

It is easy to see how these lifestyle changes of increased calorie consumption and sedentary behavior are widely accepted as major contributors to these increases in obesity.

The nutrition transition has not only resulted in obesity rates skyrocketing in developing countries but also in the development of nutrition-related noncommunicable diseases (NR-NCD), such as diabetes and cardiovascular disease. In fact, the risk of dying due to overweight- or obesity-related conditions now exceeds the risk of dying due to underweight-related conditions for 63% of the world's population (Alwan et al., 2010). The number of NR-NCD deaths is projected to increase by 15% globally between 2010 and 2020 (WHO, 2011). Developing countries are poorly prepared to manage these NR-NCD. The burden is surpassing current health care capabilities for such services as dialysis and hyperlipidemia medications. As we have learned in the United States, the emphasis needs to be on prevention of the dietary changes and obesity.

Due to the extent of the problem, the WHO Global Strategy on Diet, Physical Activity, and Health (2004) was adopted in 2004 to take actions needed to support healthy diets and regular physical activity. The Strategy calls upon all stakeholders to take action at global, regional, and local levels to improve diets and physical activity patterns at the population level. Pharmacists practicing in international communities can play a unique role in preventing obesity and obesity-related diseases (Jordan & Harmon, 2015). Through individual and community engagement, pharmacists can encourage healthy dietary and activity patterns to support health.

However, community pharmacy involvement in weight management is a very novel idea in many developing countries. The success and failure of these programs may hinge upon the beliefs of the community pharmacists and their local communities. Awad and Waheedi (2012) surveyed over 220 community pharmacies in Kuwait to gather pharmacists' perceptions of the effectiveness of obesity management programs. Kuwaiti pharmacists believed overall that obesity management programs, particularly advice on diet, exercise, and diet foods, were effective. An interesting finding was the more comfortable the pharmacists felt providing counseling to their patients, the more they believed in the effectiveness of the obesity management programs. A randomized trial conducted in Maha Sarakham province, Thailand, compared obesity interventions provided by community pharmacists with routine services provided at a primary care unit (Phimarn et al., 2013). Phimarn and colleagues found that Thai community pharmacists played a key role to help their patients to decide and engage in healthy dietary and activity patterns. Pharmacy patients not only had increased intentions to perform healthy dieting behavior; they also had higher gains in their overall and specific knowledge about the dangers of obesity and how to eat healthier.

Implications for Public Health and Pharmacy Practice

The role of pharmacists has shifted over the past several decades going from a traditional medication dispensing role to a more clinical and community role. Pharmacists have demonstrated their ability to play an integral part in patient care teams, both in the clinical and community setting. Furthermore, the Accreditation Council for Pharmacy Education (ACPE) Standards 2016 emphasizes the importance of patient-centered care, health and wellness, and population-based care (ACPE, 2015). Pharmacists' roles have also expanded to include more direct patient care, which includes disease management services. The ACPE Standards 2016 emphasizes the importance of patient-centered care, health and wellness, and population-based care (ACPE, 2015).

The importance of nutrition and the prevention of illness and disease has long been recognized and encouraged. Healthcare professionals, specifically pharmacists, play a key role in promoting healthy eating, as they will encounter nutrition issues every day with the patients they serve. Through the wide range of medical problems, weather it is in the clinical or community setting, pharmacist's need to value and understand the basics of nutrition working with the community. Healthcare costs have increased considerably, yet proper nutrition can help prevent many illnesses. With increasing public interest in nutrition, pharmacists need to be able to help guide the community in meeting their nutritional needs and goals.

With over 24 million Americans suffering from chronic diseases such as heart diseases, diabetes, and overweight/obesity, pharmacists have the opportunity to educate patients simultaneously on their medications as well as their nutrition. Pharmacists also have the opportunity to be aware of the latest interventions regarding weight loss, diabetes, and cardiovascular health. Weight loss and good nutrition can lead to decreased blood pressure, better glucose control, decreased low-density lipoprotein, and ultimately lower medication doses.

The information presented in this chapter focused on providing pharmacists an overview of the nutritional needs of people during the various stages of life. It is important for pharmacists to have a baseline understanding of these nutritional needs for any given patient population. The chapter also introduced specific strategies and programs pharmacists can refer to in order to support healthy lifestyles and public health prevention strategies focused on nutrition. As a result, the new generation of pharmacists will be equipped with the knowledge necessary not only to become medication experts but also to become a vital part in helping to support public health initiatives and providing population-based care through nutrition education.

References

Accreditation Council for Pharmacy Education. (2015). Accreditation Standards and Key Elements for the Professional Program in Pharmacy Leading to the Doctor of Pharmacy Degree. Retrieved from https://www.acpe-accredit.org/pdf/Standards2016FINAL.pdf

Alwan, A., Maclean, D. R., Riley, L. M., d'Espaignet, E. T., Mathers, C. D., Stevens, G. A., & Bettcher, D. (2010). Monitoring and surveillance of chronic non-communicable diseases: progress and capacity in high-burden countries. *Lancet, 376*(9755), 1861–1868. doi:10.1016/s0140-6736(10)61853-3

American Diabetes Association (2016). Statistics About Diabetes. Arlington, Virginia. Retrieved on www.diabetes.org/diabetes-basics/statistics

Awad, A., & Waheedi, M. (2012). Community pharmacist's role in obesity treatment in Kuwait: a cross-sectional study. *BMC Public Health, 12*, 863. doi:10.1186/1471-2458-12-863

Carlson, S. J., Andrews, M. S., & Bickel, G. W. (1999). Measuring food insecurity and hunger in the United States: development of a national benchmark measure and prevalence estimates. *Journal of Nutrition, 129*(2S Suppl.), 510s-516s.

Center for Disease Control & Prevention (2016). Chronic Disease Overview. Atlanta, GA: CDC. Retrieved from http://www.cdc.gov/chronicdisease/overview/

Center for Disease Control & Prevention (2014). National Diabetes Statistics Report, 2014. Retrieved from https://www.cdc.gov/diabetes/pubs/statsreport14/national-diabetes-report-web.pdf

Coleman-Jensen, A., Gregory, C., & Singh, A. (2014, September). *Household food security in the United States in 2013* (USDA Economic Research Report No. 173). Washington, DC: U.S. Department of Agriculture. Retrieved from http://www.ers.usda.gov/media/1565415/err173.pdfhttp://www.ers.usda.gov/media/1565415/err173.pdf

Das, J. K., Salam, R. A., Thornburg, K. L., Prentice, A. M., Campisi, S., Lassi, Z. S., . . . Bhutta, Z. A. (2017). Nutrition in adolescents: physiology, metabolism, and nutritional needs. *Annals of the New York Academy of Sciences, 1393*(1), 21–33. doi:10.1111/nyas.13330

Eckel, R. H., Jakicic, J. M., Ard, J. D., de Jesus, J. M., Houston Miller, N., Hubbard, V. S., . . . Yanovski, S. Z. (2014). 2013 AHA/ACC guideline on lifestyle management to reduce cardiovascular risk: A report of the American College of Cardiology/American Heart Association Task Force on Practice Guidelines. *Journal of the American College of Cardiology, 63*(25 Pt B), 2960–2984. doi:10.1016/j.jacc.2013.11.003

Feeding America. (2015). *Map the meal gap 2015: Highlights of findings for overall and child food insecurity.* Chicago, IL: Feeding America. Retrieved from http://www.feedingamerica.org/hunger-in-america/our-research/map-the-meal-gap/2012/2012-mapthemealgap-exec-summary.pdf

Finucane, M. M., Stevens, G. A., Cowan, M. J., Danaei, G., Lin, J. K., Paciorek, C. J., Ezzati, M. (2011). National, regional, and global trends in body-mass index since 1980: systematic analysis of health examination surveys and epidemiological studies with 960 country-years and 9.1 million participants. *Lancet, 377*(9765), 557–567. doi:10.1016/s0140-6736(10)62037-5

Gilman, S., Chokshi, D., Bowen, Rugen, & Cox, M. (2014). Connecting the dots: Intraprofessional health education and delivery system design at the Veterans Health Administration. *Academy of Medicine, 89*(8): 1113–1116.

Guo, B. (2010). Beyond the public safety net: The role of nonprofits in addressing material hardship of low-income households. *Nonprofit and Voluntary Sector Quarterly, 39*(5), 784–801. doi:10.1177/0899764009334307

Gurnani, M., Birken, C., & Hamilton, J. (2015). Childhood obesity: Causes, consequences, and management. *Pediatric Clinics of North America, 62*(4), 821–840. doi:10.1016/j.pcl.2015.04.001

Gurvey, J., Rand, K., Daugherty, S., Dinger, C., Schmeling, J., & Laverty, N. (2013). Examining health care costs among MANNA clients and a comparison group. *Journal of Primary Care & Community Health, 4*(4), 311–317. doi:10.1177/2150131913490737

Hager, E. R., Quigg, A. M., Black, M. M., Coleman, S. M., Heeren, T., Rose-Jacobs, R., . . . Frank, D. A. (2010). Development and validity of a 2-item screen to identify families at risk for food insecurity. *Pediatrics, 126*(1), e26–e32. doi:10.1542/peds.2009-3146

Iguacel, I., Fernandez-Alvira, J. M., Bammann, K., De Clercq, B., Eiben, G., Gwozdz, W., . . . Moreno, L. A. (2016). Associations between social vulnerabilities and dietary patterns in European children: the Identification and prevention of Dietary- and lifestyle-induced health EFfects In Children and infantS (IDEFICS) study. *The British Journal of Nutrition, 116*(7), 1288–1297. doi:10.1017/s0007114516003330

Jordan, M. A., & Harmon, J. (2015). Pharmacist interventions for obesity: improving treatment adherence and patient outcomes. *Integrated Pharmacy Research and Practice, 4*, 79–89. doi:10.2147/IPRP.S72206

Kaiser, M. J., Bauer, J. M., Ramsch, C., Uter, W., Guigoz, Y., Cederholm, T., . . . Sieber, C. C. (2010). Frequency of malnutrition in older adults: a multinational perspective using the mini nutritional assessment. *Journal of the American Geriatrics Society, 58*(9), 1734–1738. doi:10.1111/j.1532-5415.2010.03016.x

Lee, M. R., & Berthelot, E. R. (2010). Community covariates of malnutrition based mortality among older adults. *Annals of epidemiology, 20*(5), 371–379. doi:10.1016/j.annepidem.2010.01.008

Machen, R., Hammer, D., Odegard, P. (2007). Elective Course in Nutrition Taught by a Pharmacy Student. American Journal of Pharmacy Education, 71(4), 65.

National Heart Lung and Blood Institute. (2003, May). *Your guide to lowering blood pressure.* (NIH Publication No. 03-5232). Bethesda, MD: U.S. Department of Health and Human Services. Retrieved from https://www.nhlbi.nih.gov/files/docs/public/heart/hbp_low.pdf

Oliveira, V., & Frazão, E. (2015, January). *The WIC program background, trends, and issues, 2015 Edition* (EIB-134). Washington, DC: U.S. Department of Agriculture, Economic Research Service. Retrieved from http://www.ers.usda.gov/media/1760725/eib134.pdfhttp://www.ers.usda.gov/media/1760725/eib134.pdf

Park, H. K. (2008). Nutrition policy in South Korea. *Asia Pacific Journal of Clinical Nutrition, 17 Suppl 1*, 343–345.

Phimarn, W., Pianchana, P., Limpikanchakovit, P., Suranart, K., Supapanichsakul, S., Narkgoen, A., & Saramunee, K. (2013). Thai community pharmacist involvement in weight management in primary care to improve patient's outcomes. *International Journal of Clinical Pharmacy, 35*(6), 1208–1217. doi:10.1007/s11096-013-9851-3

Popkin, B. M., Adair, L. S., & Ng, S. W. (2012). Global nutrition transition and the pandemic of obesity in developing countries. *Nutrition Reviews, 70*(1), 3–21. doi:10.1111/j.1753-4887.2011.00456.x

Roberts, B., Povich, D., & Mather, M. (2012–2013). *Low-income working families: The growing economic gap.* Chevy Chase, MD: Working Poor Families Project. Retrieved from http://www.workingpoorfamilies.org/wp-content/uploads/2013/01/Winter-2012_2013-WPFP-Data-Brief.pdf

Ronai, C., Taylor, J. S., Dugan, E., & Feller, E. (2009). The identifying and counseling of breastfeeding women by pharmacists. *Breastfeeding Medicine, 4*(2), 91–95. doi:10.1089/bfm.2008.0122

Roth, R. (2014). Nutrition During Pregnancy and Lactation. In Brooke Wilson & Jennifer Wheaton (Eds.) In Nutrition & Diet Therapy (205–222), Clifton Park, NY: Delmar, Cengage Learning.

Sahoo, K., Sahoo, B., Choudhury, A., Sofi, N., Kumar, R. & Bhadoria, A. (2015). Childhood Obesity: Causes and consequences. Journal Family Medicine Primary Care, 4(2), 187–192.

Seligman, H. K., Laraia, B. A., & Kushel, M. B. (2010). Food insecurity is associated with chronic disease among low-income NHANES participants. *Journal of Nutrition, 140*(2), 304–310. doi:10.3945/jn.109.112573

U.S. Department of Agriculture. (2012). *Building a healthy America: A profile of the supplemental Nutrition Assistance Program.* Alexandria, VA: Author. Retrieved from https://fns-prod.azur-eedge.net/sites/default/files/BuildingHealthyAmerica.pdf

U.S. Department of Agriculture. (2016). MyPlate. [Web page]. Washington, DC: U.S. Department of Agriculture. Retrieved from http://www.choosemyplate.gov/

U.S. Department of Health and Human Services. (2010). *Healthy People 2020.* Washington, DC: U.S. Department of Health and Human Services. Retrieved from http://www.healthy people.gov/2020/http://www.healthypeople.gov/2020/

U.S. Dietary Guidelines Advisory Committee. (2015). *Dietary guidelines for Americans 2015-2020.* (8th ed.). Washington, DC: U.S. Department of Agriculture; U.S. Department of Health and Human Services. Retrieved from http://health.gov/dietaryguidelines/2015/guidelines/

U.S. Food and Drug Administration. (2016). How to understand and use the nutrition facts label. [Web page]. Silver Spring, MD: Author. Retrieved from http://www.fda.gov/Food/IngredientsPackagingLabeling/LabelingNutrition/ucm274593.htm

World Health Organization. (2016). *Global report on diabetes.* Geneva, Switzerland: Author. Retrieved from http://apps.who.int/iris/bitstream/10665/204871/1/9789241565257_eng.pdf

World Health Organization. (2011). *Global status reports on non-communicable diseases 2010: Description of the global burden of NCDs, their risk factors and determinants.* Geneva, Switzerland: WHO. Retrieved from http://whqlibdoc.who.int/publications/2011/9789240686458_eng.pdf?ua=1http://whqlibdoc.who.int/publications/2011/9789240686458_eng.pdf?ua=1

World Health Organization. (2013). *Global action plan for the prevention and control of non-communicable diseases 2013-2020.* Geneva, Switzerland: World Health Organization. Retrieved from http://www.who.int/iris/bitstream/10665/94384/1/9789241506236_eng.pdf?ua=1http://www.who.int/iris/bitstream/10665/94384/1/9789241506236_eng.pdf?ua=1

World Health Organization. (2016). Chronic diseases and health promotion. [Web page]. Geneva, Switzerland: WHO. Retrieved from http://www.who.int/chp/en/

World Health Organization, & UNICEF. (2003). *Global strategy for infant and young child feeding.* Geneva, Switzerland: World Health Organization. Retrieved from http://apps.who.int/iris/bitstream/10665/42590/1/9241562218.pdf?ua=1&ua=1http://apps.who.int/iris/bit-stream/10665/42590/1/9241562218.pdf?ua=1&ua=1

Wright, L., Corvin, J., Hoare, I., & Epps, J. (2015). Community assessment of nutritional needs and barriers to health care access in Belize. *International Journal of Nutrition and Dietetics, 2*(2), 97–114.

Wright, L., Vance, L., Sudduth, C., & Epps, J. B. (2015). The impact of a home-delivered meal program on nutritional risk, dietary intake, food security, loneliness, and social well-being. *Journal of Nutrition in Gerontology and Geriatrics, 34*(2), 218–227. doi:10.1080/21551197.2015.1022681

Xu, J., Murphy, S. L., Kochanek, K. D., & Bastian, B. A. (2016). Deaths: Final data for 2013. *National Vital Statisticss Reports, 64*(2), 1–118. http://www.cdc.gov/nchs/data/nvsr/nvsr64_02.pdfhttp://www.cdc.gov/nchs/data/nvsr/nvsr64_02.pdf

10

Financing and Insurance

SAMUEL H. ZUVEKAS, EARLE BUDDY LINGLE,

ARDIS HANSON, AND BRUCE LUBOTSKY LEVIN

Introduction

The US health care system is not a single system but is comprised of multiple systems of mixed private and public financing and insurance mechanisms in the delivery of healthcare. That structure and the costs of care differentiate it from other developed countries. The federal government reported Americans spent approximately $3.7 trillion on health care in 2015, or $9,990 per person (Centers for Medicare & Medicaid Services [CMS], 2016b). In contrast, total health expenditures for Canada reached $219.1 billion or $6,105 per Canadian in 2015 (Canadian Institute for Health Information, 2015). Comparing the per capita spending of selected nations to the United States, the Netherlands spent $5,131, France $4,361, Germany $4,920, the United Kingdom $3,364, and Israel $2,232 (Mossialos, Wenzl, Osborn, & Sarnak, 2016).

Public sources pay for most of the health care in these and other developed countries, ranging from 70% and up depending on the country. Americans, however, rely instead on a mixture of public and private health insurance coverage to pay for the bulk of the health care services they receive. In 2015, the federal government accounted for the largest share of health care spending (29%), followed by households (28%), private businesses (20%) and state and local governments (17%) (CMS, 2016b). Four federal programs, Medicare, Medicaid, the Children's Health Insurance Program (CHIP), and the Affordable Care Act (ACA) marketplace subsidies accounted for 25% or $938 billion (Center on Budget and Policy Priorities, 2016).Out-of-pocket spending by patients and families was 11%, or approximately $338 billion.

The Uninsured

Unlike other developed nations, the United States does not provide universal health care to all of its citizens. Although the federal Medicare program provides some level of coverage for adults 65 years of age and over, Americans under the age of 65 do not have guaranteed health care coverage. Approximately 55% of persons younger than age 65 were covered by private health plans in 2013 (Agency for Healthcare Research and Quality, 2017). The passage of the ACA extended Medicaid coverage to many low-income individuals in states with incomes at or below 138% of the federal poverty level (FPL) that chose to offer extended Medicaid coverage and provides marketplace subsidies for individuals below 400% of poverty (Office of the Assistant Secretary for Planning and Evaluation, 2017). Since the ACA-extended Medicaid coverage provisions went into effect in 2014 (with a few states expanding earlier), the number of uninsured nonelderly Americans now stands at 28.5 million, a decrease of nearly 7.4 million individuals (Cohen, Martinez, & Zammitti 2016).

Many of the remaining 28 million uninsured US adults live in states that did not expand Medicaid. Many of the uninsured are very poor. An estimated 39% of uninsured adults have incomes below the FPL. This is twice the rate of their overall representation in the adult population (Collins, Gunja, Doty, & Beutel, 2016). Further, not all workers offered employer-sponsored coverage can afford to pay the premiums or are eligible for the major public insurance programs. Other uninsured individuals are young and relatively healthy and do not elect to enroll in health insurance coverage even when offered.

The most common reason cited for being uninsured is that it is too expensive to carry health insurance (Collins et al., 2016). From 2006 to 2016, not only did total premiums for family coverage increase by 58%, but the worker's share increased by 78%, far outpacing wage growth (Henry J. Kaiser Family Foundation, 2016c). Of uninsured adults who are aware of the marketplaces or who have tried to enroll for coverage, affordability concerns is the major reason for not signing up. The uninsured pay for health care out of their own pockets or rely upon the public health insurance system. To understand better the financing of US health care, the next section describes major government health care programs, funding, and how public and private payers actually pay health care providers to deliver their services.

The Public Health Insurance System

Federal, state, and local governments play three major roles in the provision of health care: (1) regulate the health care marketplace, (b) mandate the provision of services by others for the public good, and (c) purchase services for the public good. Two examples are the U.S. Food and Drug Administration (FDA) and the National Institutes of Health (NIH). The FDA regulates pharmaceuticals and food due to safety concerns that the market did not adequately address. The NIH develops new medical treatments diseases. Other types of health care services that are in the public interest, such as disease prevention, generally are not provided in a normal market setting—hence the passage of regulations to mandate the purchase or provision of specific services or the assumption of the government to provide these services directly.

Government health insurance includes federal programs such as Medicare, Medicaid, CHIP, health insurance marketplaces, individual state health plans, TRICARE, Civilian Health and Medical Program of the Department of Veterans Affairs (VA), and care provided by the VA and the military.

Health insurance marketplaces, also called "health exchanges," are organizations established in each state to assist individuals with the purchase of health insurance in accordance with the provisions of the ACA. These marketplaces are open each year during an annual open enrollment period during which time individuals can enroll in a plan, switch plans, or request cost assistance. The ACA requires all Americans to have minimum essential health insurance coverage, which is found in all marketplace plans. Next, we examine the two largest programs, Medicare and Medicaid.

MEDICARE

Authorized under amendments to the Social Security Act of 1965, Medicare is a national health insurance program for the aged (65 years or older). In addition, certain categories of persons with disabilities and persons with end-stage renal disease are eligible for Part A and Part B after receiving disability benefits from Social Security for 24 months. Medicare uses a social insurance model. Benefits and eligibility requirements are defined by statute, a defined population is served, the program is funded by special taxes, the program is administered centrally (by the federal government) with national uniform rules, and beneficiaries receive care regardless of their ability to pay. There are three primary funding sources for Medicare: (a) general revenues (41%), (b) payroll taxes (38%), and (c) beneficiary premiums (13%) (Cubanski & Neuman, 2016).

The current Medicare program consists of four parts: A, B, C, and D. The first part, Medicare Part A (the Hospital Insurance Program), covers inpatient hospital services, skilled nursing facility benefits, home health visits, hospice care, lab tests, and surgery. Most persons age 65 or older are automatically entitled to these benefits. In addition, persons under 65 who receive Social Security cash payments due to a disability (noted earlier) and persons with end-stage renal disease are automatically entitled to these benefits. Part A is financed by a 2.9% payroll tax paid equally by employers and employees (1.45% each) (Cubanski & Neuman, 2016).

Medicare Part B (the Supplementary Medical Insurance Program) pays for physician services, outpatient hospital services, cancer screenings, lab procedures, and durable medical equipment. Although Part B is voluntary for Part A–eligible people, approximately 95% of Part A beneficiaries are also enrolled in Part B. Part B is funded by general revenues (73%), beneficiary premiums (25%), and interest and other sources (2%) (Cubanski & Neuman, 2016). Medicare Part B premiums cover 25% of total Part B costs.

Medicare Part C, also called Medicare Advantage, is not financed separately. Individuals enrolled in Medicare Advantage receive Part A and Part B benefits through privately administered plans. Typically, they pay monthly premiums for additional benefits covered by their plan, in addition to the Part B premium. Approximately 31% of the Medicare population participates in Part C programs (Cubanski & Neuman, 2016, July). Medicare-managed care plans include health maintenance organizations (HMOs), provider-sponsored organizations, preferred provider organizations, private fee-for-service plans, special needs plans, and Medicare Medical Savings Account plans.

Medicare Part D, the outpatient prescription drug benefit, began in 2006. Part D is financed mostly by general revenues (76%), beneficiary premiums (14%), and state payments for dually eligible beneficiaries (10%) (Cubanski & Neuman, 2016). Prescription drug coverage is provided through private, stand-alone prescription drug plans, including some Medicare cost plans, some Medicare private fee-for-service plans, and Medicare Medical Savings Account plans, as well as through Medicare Advantage plans with integrated benefits including drug coverage. Part D plans vary in benefit design, cost-sharing amounts, utilization management tools (i.e., prior authorization, quantity limits, and step therapy), and formularies.

Formularies must provide drug classes for all disease states including six "protected" classes (immune suppressants, antidepressants, antipsychotics, anticonvulsants, antiretrovirals, and antineoplastics). Individuals enrolled in Medicare drug plans have access to a free medication therapy management (MTM) program. The MTM program provides a written medication review, an action plan that recommends how to make the best use of medications, and a personal medication list.

In 2016, an estimated 2 million beneficiaries had drug coverage through employer-sponsored retiree plans, employer plans for active workers, Federal Employees Health Benefits, TRICARE, and Veterans Affairs (Henry J. Kaiser Family Foundation, 2016b). Medicare recipients without prescription drug coverage can purchase coverage for a monthly premium that provides an estimated 50% discount on their drug costs. Yet an estimated 13% of Medicare beneficiaries lack drug coverage.

The solvency of the Medicare program continues to be of concern. The Boards of Trustees of the Federal Hospital Insurance Trust (FHI) and Federal Supplementary Medical Insurance Trust Funds (2016) project that Medicare's current costs at 3.6% of gross domestic product (GDP) will increase to 5.6% in 2040 and to 6.0% in 2090.

Without adherence to the Medicare Access and CHIP Reauthorization Act of 2015 (MACRA)[1] and ACA cost-reducing measures, projected costs would rise even higher to 6.2% of GDP in 2040 and to 9.1% in 2090.

Over the past five years, Part B and Part D costs have averaged annual growth of 5.6% and 7.7%, respectively, compared to the average GDP growth of 3.7%. Estimated growth rates over the next five years for Parts B and D are 6.9% and 10.6%, respectively, with a projected average annual rate of growth for the US economy of 5.0% during this period. Since premium income and general revenue income are reset each year to cover expected costs, Part B and Part D accounts in the trust fund are adequately financed. However, the financing needs to increase faster than the economy to cover expected expenditure growth. The trustees also project that FHI (Medicare) tax income and other dedicated revenues will fall short of FHI expenditures in the future.

The Patient Protection and ACA, as amended by the Health Care and Education Reconciliation Act of 2010, contained approximately 165 provisions affecting the Medicare program, including cost-reduction measures, improved benefits, fraud and abuse reduction, and alternative provider payment mechanisms. The projections created by the Boards of Trustees (2016) assume substantial long-term reduction in per capita health expenditure growth rates and substantial savings from the cost reduction provisions of the ACA and MACRA. While the Boards expect smaller deficits from 2016 to 2021 with continued recovery from the 2007–2009 recession, there are concerns about ratio of workers to beneficiaries (i.e., the aging of the baby boom population), future economic conditions (recession), and significant declines in the fertility rates. Two other major concerns address the transition of health care to more efficient and productive models of care delivery commensurate with economy-wide productivity, and provider reimbursement rates, as currently negotiated, would result in a decrease in the quality and availability of care over time compared to services received by recipients with private insurance (Boards of Trustees, 2016).

MEDICAID

Representing one-sixth of the national health economy, Medicaid has the largest health program enrollment (68.9 million; 20%) and has the second largest health program expenditures ($554 billion) (Truffer, Wolfe, & Rennie, 2016). Medicaid serves as a safety net for the nation's most vulnerable populations. Children account for the largest number of beneficiaries (29.6 million, or 43.0%) (CMS, 2015). Unlike

---

[1] MACRA (Public Law 114-10) repealed and replaced Medicare's Sustainable Growth Rate formula. MACRA will establish new payment systems designed to reward quality over quantity of physician services.

Medicare, Medicaid is not a social insurance program. It does not have any dedicated revenue source at the federal level, such as the Medicare Hospital Insurance payroll tax, or a trust fund approach to financing. It has a very small amount of premium revenue from enrollees and certain other sources of state revenue (such as some provider taxes) (CMS, 2015; Truffer et al., 2016).

State and federal governments administer Medicaid jointly. The federal government will match all Medicaid expenditures at the appropriate federal matching assistance percentage (FMAP) rate for that state. Although a state can choose if it wants to participate in the program, all 50 states and the District of Columbia participate in Medicaid. Once a state decides to provide services under Medicaid, federal regulations require that states offer certain services, identify population groups eligible for benefits, and specify reimbursement.

State and federal funds also finance Medicaid jointly. Since the federal government's share of traditional Medicaid is based on a state's per capita income as compared to the national average, state dollars vary widely. The federal share may range from 50% to 77%, but the average federal contribution is 57%. US territories also receive base funding for Medicaid under Section 1108 of the Social Security Act. Puerto Rico, for example, received an additional $5.4 billion in Medicaid funding from 2011 to 2019 under Section 2005 of the ACA (CMS, 2017d).

In order to qualify for Medicaid benefits, recipients must meet certain eligibility criteria (CMS, 2017b). Since each state sets income and asset limits for qualification, states vary widely in coverage. A beneficiary must meet criteria for being categorically needy or medically needy or specific income requirements. Some states opt to provide services to individuals receiving home- and community-based services and to children in foster care who may not be eligible otherwise.

Federal regulations require states to provide a basic set of services that are medically necessary. These services may include inpatient and outpatient hospital services, physician services, laboratory and X-ray services, nursing home care, and home health care. Optional services include outpatient prescription drugs, dental care services, vision care, and intermediate-care facilities.

All 50 states and the District of Columbia offer outpatient prescription drug services, which are the most utilized Medicaid service. States may use managed care plans to provide and coordinate benefits, participate in demonstration projects, develop alternative benefit plans, or apply for waivers to have more flexibility in developing specialized benefit packages for specific populations (Truffer et al., 2016).

One particular financing problem in the Medicaid program is the expenditure for long-term care, whether it is institutional care or community-based care. As the US population increases in age, number of chronic diseases, and level of disability, while at the same time decreases in levels of daily functioning, higher costs can be expected. Medicaid is the only public health insurance program that pays for such care. Long-term care was responsible for approximately 25% ($116 billion) of total Medicaid expenditures in 2014 (Truffer et al., 2016).

Persons who are eligible for both Medicare and Medicaid are said to be "dually eligible." Within the CMS, the Medicare-Medicaid Coordination Office manages care for individuals who are eligible for both Medicaid and Medicare, including improving access and quality of care, simplifying administrative processes, and eliminating regulatory conflicts and cost-shifting among the two agencies. In some cases, Medicare provides the primary coverage for hospital insurance (Part A) and state Medicaid programs pay the premiums for supplemental medical insurance (Part B) so that Medicare will also cover those services. In addition, state Medicaid programs may pay the patient cost sharing and may provide the services Medicare does not, such as outpatient prescription drugs and long-term care.

Medicaid Expansion

The ACA provided for the expansion of Medicaid eligibility to almost all persons under the age 65 who are living in families with incomes below 138% of the FPL who are citizens or eligible legal residents, comparable to the national minimum Medicaid income eligibility levels for children. The intent of the expansion was to create a nationwide base of coverage for adults who are ineligible for Medicaid but earn too little to qualify for premium tax credits to be eligible for marketplace coverage. Approximately 4 million poor uninsured adults fall into a coverage gap as a result of these limited eligibility levels (Garfield & Damico, 2016).

States who opted to expand eligibility included adjustments to reflect a higher level of acuity or morbidity, increased capitation rates for newly eligible adults, who may create a higher demand than usual for additional services (pent-up demand), and made adjustments for adverse selection in case the new enrollees would have the greatest health care needs. The CMS estimate the effects of pent-up demand and adverse selection will diminish a few years after the expansion is implemented (Truffer et al., 2016).

With the implementation of the Medicaid eligibility expansion under the ACA, an additional 9 million persons became eligible for services and supports. In 2015, state and local Medicaid expenditures grew 4.9% compared to federal Medicaid expenditures, which increased 12.6%. The increased federal spending was driven largely by newly eligible enrollees under the ACA, which were financed fully by the federal government.

In the 2012 ruling *National Federation of Independent Business (NFIB) v. Sebelius*, the Supreme Court ruled that a state may not lose federal funding for its existing program if the state does not implement the Medicaid eligibility expansion under the ACA. As of January 1, 2017, 19 states (Alabama, Florida, Georgia, Idaho, Kansas, Maine, Mississippi, Missouri, Nebraska, North Carolina, Oklahoma, South Carolina, South Dakota, Tennessee, Texas, Utah, Virginia, Wisconsin, and Wyoming) had not adopted Medicaid expansion (Henry K. Kaiser Family Foundation, 2017a).

STATE CHILDREN'S HEALTH INSURANCE PROGRAM

Historically, Medicaid served children in families who were eligible for cash assistance through the federal welfare program. With the enactment of the State Children's Health Insurance Program as part of the Balanced Budget Act of 1997, Medicaid programs expanded their eligibility guidelines to add more low-income children. In 2009, President Obama signed the Children's Health Insurance Program Reauthorization Act (Pub. L. No. 111–3), which provided significant new funding, programmatic options, and incentives to identify, enroll, and retain health coverage for uninsured children who are eligible for but not enrolled in Medicaid or CHIP. More recently, the Medicare and CHIP Reauthorization Act of 2015 renewed funding for CHIP through fiscal year 2017. A joint federal–state program, CHIP is a state- and territory-administered program, as each state and territory sets its own guidelines regarding CHIP eligibility and services.

According to the Medicaid and CHIP Payment and Access Commission (2017), 8.4 million children received CHIP services in 2015, with a cost of $13.7 billion ($9.7 billion federal, $4.0 billion state). Since the U.S. Congress is working on proposals to repeal the ACA, which would damage the exchange market and change the structure and financing of the Medicaid program, the Commission recommends an extension of CHIP funding through fiscal year 2022.

DEPARTMENT OF VETERANS AFFAIRS

The VA provides programs for medical care and financial assistance for military veterans and their families subject to eligibility rules. The president's 2017 budget and 2018 advance appropriations requested $182.3 billion for the VA in 2017, with $65 billion allocated for medical care and an additional $7.2 billion allocated for the VA Care in the Community program, which covers medical procedures for veterans by non-VA providers (U.S. Department of Veterans Affairs, 2017).

The VA's comprehensive and integrated health care system is the largest in the United States with at least one medical center in each state, as well as in Puerto Rico and the District of Columbia. The VA health care system also includes 21 Veterans Integrated Service Networks (regional systems of care), 168 VA medical centers, 1,053 outpatient sites of care, over 800 community-based outpatient clinics, 135 skilled nursing facilities, 48 residential rehabilitation treatment programs, 278 vet centers across all 50 states, Guam, Puerto Rico, the U.S. Virgin Islands, and Washington, DC. The VA's standard medical benefits package includes preventive care services, ambulatory (or outpatient) diagnostic and treatment services, inpatient hospital diagnostic and treatment services including surgery, as well as medication and supplies.

TRICARE

TRICARE is the U.S. Department of Defense's health care program. Persons eligible for benefits under TRICARE include active duty military personnel, retirees, and their families. Individuals who are eligible may receive health care through TRICARE Prime (a managed care option), TRICARE Extra (a preferred provider option), or TRICARE Standard (a fee-for-service option) (Defense Health Agency, 2016). TRICARE coverage meets the minimum essential coverage requirement under the ACA.

INDIAN HEALTH SERVICE

The Indian Health Service (IHS) is an agency within the U.S Department of Health and Human Services (DHHS). Comprised of three components, the IHS directs health care services, tribally operated health care services, and urban Indian health care services and resource centers. The IHS provides health care for members of 567 federally recognized tribes, comprising approximately 2.2 million Native Americans and Alaska Natives (Indian Health Service, 2016). The tribes administer over 60% of the IHS appropriation primarily through self-determination contracts or self-governance compacts. Fiscal year 2016 IHS budget appropriation was $4.8 billion (IHS, 2016).

Twelve area offices and 170 IHS and/or tribally managed services administer IHS services. The IHS health care system consists of 26 hospitals, 59 health centers, and 32 health stations. In addition, Native American tribes and Alaska Native corporations provide care through 19 hospitals, 284 health centers, 28 residential treatment centers, 79 health stations, and 163 Alaska village clinics (IHS, 2016). In addition to IHS and tribal health services, more than 1 million Native Americans and Alaska Natives are enrolled in coverage through Medicaid and CHIP (CMS, 2017a).

The 1976, the Social Security Act was amended by the Indian Health Care Improvement Act (IHCIA). This permitted reimbursement by CMS for services provided to Native Americans and Alaska Natives in IHS and tribal health care facilities. The IHICA also created a 100% FMAP for Medicaid services provided through an IHS or tribal facility. In 2009, Section 5006 of the American Recovery and Reinvestment Act formally required states to consult with tribal communities on Medicaid and CHIP policy matters and to describe the process by which they sought advice from Native American health programs and urban Native American organizations (CMS, 2017a).

WORKERS COMPENSATION

Another method of financing health care involves states workers' compensation programs. These programs are financed by employer premiums that provide reimbursement to workers for health care when they are injured on the job or for occupational disease resulting from a specific accidental occurrence while employed. The U.S. Department of Labor also administers four disability compensation programs for federal workers or their dependents who receive an injury at work or who acquire an occupational disease.

The Health Care Safety Net

Many uninsured and other Americans with difficulties obtaining health care rely on what is called the "health care safety net" for their medical needs. Although often called a "system," the safety net is more of a patchwork of public, private, and philanthropic providers and programs that varies considerably from state to state. The Institute of Medicine (2000, p. 21) defines core safety net providers as having "two distinguishing characteristics: 1) by legal mandate or explicitly adopted mission, they maintain an "open door," offering access for services to patients regardless of their ability to pay; and 2) a substantial share of their patient mix is uninsured, Medicaid, and other vulnerable populations." The core health care safety net providers, under the Institute of Medicine definition, also include state and local public health clinics and many private nonprofit charitable organizations. However, hospitals, doctors, and other providers also provide a substantial amount of charitable care informally.

Some 21 million Americans rely on community-based federally qualified health centers (FQHCs) to serve their primary health care needs (Henry J. Kaiser Family Foundation, 2017b). FQHCs serve designated medically underserved areas or medically underserved populations with a lack of access to primary care services (CMS, 2016a). FQHCs include a variety of facilities, including community health centers, health care for the homeless centers, migrant health centers, public housing primary care centers, and outpatient health programs or facilities operated by tribes, tribal organizations, or urban Native American organizations (CMS, 2016a).

Although Congress established federal grants in 1964 to address safety net concerns, FQHCs and a number of other centers also depend on Medicaid and other state and local funding sources. Community mental health centers and substance abuse treatment facilities similarly depend on a variety of federal, state, and local funding sources to provide treatment to individuals with chronic mental illnesses and individuals with substance use disorders.

State and local public hospitals as well as university teaching hospitals are critical components of the health care safety net. These hospitals finance services through a variety of federal, state, and local funding sources. Additional payments from the Medicaid and Medicare Disproportionate Share Hospital program are an especially important source of funding for these hospitals serving large proportion of low-income populations (Neuhausen et al., 2014).

However, with reduced federal and state expenditures for health care safety net programs and the closing of state hospitals, there has been a slow and incremental decay in the "publicly funded urban health care safety net" (Kulesher, 2015). Although the federal government spends more than $20 billion to support the cost of uncompensated care, some estimates suggest that amount only covers half of the total cost of uncompensated care. Further, uncompensated care comprises approximately one-third of the medical costs of persons who are uninsured. Hence, there is also concern that if more individuals lose their health insurance, the safety net will continue to decline, increasing the costs to state and federal governments of uncompensated care. It is estimated, even with the implementation of the ACA, there may be in excess of 40 million individuals without insurance in the United States when adding in the uninsured, undocumented residents, and persons unwilling to purchase health insurance (Kulesher, 2015).

Paying for Health Care

Prior to the 1960s, traditional fee-for-service (FFS) was the most common form of health care insurance reimbursement. Under FFS, providers are paid by a payer for each service given by the provider. Traditionally, doctors or hospitals set their own fees, but that is rarely the case today as insurers have sought to control costs either through negotiated fees or through directly setting fees. Since the 1960s, new types of payment systems, such as capitation, also emerged as public and private insurers attempted to control health care costs.

However, FFS still remains the dominant payment mechanism in the United States with approximately 95% of all physician visits paid under some form of FFS (Zuvekas & Cohen, 2016). A major problem with FFS is that it provides little or no incentives for providers to economize on the quantity of health care services. In fact, quite the opposite occurs.

Today, state and federal Medicaid and Medicare programs set the fees they are willing to pay for each service in an attempt to control rising health care costs (Zuvekas & Cohen, 2016). Physicians who accept Medicaid patients then are reimbursed a set amount. Because Medicaid fees are often low, many physicians do not take Medicaid patients. The Medicare program also sets fees for physician and other services. In contrast to the Medicaid program, nearly all physicians accept Medicare patients. In part, this is because Medicare fees are generally higher than Medicaid fees but also because Medicare patients also account for a greater proportion of medical spending. Private plans generally negotiate fees with providers they contract with as part of their networks, with these negotiated fees generally higher than Medicare fees.

CAPITATION/PROSPECTIVE PAYMENT

The search for controlling health care costs led to the introduction of another type of financing system, called *capitation* financing, which includes plan capitation and provider capitation. Under a *capitation plan*, a public program (e.g., Medicaid) or a private entity pay a set fee for each person covered for a specified period to a health care plan. For example, the CMS, a state, and a health plan will enter into a three-way contract in order to provide comprehensive, coordinated care to recipients. The health care plan then determines which services it will deliver and how it will pay its health care providers. Since the health plan now is *at risk* for the services delivered, there is a strong financial incentive to control service use. Under *provider capitation*, providers receive a fixed amount for each person assigned to them. Similar to plan capitation, the risk shifts to the provider, providing an incentive for efficient treatment. However, provider capitation is more limited due to provider resistance to risk shifting, administrative costs for capitated payments, and the difficulty in determining capitation rates for specialty services.

Here, however, is a conundrum. FFS contains incentives to overprovide care (more cost), whereas capitation contains incentives to underprovide health care services (less costs). While capitation has been shown to reduce the costs of care, there is concern that the quality of care may suffer, leading to poorer patient outcomes (Barham & Milliken, 2015; Flodgren et al., 2011; Zuvekas & Cohen, 2010; Zuvekas & Hill, 2004).

LINKING PAYMENT TO QUALITY/OUTCOMES

Pay-for-performance (P4P) programs links payment to performance benchmarks such as quality of care delivered or improvements in health outcomes. It is a very popular concept among policymakers and public/private payers who want to know the benefits received for the money invested into health care systems. Approximately half of the HMOs in the United States, most state Medicaid, programs, and the Medicare hospital P4P program use P4P incentives. However, the published literature shows mixed evidence that P4P is effective in improving health care (Mendelson et al., 2017). Further, there are no national P4P design guidelines, leading to significant heterogeneity in program design across providers (Mehrotra, Sorbero, & Damberg, 2010). An investigation of the use of P4P in safety net settings identified two potential barriers to such programs: complex patient care requirements and limited motivational effects from financial incentives (Young et al., 2010).

A major emphasis for the CMS is basing reimbursement of services upon quality, such as its goal to base all Medicare fee-for-service payments on quality or value by the end of 2018 (Staff, 2015). Accountable care organizations (ACOs), for example, are groups of providers who join as a practice and are accountable for both the quality and cost of the care they deliver to their Medicare patients. ACOs also use bundled payments, which ties reimbursement of providers to identified metrics of quality. When *The Lancet* ACO reaches its benchmarks for delivery of quality care and cost savings, it shares in the savings it achieves for the Medicare program. CMS is also examining social risk factors in Medicare payment programs mandated through the Improving Medicare Post-Acute Care Transformation Act (IMPACT) Act (Committee on Accounting for Socioeconomic Status in Medicare Payment, 2016). The IMPACT Act (Pub. L. 113-185) requires postacute care providers to compile and submit quality, performance, and resource use data and standardizes data collection and data sharing among postacute providers. CMS's eventual aim is to take these data and make them publicly available to improve care.

Adverse and Favorable Risk Selection

Risk selection is a continuing problem for health care services plan providers. Inevitably, some individuals will be more at risk from diseases, will require more costly health care, and are more likely to purchase insurance to cover the costs of anticipated care. As insurers want to keep their payouts low, guaranteed availability of insurance is problematic for them. *Adverse selection* occurs when unfavorable risks (sicker than average individuals) are in an insurance pool; *favorable selection* results when better risks are in an insurance pool. Adverse selection can take place between insurers, between benefit plans, and between markets (public or private).

Concerns about adverse selection were central in the creation of the Medicare program. This is why hospital insurance (Medicare Part A) is mandatory for all eligible Americans 65 and over. Although Medicare Part B (outpatient coverage) is voluntary, to counter incentives for adverse selection Americans who enroll after the age of 65 pay a permanent 10% higher penalty premium for Part B for each year they delayed enrollment. Substantial penalties also are mandated for late enrollment in the Medicare Prescription Drug Program (Part D).

Clearly, insurers, managed care plans, and providers have powerful financial incentives to attract favorable risks and discourage poor risks. Payments are often set at the *average* cost. Hence, the potential for risk selection is significant. Consider that the healthiest 50% of the population account for 2.8% of all health care spending, with an annual mean expenditure of $264 (Mitchell, 2016). Then consider that 1% of the population accounts for 22.8% of all health care costs in the United States with an annual mean expenditure of $107,208 and the top 5% account for over half of health care spending, with an annual mean expenditure of $47,498 (Mitchell, 2016).

RISK SELECTION AND QUALITY

Risk selection also creates problems for determining which hospitals, doctors, nursing homes, and other providers deliver the best quality of health care. For example, if one wanted to know which local hospital was best at treating breast cancer, one might look at the mortality rates for breast cancer patients at each treatment center. However, mortality rates may not be a good indicator of excellent treatment. An excellent hospital may have higher mortality rates if it accepts the sickest patients, while a hospital with lower mortality rates may actually be treating far less seriously ill patients.

RISK ADJUSTMENT

Risk adjustment, sometimes called case-mix adjustment, allows plans to adjust payments to reflect how a hospital or treatment facility distributes risks. In a perfect risk-adjusted world, Hospital A would be paid more if they treated sicker than average patients and Hospital B would be paid less if they treated healthier than average patients. Payments to competing health insurance plans would be risk adjusted in the same way. In the real world, however, accurate risk adjustment is difficult to achieve. Part of the issue is data. Most risk adjustment models use limited health information along with age, sex, and other demographic characteristics, thereby providing less than accurate predictive models. Despite its limitations, risk adjustment is widely used to set capitation and reimbursement rates.

Financing Pharmacy in the Public Health System

In 2015, retail prescription drug spending increased by 9.0% to $324.6 billion (CMS, 2016b). Medicare and Medicaid prescription drug spending in 2015 increased at double-digit rates in 2015, 11.0% and 13.6%, respectively (Martin, Hartman, Washington, & Catlin, 2017). The growing trend in public coverage of pharmaceuticals is evident considering that government programs have added in additional prescription drug benefits with the passage of the ACA.

MEDICAID

The Medicaid program has the largest public drug benefit program. Although Medicaid spent approximately $42 billion on prescription drugs in 2014, with collected rebates, net drug spending was $22 billion (Medicaid and CHIP Payment and Access Commission, 2016). Medicaid prescription drug spending increased 24.3% in 2014 (Martin, Hartman, Benson, & Catlin, 2016) due to coverage expansions under the ACA and new specialty drugs to treat conditions such as hepatitis C

(Keehan et al., 2015). With the expansions of coverage through Medicaid and the health insurance marketplaces, the financing of health care shifted further toward the federal government in 2014 (Keehan et al., 2015). However, it is important to remember that the Medicaid drug benefit program is comprised of 51 discrete programs (the 50 states plus the District of Columbia).

STATE PHARMACY ASSISTANCE PROGRAMS

Most states have enacted laws to provide additional pharmaceutical insurance coverage or assistance to low-income and medically needy senior citizens and individuals with disabilities who do not qualify for Medicaid through State Pharmacy Assistance Programs (SPAPs) (National Council of State Legislators, 2016). SPAPs either provide drug benefits directly to recipients or offer discounted prescription drug programs. In the discounted programs, the states negotiate or mandate lower prescription drug prices for recipients. Although state governments fund SPAPs entirely, a few SPAPs qualify to receive federal matching funds. Some states also offer programs to help individuals with certain illnesses, such as HIV/AIDS or end-stage renal disease, pay for their prescription drugs. The states that do offer SPAPs coordinate their programs with Medicare's Part D benefit. The Medicare Part D drug benefit allows SPAPs to supplement the Part D drug benefit recipients by helping to pay premiums or contributing to a recipient's cost sharing.

MEDICARE

The ACA closed the Medicare prescription drug coverage gap (aka "donut hole") that resulted from the Medicare Modernization Act. The Medicare Part D coverage gap is the period of time when the consumer pays for prescription medication costs that lie between the initial coverage limit and the catastrophic-coverage threshold. The ACA provides enrollees with a 55% discount on brand-name pharmaceuticals once they reach the Medicare prescription drug "donut hole" and a separate 35% discount on generic drugs. The CMS expects that the coverage gap should phase out by 2020.

Medicare beneficiaries do not receive the same drug benefit as Medicaid beneficiaries. Although the benefit varies among the different plans, it must be actuarially similar in terms of the value of the benefit provided. This means that different beneficiaries within the same family may have different drug benefits concerning cost-sharing and drug coverage policies. As mentioned earlier, administrators of the Medicare drug benefit plans must provide MTM programs to Medicare beneficiaries with multiple chronic diseases, multiple covered drugs, and annual drug costs exceeding $4,000. This is an excellent opportunity for pharmacists to become involved with patient care, as they would be the community providers and information sources regarding medication.

SYSTEM STABILITY

Rapidly escalating costs threaten the stability of the US health care systems. In 2014 and 2015, while growth in GDP averaged 4.0%, health spending increased at an average annual rate of 5.5%. However, three factors contributed to this increase: the addition of millions of people who gained health insurance coverage after 2013, the rapid growth in retail prescription drug spending, and postrecession recovery (Martin et al., 2017). Other explanations include increasingly complex payment and financing incentives, the aging of the US population, medical malpractice liability, societal expectations, and technological innovation (Freedman, 2012; Glied & Little, 2003; Newhouse, 1992; Okunad & Murthy, 2002; Serra-Sastre & McGuire, 2012). In part, we may be spending more on medical care simply because we can do a lot more.

Increasing health care spending puts pressure on everyone. Common responses include increasing the amount employees must pay for health insurance coverage, increasing the amount that people pay out of pocket for health care services, or dropped health insurance coverage altogether. Any of these actions increase the reliance on public sector and safety net providers (Fan, Anderson, Foley, Rauser, & Silverstein, 2011; Vistnes, Zawacki, Simon, & Taylor, 2012).

Rising health care spending puts strong pressure on federal, state, and local governments. Not only is net Medicare spending projected to increase from $591 billion in 2016 to $1.1 trillion in 2026, but also long-term spending projections estimate that net Medicare spending will grow from 3.2% of GDP in 2016 to 3.9% in 2026, 5.0% in 2036, and 5.7% in 2046 (Congressional Budget Office, 2016). Declining employer-based coverage and limited public funding may lead to a growing number of uninsured people, higher costs when they do need medical care, and additional strain both on families and the publicly financed health care safety net.

Reforming the Healthcare System

The emergence of Medicare, Medicaid, and other public programs during the 1960s greatly increased the capacity of the US health care system. At the same time, these public programs have created tensions among policymakers and insurers in their attempts to address the programs' original mandates and increasing pressures to contain costs. As federal, state, and local budgets are reduced, they restrain reimbursement rates with adverse consequences on how providers serve populations in public programs (Lingle & Zuvekas, 2008). Medicare, as the nation's single largest health care purchaser, has altered the delivery of health care for all Americans by its decisions on what services to cover and how much it pays. After the enactment of the ACA, there were numerous expectations on how the ACA would affect insurance providers, uninsured populations, and state bureaucracies.

The institutional design of the ACA's regulatory reforms of the insurance market equally affected coverage and delivery of services as has its opportunities for Medicaid expansions at the state level. However, due to the complex federal–state design of the law, governing authority did not reside within DHHS. Instead, governing authority went to a number of players, including state governors, legislatures, and regulatory agencies, all of whom had to collaborate with DHHS to negotiate the rules for the new system state by state. The inability of DHHS to promulgate fully formed homogenous administrative rules and routines to the states (National Association of Insurance Commissioners [NAIC], 2011) led to both difficulties in implementation and confusion in the public's understanding of the ACA.

The creation of the new health insurance exchanges (HIEs), for example, which permit individuals to buy quality health coverage at low costs, was an expectation of the ACA, not a requirement. Three requirements of the federal HIEs are (a) to be a state-established governmental agency or nonprofit entity, (b) to consult with stakeholders in carrying out required HIE activities, and (c) to be financially self-sustaining (ACA, § 1311(d)). Existing state insurance exchanges could serve as models for the federal HIEs. The NAIC (2011) identified Massachusetts and Utah as good models for a state-established governmental agency (i.e., quasi-governmental agency or independent public entity); however, it was unable to identify an existing model for "a nonprofit entity that is established by a State" (NAIC, 2011, p. 2). The NAIC advised states to reflect carefully upon their exchange governance structures, considering the "hundreds, if not thousands, of structural and operational issues" they will have to address to meet the ACA requirements (NAIC, 2011, p. 5).

A second example of federal–state complexity is Medicaid expansion, which was to decrease the number of uninsured individuals in each state and reduce the wide variation in state Medicaid rules governing coverage. However, the 2012 Supreme Court ruling on the ACA substantiated a state's rights to not participate in Medicaid expansion with no loss of current federal funding.

In March 2017, the new presidential administration prepared its strategy to address the costs of health care in the United States. The American Health Care Act (H.R. 1628), which would repeal the ACA enacted under President Obama, was passed by the House of Representatives. It is currently under review by the Senate. The House of Representatives has also introduced legislation to reduce the costs of care, including H.R. 372, which limits the McCarran-Ferguson antitrust exemption for health insurers, and H.R. 1101, which exempts association health plans from the state licensing and financial requirements imposed on traditional insurers. All three proposals have come under intense scrutiny, with widely varying reports on the impact of each on health insurance markets and the insured/uninsured populations (American Academy of Actuaries, 2017; America's Health Insurance Plans, 2017; Congressional Budget Office, 2017).

Implications for Public Health and Pharmacy Practice

Although the ACA expanded health care and medication insurance coverage through Medicaid expansion and health plan subsidies, what does that mean for those who were uninsured? Mahendraratnam, Dusetzina, and Farley (2017) determined that Medicaid expansion offers vulnerable patients, who were previously uninsured, increased access to coverage and care, particularly to prescription drugs. Increased utilization in expansion states suggests that the drops in per member per quarter (PMPQ) utilization may be partially attributable to successful risk-pooling. Increased PMPQ reimbursement may be due to new enrollment as well as changes in product mix, risk pool composition, and drug pricing (Mahendraratnam et al., 2017).

A second study by Ngorsuraches and Mort (2016) examined the value of health plan subsidies, including cost-sharing for prescription drugs in the health insurance marketplace. The value of subsidies varied widely across geographic areas with different numbers of health plans. Further, although plans may have the same actuarial value, each plan has specific features that differentiate it from other plans, which needs careful examination to meet enrollee (patient) needs. They suggest it may not be feasible to reduce variations in health insurance plans unless new cost-saving features are adopted, such as a maximum out-of-pocket spending for drugs (Ngorsuraches & Mort, 2016).

In terms of implications for pharmacy, the ACA extended health insurance benefits to almost 23 million people and provided financial assistance to individuals living on up to 400% of the poverty level. This should function to expand the pharmacy market. Another important factor is CMS Triple Aim goals of improving patient care quality and satisfaction, improving population health, and reducing costs, which come from increased coverage and utilization and decreased downstream costs for morbidity. One of the most immediate and direct impacts of recent policy changes was through reductions in payment updates to providers and Medicare Advantage, which produced short-term federal savings of $68 billion between 2011 and 2016 (Henry J. Kaiser Family Foundation, 2016a). Also important are the mandated changes to Medicare in the MACRA, which further move Medicare toward alternative payment models, such as risk-sharing arrangements or reimbursement tied to quality measures (CMS, 2017c). The private and public sector continue to experiment with payment methods.

Collins et al. (2016) determined a number of factors contribute to continued high rates of uninsured individuals. These include the lack of Medicaid expansion in 19 states, which make up 51% of the remaining uninsured in the nation; lack of awareness of marketplaces among some demographic groups; plan selection, affordability, and subsidy eligibility; lack of assistance; and exclusion of undocu-mented immigrants from coverage expansions.

While policy recommendations regarding universal coverage are beyond the scope of this chapter, it is important to note that the escalation of the cost of health care will likely continue absent resolution of inequities in health care, high admin-istrative costs, lack of cost controls, and inadequate risk adjustment models. Prices remain a significant driver of health care costs in the United States, with increasing scrutiny on the costs of medications.

Authors' Note

The views expressed here are those of the authors, and no official endorsement by the U.S. Agency for HealthCare Research and Quality or the U.S. Department of Health and Human Services is intended or should be inferred.

References

Agency for Healthcare Research and Quality. (2017). Ever have private insurance during 13? MEPS: Medical Expenditure Panel Survey. [Database query]. Rockville, MD: Author. Retrieved from https://meps.ahrq.gov/mepsweb/data_stats/MEPSnetHC.jsp

American Academy of Actuaries. (2017, March 8). Re: Markup of H.R. 1101, the Small Business Health Fairness Act of 2017. Washington, DC: Author. Retrieved from https://www.actuary. org/files/publications/AHPs_HR1101_030817.pdf

America's Health Insurance Plans. (2017, February 16). Statement on "The Unintended Consequences and Harmful Impact of Repealing the McCarran-Ferguson Act's Antitrust Exemption" submitted to the House Committee on the Judiciary Subcommittee on Regulatory Reform, Commercial and Antitrust Law. Washington, DC: Author. Retrieved from https://www.ahip.org/wp-content/uploads/2017/02/statement-for-House-Judiciary-Hearing-on-McCarran-Ferguson-02-16-17final.pdf

Barham, V., & Milliken, O. (2015). Payment mechanisms and the composition of physician prac-tices: Balancing cost-containment, access, and quality of care. Health Economics, 24(7), 895–906. doi:10.1002/hec.3069

Boards of Trustees of the Federal Hospital Insurance, and Federal Supplementary Medical Insurance Trust Funds. (2016). 2016 annual report of the Boards of Trustees of the Federal Hospital Insurance and Federal Supplementary Medical Insurance Trust Funds. Washington, DC: Author. Retrieved from https://www.cms.gov/Research-Statistics-Data-and-Systems/Statistics-Trends-andReports/ReportsTrustFunds/Downloads/TR2016.pdf

Canadian Institute for Health Information. (2015, October). National health expenditure trends, 1975 to 2015 report Ottawa, ON: Author. Retrieved from https://secure.cihi.ca/free_prod-ucts/nhex_trends_narrative_report_2015_en.pdf

Center on Budget and Policy Priorities. (2016, March 4). Where do our federal tax dollars go? (Policy Basics). Washington, DC: Author. Retrieved from http://www.cbpp.org/sites/default/files/atoms/files/4-14-08tax.pdf

Centers for Medicare & Medicaid Services. (2015, December). 2015 CMS statistics (CMS Pub. No. 03512). Washington, DC: U.S. Department of Health and Human Services Retrieved from https://www.cms.gov/Research-Statistics-Data-and-Systems/Statistics-Trends-and-Reports/CMS-Statistics-Reference-Booklet/Downloads/2015CMSStatistics.pdf

Centers for Medicare & Medicaid Services. (2016a). *Federally qualified health center.* Baltimore, MD. Retrieved from https://www.cms.gov/Outreach-and-Education/Medicare-Learning-Network-MLN/MLNProducts/downloads/fqhcfactsheet.pdf

Centers for Medicare & Medicaid Services. (2016b). *National health expenditures, 2015 highlights.* Baltimore, MD: Author.

Centers for Medicare & Medicaid Services. (2017a). Indian health and Medicaid. Baltimore, MD Author. Retrieved from https://www.medicaid.gov/medicaid/indian-health-and-medicaid/index.html

Centers for Medicare & Medicaid Services. (2017b). *List of Medicaid eligibility groups: Mandatory categorically needy.* Washington, DC: Author. Retrieved from https://www.medicaid.gov/medicaid-chip-program-information/by-topics/waivers/1115/downloads/list-of-eligibility-groups.pdf

Centers for Medicare & Medicaid Services. (2017c, January 18). New participants join several CMS alternative payment models [Press release]. Retrieved from https://www.cms.gov/Newsroom/MediaReleaseDatabase/Press-releases/2017-Press-releases-items/2017-01-18.html

Centers for Medicare and Medicaid Services. (2017d). Puerto Rico. Washington, DC: Author. Retrieved from https://www.medicaid.gov/medicaid/by-state/puerto-rico.html

Children's Health Insurance Program Reauthorization Act, Pub. L. No. 111-3 (2009). Retrieved from https://www.gpo.gov/fdsys/pkg/PLAW-111publ3/pdf/PLAW-111publ3.pdf

Cohen, R. A., Martinez, M. E., & Zammitti, E. P. (2016). *Health insurance coverage: Early release of estimates from the National Health Interview Survey, 2015.* Atlanta, GA: Centers for Disease Control and Prevention, Division of Health Interview Statistics. Retrieved from https://www.cdc.gov/nchs/data/nhis/earlyrelease/insur201605.pdf

Collins, S. R., Gunja, M. Z., Doty, M. M., & Beutel, S. (2016). *Who are the remaining uninsured and why haven't they signed up for coverage? Findings from the Commonwealth Fund Affordable Care Act Tracking Survey, February–April 2016* (Tracking Trends in Health System Performance, no. 24). Washington, DC: Commonwealth Fund. Retrieved from http://www.commonwealthfund.org/~/media/files/publications/issue-brief/2016/aug/1894_collins_who_are_remaining_uninsured_tb_rev.pdf

Committee on Accounting for Socioeconomic Status in Medicare Payment. (2016). *Accounting for social risk factors in Medicare payment: Criteria, factors, and methods.* Washington, DC: National Academies Press. Retrieved from https://www.nap.edu/catalog/23513/accounting-for-social-risk-factors-in-medicare-payment-criteria-factors

Congressional Budget Office. (2016, July). *The 2016 long-term budget outlook.* Washington, DC: Author. Retrieved from https://www.cbo.gov/sites/default/files/114th-congress-2015-2016/reports/51580-ltbo-2.pdf

Congressional Budget Office. (2017, May). *H.R. 1628, American Health Care Act of 2017.* Washington, DC: Congressional Budget Office, Joint Committee on Taxation. Retrieved from https://www.cbo.gov/system/files/115th-congress-2017-2018/costestimate/hr1628as-passed.pdf

Cubanski, J., & Neuman, T. (2016, July). *The facts on Medicare spending and financing.* (Issue Brief). Menlo Park, CA: Henry K. Kaiser Family Foundation. Retrieved from http://files.kff.org/attachment/Issue-Brief-The-Facts-on-Medicare-Spending-and-Financing

Defense Health Agency. (2016, August). *TRICARE® choices in the United States: Handbook.* Falls Church, VA: Author. Retrieved from http://www.tricare.mil/~/media/Files/TRICARE/.../Handbooks/Choices_HB.pdf

Fan, Z. J., Anderson, N. J., Foley, M., Rauser, E., & Silverstein, B. A. (2011). The persistent gap in health-care coverage between low- and high-income workers in Washington State: BRFSS, 2003–2007. *Public Health Reports, 126*(5), 690–699.

Flodgren, G., Eccles, M. P., Shepperd, S., Scott, A., Parmelli, E., & Beyer, F. R. (2011). An overview of reviews evaluating the effectiveness of financial incentives in changing healthcare professional behaviours and patient outcomes. *Cochrane Database of Systematic Reviews, 7,* Cd009255. doi:10.1002/14651858.cd009255

Freedman, S. (2012). Health insurance and hospital technology adoption. *Advances in Health Economics and Health Services Research, 23,* 177–198.

Garfield, R., & Damico, A. (2016, October). *The coverage gap: Uninsured poor adults in states that do not expand Medicaid* (Issue Brief). Menlo Park, CA: Henry J. Kaiser Family Foundation. Retrieved from http://files.kff.org/attachment/Issue-Brief-The-Coverage-Gap-Uninsured-Poor-Adults-in-States-that-Do-Not-Expand-Medicaid

Glied, S., & Little, S. E. (2003). The uninsured and the benefits of medical progress. *Health Affairs, 22*(4), 210–219.

Henry J. Kaiser Family Foundation. (2016a, May). *Medicare Advantage* (Fact sheet). Menlo Park, CA: Author. Retrieved from http://files.kff.org/attachment/Fact-Sheet-Medicare-Advantage

Henry J. Kaiser Family Foundation. (2016b, September). *The Medicare Part D prescription drug benefit.* (Fact sheet). Menlo Park, CA: Author. Retrieved from http://files.kff.org/attachment/Fact-Sheet-The-Medicare-Part-D-Prescription-Drug-Benefit

Henry J. Kaiser Family Foundation. (2016c, September). *2016 employer health benefits survey.* Washington, DC: Author. Retrieved from http://kff.org/report-section/ehbs-2016-summary-of-findings/

Henry J. Kaiser Family Foundation. (2017a). Patients served by federally funded federally qualified health centers. Menlo Park, CA: Author. Retrieved from http://kff.org/other/state-indicator/total-patients-served-by-fqhcs/?currentTimeframe=0

Henry K. Kaiser Family Foundation. (2017b). Status of state action on the Medicaid expansion decision. Menlo Park, CA: Author. Retrieved from http://kff.org/health-reform/state-indicator/state-activity-around-expanding-medicaid-under-the-affordable-care-act/?currentTimeframe=0

Indian Health Service. (2016, September). *IHS 2016 profile.* Rockville, MD: Author Retrieved from https://www.ihs.gov/newsroom/includes/themes/newihstheme/display_objects/documents/factsheets/Profile2016.pdf.

Institute of Medicine. (2000). *America's health care safety net: Intact but endangered.* Washington, DC: National Academy Press. Retrieved from https://www.nap.edu/catalog/9612/americas-health-care-safety-net-intact-but-endangered

Keehan, S. P., Cuckler, G. A., Sisko, A. M., Madison, A. J., Smith, S. D., Stone, D. A., . . . Lizonitz, J. M. (2015). National health expenditure projections, 2014–24: Spending growth faster than recent trends. *Health Affairs, 34*(8), 1407–1417. doi:10.1377/hlthaff.2015.0600

Kulesher, R. (2015). Transformation of the urban health care safety net: The devolution of a public responsibility. *The Health Care Manager, 34*(4), 279–287. doi:10.1097/hcm.0000000000000076

Lingle, B., & Zuvekas, S. H. (2008). Financing. In B. L. Levin, P. D. Hurd, & A. Hanson (Eds.), *Introduction to public health in pharmacy* (pp. 175–204). Sudbury, MA: Jones & Bartlett.

Mahendraratnam, N., Dusetzina, S. B., & Farley, J. F. (2017). Prescription drug utilization and reimbursement increased following state Medicaid expansion in 2014. *Journal of Managed Care & Specialty Pharmacy, 23*(3), 355–363. doi:10.18553/jmcp.2017.23.3.355

Martin, A. B., Hartman, M., Benson, J., & Catlin, A. (2016). National health spending in 2014: Faster growth driven by coverage expansion and prescription drug spending. *Health Affairs, 35*(1), 150–160. doi:10.1377/hlthaff.2015.1194

Martin, A. B., Hartman, M., Washington, B., & Catlin, A. (2017). National health spending: Faster growth in 2015 as coverage expands and utilization increases. *Health Affairs, 36*(1), 166–176. doi:10.1377/hlthaff.2016.1330

Medicaid, and CHIP Payment and Access Commission. (2016, January). *Medicaid spending for prescription drugs* (Issue Brief). Retrieved from https://www.macpac.gov/wp-content/uploads/2016/01/Medicaid-Spending-for-Prescription-Drugs.pdf

Medicaid, and CHIP Payment and Access Commission. (2017, January). *Recommendations for the future of CHIP and children's coverage.* Washington, DC: Authors. Retrieved from https://www.macpac.gov/wp-content/uploads/2017/01/Recommendations-for-the-Future-of-CHIP-and-Childrens-Coverage.pdf

Mehrotra, A., Sorbero, M. E., & Damberg, C. L. (2010). Using the lessons of behavioral economics to design more effective pay-for-performance programs. *American Journal of Managed Care, 16*(7), 497–503.

Mendelson, A., Kondo, K., Damberg, C., Low, A., Motuapuaka, M., Freeman, M., . . . Kansagara, D. (2017). The effects of pay-for-performance programs on health, health care use, and processes of care: A systematic review. *Annals of Internal Medicine, 166*(5), 341–353. doi:10.7326/m16-1881

Mitchell, E. M. (2016). *Concentration of health expenditures in the U.S. civilian noninstitutionalized population, 2014* (Medical Panel Expenditure Panel Survey, Statistical brief #497). Rockville, MD: Agency for Healthcare Research and Quality. Retrieved from https://meps.ahrq.gov/data_files/publications/st497/stat497.shtml

Mossialos, E., Wenzl, M., Osborn, R., & Sarnak, D. (Eds.). (2016). *2015 international profiles of health care systems.* New York: Commonwealth Fund.

National Association of Insurance Commissioners. (2011). *Health insurance exchanges under the Affordable Care Act: Governance options and issues.* Washington, DC: Author. Retrieved from http://www.naic.org/store/free/HIE-OP.pdf

National Council of State Legislators. (2016). State pharmaceutical assistance programs. Denver, CO: Author. Retrieved from http://www.ncsl.org/research/health/state-pharmaceutical-assistance-programs.aspx

Neuhausen, K., Davis, A. C., Needleman, J., Brook, R. H., Zingmond, D., & Roby, D. H. (2014). Disproportionate-share hospital payment reductions may threaten the financial stability of safety-net hospitals. *Health Affairs, 33*(6), 988–996. doi:10.1377/hlthaff.2013.1222

Newhouse, J. P. (1992). Medical care costs: How much welfare loss? *The Journal of Economic Perspectives, 6*(3), 3–21.

Ngorsuraches, S., & Mort, J. R. (2016). Examining the value of subsidies of health plans and cost-sharing for prescription drugs in the health insurance marketplace. *American Health & Drug Benefits, 9*(7), 368–377.

Office of the Assistant Secretary for Planning and Evaluation. (2017). *2016 poverty guidelines.* Washington, DC: U.S. Department of Health and Human Services. Retrieved from https://aspe.hhs.gov/poverty-guidelines

Okunad, A. A., & Murthy, V. N. (2002). Technology as a "major driver" of health care costs: A cointegration analysis of the Newhouse conjecture. *Journal of Health Economics, 21*(1), 147–159.

Serra-Sastre, V., & McGuire, A. (2012). Technology diffusion and substitution of medical innovations. *Advances in Health Economics and Health Services Research, 23,* 149–175.

Staff. (2015). Game changer: HHS sets goals for basing payments on quality. *Hospital Case Management, 23*(4), 45–47.

Truffer, C. J., Wolfe, C. J., & Rennie, K. E. (2016). *2016 actuarial report on the financial outlook for Medicaid.* Washington, DC: Department of Health & Human Services, Centers for Medicare & Medicaid Services. Retrieved from https://www.cms.gov/Research-Statistics-Data-and-Systems/Research/ActuarialStudies/Downloads/MedicaidReport2016.pdf

U.S. Department of Veterans Affairs. (2017). *Budget in brief.* Washington, DC: Author. Retrieved from https://www.va.gov/budget/docs/summary/Fy2017-BudgetInBrief.pdf

Vistnes, J., Zawacki, A., Simon, K., & Taylor, A. (2012). Declines in employer-sponsored insurance between 2000 and 2008: Examining the components of coverage by firm size. *Health Services Research, 47*(3 Part 1), 919–938. doi:10.1111/j.1475-6773.2011.01368.x

Young, G., Meterko, M., White, B., Sautter, K., Bokhour, B., Baker, E., & Silver, J. (2010). Pay-for-performance in safety net settings: Issues, opportunities, and challenges for the future. *Journal of Healthcare Management 55*(2), 132–141; discussion 141–132.

Zuvekas, S. H., & Cohen, J. W. (2010). Paying physicians by capitation: Is the past now prologue? *Health Affairs, 29*(9), 1661–1666. doi:10.1377/hlthaff.2009.0361

Zuvekas, S. H., & Cohen, J. W. (2016). Fee-for-service, while much maligned, remains the dominant payment method for physician visits. *Health Affairs, 35*(3), 411–414. doi:10.1377/hlthaff.2015.1291

Zuvekas, S. H., & Hill, S. C. (2004). Does capitation matter? Impacts on access, use, and quality. *Inquiry, 41*(3), 316–335.

11

Pharmacoeconomics

SCOTT K. GRIGGS AND PETER D. HURD

Pharmacoeconomics and the applications of pharmacoeconomics principles are important components of public health pharmacy today much as they were when the first edition of this book was published (Shaw & Delate, 2008). While a pharmacoeconomic justification is often provided in dollars spent or lives saved, the implications for the health of a community can be just as important, and the United States' response to the Zika virus illustrates both the costs and the politics of public health.

Zika was categorized as a Public Health Emergency of International Concern in February of 2016 by the World Health Organization (WHO) as the WHO reacted to the number of babies being born at the start of 2016 with very small heads (microcephaly) (Chan, 2017). The impact of a mosquito bite for a pregnant mother was devastating, and continued study led to the discovery of a cluster of symptoms referred to as Congenital Zika Syndrome (CZS). While the virus was identified in 1947, the disease had little impact in the Americas until 2015 (Chan, 2017). In the United States, President Obama requested funding in February of 2016 to deal with the impending threat for the southern United States, but because of political disagreements in Congress, funding was not approved until September of 2016 (Greer & Singer, 2017). As this chapter points out, during that time budgets meant for other national or state or local priorities had to be shifted to combatting mosquitos and a season of mosquito control was underfunded (the gap between February and August). While the economic costs of prevention for a population and healthcare for those born with CZS is significant, the balance with human suffering is clearly illustrated in the Zika example and can be an important part of a pharmacoeconomic analysis.

Why Are Pharmacoeconomic Evaluations Important?

The United States has the most expensive health care and, not surprisingly, ranks first in total pharmaceutical spending in the world; however, this high price tag does not necessarily result in the world's best health care outcomes. In 2015, health care spending in the United States reached $3.21 trillion, which equates to $9,990 per person (17.8% of gross domestic product [GDP]), with retail prescription medications accounting for approximately 10% ($324.6 billion) of that total (Centers for Medicare & Medicaid Services [CMS], 2016). With respect to volume, approximately 4.4 billion total prescriptions were dispensed in 2015 (QuintilesIMS, 2016). Future increases in health care (and prescription) expenditures are predicted to be due, in part, to the aging of the US population, the higher percentage of individuals covered by health insurance, as well as rising health care and medication costs; thus increases in both health care utilization and health care costs are responsible for the creation of this perfect storm. Accordingly, 10-year projections (2016–2025) estimate that US health care spending will increase to $5.55 trillion, or $15,800 per person (19.9% of GDP), by 2025, which is an average growth rate of 5.6%. Prescription drug spending is projected to rise even more rapidly, at 6.3%, during this 10-year period. Reasons for the growth in prescription expenses include a predicted increase in the use of high-cost specialty medications such as biologics as well as an increased overall utilization, driven by demographics and insurance coverage expansion (CMS, 2016).

Global expenditures for medicines are expected to reach $1.4 trillion by 2020, an increase of $349 billion, or about 30%, from 2015 (QunitilesIMS, 2015). The primary drivers for this growth are increased access to pharmaceuticals in emerging countries, increased utilization of branded medications in developed markets, and increased use of less expensive generics after patent expiration. Global medicine use in 2020 will reach an astonishing 4.5 trillion doses, corresponding to a 24% increase from 2015. Better access to medications globally will lead to the consumption of greater than one dose per person per day by more than half of the world's increasing population (7.6 billion in 2020). Notably, India, China, Brazil, Indonesia, and Africa will account for a majority of the projected global volume increase between 2015 and 2020 (QunitilesIMS, 2015).

Given the significant and growing cost of health care and medications, decision-makers are faced with the difficult dilemma of optimizing resources efficiently (i.e., the best bang for the buck) and effectively (relating to outcomes in the real world). With limited resources (e.g., time, money, labor, land, and knowledge), difficult choices must be made as to how best to achieve the goals of the organization or project. In order to achieve value in health care, and more specifically pharmaceuticals, decision-makers, health care professionals, and payers must better understand the relationship between costs (inputs) and outcomes. Costs are the resources (inputs) used in the creation or production of a good or service.

Pharmacoeconomics Defined

Pharmacoeconomics is a term that describes the identification, measurement, and evaluation of the costs as well as the consequences of the pharmaceutical product or service (Bootman, Townsend, & McGhan, 2005). The evaluation requires that two or more choices, or alternatives, be compared. To be a true pharmacoeconomic analysis, both the costs and the outcomes of the intervention (i.e., the medication or pharmacy service) must be considered and compared. In broad terms, pharmaco-economics encompasses the fields of health care economics as well as clinical and/ or humanistic pharmacy outcomes research via the evaluation of the *economic, clin-ical,* and *humanistic outcome* dimensions (ECHO) (Rascati, 2014). While the field of pharmacoeconomics is somewhat new, with the term *pharmacoeconomics* first appearing in the 1980s (Townsend, 1986), there has been a remarkable growth in the number of pharmacoeconomic studies published since its inception.

The economic evaluation of pharmaceuticals developed from the need to bet-ter understand a medication's relative worth or value. Value encompasses both the cost as well as the benefit of the intervention. While this term can be somewhat subjective—that is, what may be a value to one may not be to another—the impor-tance of this method of evaluating various alternatives, due to the rising costs of medications, is increasing rapidly. A primary goal, therefore, of pharmacoeconomic evaluation is to assist and inform decision-making based upon relevant alternatives (e.g., reviewing inclusion in a formulary review, developing treatment guidelines, or designing prescription benefit programs).

Pharmacoeconomic Cost Terms and Categories

Costs are computed to approximate the magnitude of resources (inputs) consumed when creating a product or service (Box 11-1). If a resource, such as time, is used for one task, it is no longer available for use on another task. The term *opportunity cost* describes the value of a resource in its next best use. This implies a choice between desirable yet mutually exclusive results and is not necessarily restricted to mone-tary or financial costs (e.g., time). The *price* or the amount charged (not the same as cost) is the amount of money that a consumer (or payer) is asked to pay for the product or service. The *amount of reimbursement* is the amount that is actually paid. The business, therefore, hopes that the reimbursed amount is greater than its cost to produce it.

Box 11-1 **Types of Costs**

Opportunity Cost
Price
Reimbursement Amount
Fixed Cost
Variable Cost
Average Cost
Incremental Cost

Economic evaluations use the terms *fixed* and *variable costs*. A *fixed cost* is a cost that does not change based upon either an increase or a decrease in production. An example of a fixed cost is the insurance on the physical building of a business, such as a pharmacy; the cost of the insurance is not dependent on the number of prescriptions or services rendered. A *variable cost* is affected by a change in volume. In a pharmacy, as the volume of prescriptions increases, the number of labels and vials would likewise increase.

An understanding of average and incremental (marginal) costs are fundamental to pharmacoeconomic analysis. The *average cost* is simply the total costs divided by the total units. If a bottle of #100 pills costs $50, the average cost would be $50 ÷ 100 = $0.50 per pill. *Incremental costs* (synonymous with marginal costs) are calculated between two alternatives such that the change in total costs is divided by the change in units (e.g., outcomes). If we compare two medications, where Drug A costs $80 with a 76% cure rate and Drug B costs $65 with a 64% cure rate, we find the difference in costs (numerator) and divide by the change in cure rate (denominator)—yielding $125 per added cure (($80 − $65) ÷ (0.76 − 0.64) = $15/ 0.12 = $125 per added cure). In this way, pharmacoeconomic evaluations can measure the average costs as well as the incremental costs between alternatives.

In an effort to categorize costs included in pharmacoeconomic analyses, four classifications are often used: direct medical, direct nonmedical, indirect, and intangible (Table 11-1). *Direct medical costs* are resources consumed to directly provide medical treatment. Examples include medications, hospitalizations, physician visits, ambulance service, and laboratory tests. *Direct nonmedical costs* are nonmedical resources consumed by the patient and/or family associated with treatment. Examples could include travel costs to receive medical care as well as food and lodging. In both of these first two cost classifications, the resources are "directly" related to care, and thus there is a direct transfer of money. *Indirect costs*, however, relate to loss of productivity due to illness or death. The lost productivity could be for the patient, a family member, or an unpaid caregiver. Finally, *intangible costs* are costs that are associated with pain, suffering, anxiety, and fatigue due to illness or as a result

Table 11-1 **Factors Leading to Increased Drug Prices**

Drug Shortages	Raw materials, plant closings, business decisions to
Decreased Competition	stop production
Specialty Medications	Mergers, acquisitions of companies or of products
Advertising	Commercial trends
Research and Development	Direct to consumer advertising
	Increasing costs and time necessary

of the treatment. Different costs may be incurred based upon many factors, including the patient's condition, treatment, employment, and location. Furthermore, it is possible that all four types of costs may be included in a pharmacoeconomic study.

In an article that reviewed the literature to explore ways to reduce drug costs in acute care settings, McConnell and colleagues (2017) discussed a number of factors that are leading to increased costs of medications. Some of the factors, such as drug shortages, can be caused by business decisions (a company decides to cease production of a particular product), regulation problems (a production line is shut down until a manufacturing issue is changed to meet regulations), or changes in demand for the product. Another factor would be specialty drugs, which are high in cost and can require special administration or special handling or have limited availability. The increase in the number of these specialty products is part of the increasing costs of medications in general.

McConnell et al. (2017) searched PubMed for terms such as *cost control* or *cost savings* through March 2016. They identified four major steps for the in-patient hospital setting: (a) develop an interdisciplinary oversight committee, (b) develop a process to identify opportunities, (c) implement strategies, and (d) assess outcomes. This would, of course, be a circular process and would continue as new products reached the market. Physicians need to be on board and willing to work to reduce costs, and patients preferences need to be aligned with treatments. Purchasing, utilization, and cost data need to be included in regular reports and become a part of the decision-making process. Inventory control, waste reduction, evidence-based medicine decisions, therapeutic interchanges, and drug restrictions are just a few of the suggestions to reduce costs. Cost control, like many public health endeavors, can require a group of cooperating individuals with a well-constructed plan and an effective assessment strategy.

Comparing Pharmacoeconomic Methodologies

A true pharmacoeconomic analysis must consider and compare both the costs and the consequences of the intervention (i.e., the medication or pharmacy service).

Table 11-2 **Comparison of Different Pharmacoeconomic Methodologies**

Method	Measurement	Assumptions	Example
Cost-Minimization Analysis	Dollars or other monetary cost equivalent	Outcomes other than cost are assumed to be equal	Comparing the same medication from two or more generic manufacturers
Cost-Effectiveness Analysis	Outcomes in the same natural units (blood pressure or life-years gained or symptoms) and costs	Decision-maker can determine the value of the incremental cost-effectiveness ratio	Comparison of two drugs with different costs and different impacts on the same outcome
Cost-Utility Analysis	Similar to cost-effective analysis but using quality-adjusted life-years	Analysis assesses utility and years of life saved	Comparison of two drugs that differ on quantity and quality of life
Cost-Benefit Analysis	Costs and outcomes are measured in dollars (or other monetary equivalent)	An economic value can be placed on medical outcomes like quality of life or decreased suffering	Comparison of two programs with different outcomes (e.g., flu vaccination and smoking cessation) by converting to dollar measures

There are four basic types of pharmacoeconomic approaches: (a) cost minimization, (b) cost effectiveness, (c) cost utility, and (d) cost benefit. Each of these four types of pharmacoeconomic analyses measures the costs in monetary units (e.g., US dollars); they differ, however, in the measurement of their outcomes (Table 11-2).

COST-MINIMIZATION ANALYSIS

The most basic of the pharmacoeconomic study designs is the cost-minimization analysis (CMA). The costs are measured in monetary units while *the outcomes are assumed to be equal.* CMAs are limited by this very important assumption. The primary application of this study design is in comparing two (or more) generic medications (i.e., drugs consisting of the same chemical entity and the same chemical properties but manufactured by different companies) at the same dose that are rated as equivalent by the Food and Drug Administration. Another potential use of the

CMA is where the same medication (same dose) is given to the patient in different settings (e.g., home versus clinic versus hospital); a specific example would be influenza vaccinations administered in a community pharmacy versus a clinic or physician's office (Rascati, 2014). If the outcomes are assumed to be equal but are not in fact measured, the study would be described as a cost analysis; in this case, the evaluation becomes merely a comparison of the respective costs, which is not a true pharmacoeconomic analysis. Last, some may consider CMAs as a type of cost-effectiveness analysis, whereby clinical outcomes are measured, and one cannot know a priori (before) that the outcomes are indeed equivalent.

COST-EFFECTIVENESS ANALYSIS

Cost-effectiveness analyses (CEA) are the most common pharmacoeconomic studies due to their measurement of *outcomes in natural units* (such as blood glucose, peak flow, life years gained, blood pressure, HgA1C, etc.). A benefit on this type of analysis is that it is most familiar to clinicians and practitioners, as it measures outcomes in clinical units. A disadvantage of this method is that the outcomes must be measured in the *same* clinical units or scale, such as serum cholesterol levels or mm Hg. Therefore, a cost-effectiveness analysis cannot compare dissimilar outcomes. Additionally, only one outcome can be measured at a time, for example percentage cured versus percentage cured, or symptom-free days versus symptom-free days.

When comparing more than one alternative in a cost-effectiveness analysis, the incremental cost-effectiveness ratio (ICER) is used:

$$\textbf{ICER} = \Delta\textbf{costs} \div \Delta\textbf{outcomes}$$

In an example where two medications are being compared, Drug A costs $200 and has a 78% success rate while Drug B costs $360 and has an 86% success rate. In this case, the difference in costs equals –$160 ($200 – $360) and the difference in outcomes is –8% success rate (78% – 86%). By dividing –$160 by –8% success rate, the result of this ICER is $20 per additional successful treatment. It is then up to the decision-maker (e.g., the patient or payer) to determine if the extra effectiveness (improvement in success rate) is worth the extra cost. Some may deem this extra cost worth it, while others may not.

COST-UTILITY ANALYSIS

Cost-utility analysis (CUA), sometimes considered a subtype of CEA, most commonly measures outcomes in quality-adjusted life-years (QALYs). A utility may be thought of as a preference or value for a health state, measured between 0.0 and 1.0, where zero represents death and 1.0 represents perfect health. To calculate the QALYs, the utility measure is multiplied by the years of life saved. If, for example, the utility score is 0.75 and the years of life saved is 4.0, the resulting QALYs would be 3.0 QALYs (0.75 utility × 4 years = 3.0 QALYs). Similar to the aforementioned CEA, the CUA compares two alternatives via the incremental cost-utility ratio (ICUR), where the outcome measure is the QALY. Thus the ICUR is simply Δ costs ÷ Δ QALYs (Griggs, 2017).

COST-BENEFIT ANALYSIS

The fourth type of pharmacoeconomic analysis is the cost-benefit analysis (CBA), which measures both costs and *outcomes in dollars* (or monetary unit). By converting outcomes into dollars, comparisons can now be made between alternatives that are very different. A vaccination program could be compared to an HIV awareness program or a diabetes education initiative with a cancer screening. Additionally, multiple interventions (more than two) can be compared at the same time, with the option that yields the highest benefit to cost ratio being preferred. A drawback of the CBA is that it can be difficult and controversial to place an economic value on medical outcomes such as human life, pain, suffering, satisfaction, anxiety, fatigue, and quality of life. Additionally, CBAs tend to favor those who are employed (versus children, elderly, or the unemployed) and those who are wealthier (as they have a greater ability to pay when valuing healthcare options).

Steps in Conducting a Pharmacoeconomic Evaluation

When evaluating pharmacoeconomic literature, there is not just one, specific, accepted methodology. Instead there may be various criteria depending on the type of question being considered. Nevertheless, conducting a pharmacoeconomic evaluation contains a number of essential elements—five are listed here.

The first step is to determine if there is one or more clearly defined research questions or objectives. This purpose or objective statement is usually found toward the beginning of the article. An example of an objective statement might be: "The purpose of this study is to evaluate the cost-effectiveness of metformin versus acarbose versus lifestyle modification in type 2 diabetes mellitus." Additionally, the type of study, described earlier as CMA, CEA, CUA, or CBA, is commonly stated in the purpose statement.

The second step is to ascertain if appropriate comparators (alternatives) were considered. While a degree of medical knowledge is helpful, the most clinically appropriate therapy (or therapies) should be considered. We see in the previous purpose statement that two medications are being evaluated along with a nonmedication option. It is also possible that one of the choices is to do nothing. The alternatives should be described in enough detail so that the study could be replicated.

A third critical step is to identify the perspective of the analysis. Pharmacoeconomic studies may take the perspective of the patient, the payer (e.g., the health insurer or government), the provider (e.g., health system, hospital, or clinic), the employer, or society. In essence, the perspective of the study determines whose costs are being assessed and which costs are considered relevant (Bootman, 2005). From the patient's perspective, his or her out-of-pocket expenses (e.g., copayments, deductibles, coinsurance, and transportation costs) would be important, but these would not be the relevant costs for private insurance payer. Some studies incorporate more than one perspective, depending on the research question(s) presented. Using a patient perspective (outcome preference), for example, may make it more difficult to show that a novel treatment modality is cost-effective when compared to older, less expensive therapies. A patient perspective can be justified for a constrained condition and selected treatments. However, from a public health perspective, the population (societal) perspective is preferred, especially when evaluating the cost-effectiveness of novel health care technologies with disease-targeted preference-weighted indices (Shaw, 2011).

The fourth step is to confirm whether relevant costs are included or are missing. The appropriate costs, based upon the three previous steps, must be identified, measured, and valued. If the study extends more than a year into the past, *adjustment* (or standardization) is utilized to bring past costs to a single point in time. This ensures that costs are valued at one point in time, even though they may have been collected in different years. In general, goods and services, including health care, become more expensive over time. There is a time preference for money such that a dollar today is worth more than a dollar tomorrow. Thus, in the event that a study extends into the future, *discounting* brings future costs to the present. The *discount rate* (e.g., 3%) is used in the calculation to approximate the cost of capital and can be varied up and down (e.g., 0% to 6%) via a sensitivity analysis. Sensitivity analyses test assumptions or items of uncertainty, such as the discount rate, in order to determine how confident we are in the estimate(s).

The fifth and final step would be to confirm that the outcome(s) are correctly identified and measured. The outcome(s) of the study depend upon the study design, the comparators, and the time frame of the project. Outcomes may range from symptom-free days (e.g., seasonal allergies) to reduction in mm Hg (e.g., hypertension) to QALYs (e.g., both quantity and quality of life for a cancer treatment).

The importance of accurate reporting of economic evaluations cannot be stressed enough, especially in the contribution of real-world evidence to the larger clinical and policy decision-making process. However, as discussed already, there are numerous methodological challenges to trial-based evaluations. The collection of reliable data on resource use and cost, choice of health outcome measure, calculating minimally important differences, dealing with missing data, extrapolating outcomes and costs over time, and the analysis of multinational trials add levels of complexity to the selection, modeling, and extrapolation of these studies. In 2013, the International Society for Pharmacoeconomics and Outcomes Research published the Consolidated Health Economic Evaluation Reporting Standards (CHEERS) (Husereau et al., 2013). The CHEERS Good Reporting Practices Task Force intends for the CHEERS guidelines to help standardize the reporting of health economic evaluations and to assist editors and peer reviewers in the assessment of economic evaluations. Using a checklist framework, the 24-item CHEERS guideline also explains the rationale for why and how specific elements of economic evaluations should be reported. There are additional studies and proposed guidelines on how to conduct specialty economic evaluations, such as those that are done in concert with randomized trials (Hughes et al., 2016; Petrou & Gray, 2011; Thorn, Noble, & Hollingworth, 2014) or "mapping" preference-based outcomes measures, such health utility values, using data on other indicators or measures of health (Petrou et al., 2015).

Decision Analysis in Pharmacoeconomic Studies

Decision analysis is a systematic approach to comparing two or more decision options under conditions of uncertainty (Bootman, 20005). Prospective studies—research investigations that are conducted into the future—such as randomized control trials may take months or even years to perform and are very expensive. Decision analysis, on the other hand, uses analytic models, called decision trees, to more quickly and less expensively compare various alternatives. This technique provides a formal, transparent, and orderly approach for the decision-maker to identify the preferred course of action. One benefit of decision analysis is the ability to perform sensitivity analyses on the constructed model. Sensitivity analyses allow researchers to alter probabilities within the decision tree, such as side effects, cure rates, and costs, to very quickly determine the impact of changes where there is uncertainty. The ability of decision analysis, with the use of computer programs such as TreeAge Software©, to evaluate multiple decision options when collection of the data is not feasible, too expensive, or would take too long has made this technique more common in recent years. While simple decision trees are useful in comparing less complicated decision options, *Markov models* allow for the more accurate representation of more complex or chronic disease conditions, such as HIV, diabetes, cancer, or multiple sclerosis. Markov models add a time component to the decision model that permits the patient to move back and forth between heath states, such as well, sick, and dead. By allowing time intervals, called cycles, Markov models more closely represent many of the disease conditions that health care providers and patients experience.

Implications for Public Health and Pharmacy Practice

Globally, more health care providers (physicians, pharmacists, and hospital systems) are being reimbursed in a fundamentally different way. *Volume-based* health care reimbursement is being transformed into a *value-based* reimbursement system, where both costs and outcomes associated with patient care will be closely analyzed. Value-based pricing may be one of the methods to control medication costs in the future, and the CMS is considering this approach in 2017. While one can prove value in many ways, the drug cost to the insurer is tied to some type of performance that demonstrates the value of using the drug. Perhaps the drug has the desired outcomes such as a cure of the disease, or the drug may decrease the number of patients who require hospital care, the death rates might be shown to decrease, or the drug compares favorably to other drugs in the appropriate treatment category (e.g., cholesterol or a cancer treatment). For example, the rate of success can be used to determine the percentage of the drug price to be paid (put simply: a 75% cure rate would mean that the price of the drug is only 75% of what the manufacturer was charging—of course this is too simple for most health care situations). The challenge for this approach is largely in the formula that would determine reimbursement, the manner in which things can be quantified, and the large number of insurance companies that might differ on how agreements are to be made and modified.

Glode and May (2017) included value-based pricing as an intervention that could help control costs in their review of the rising costs of cancer pharmaceuticals and the interventions that could control such costs. Factors that contribute to rising costs included the high cost of cancer research and product development, the length and cost of clinical trials, and the nature of the marketplace where many economic principles may not apply (supply and patient demand, lack of choices, new drugs with unique values, etc.). Interventions to control cost included streamlining the research and approval process, changes in the marketplace, government involvement in negotiating pharmaceutical prices, value-based pricing, guidance to patients/providers making treatment decisions, resources to address costs, and clinical pathways based on evidence-based tools for treatment planning.

The chapter began with an example of the costs and politics of fighting Zika virus and ends with a contrast of costs and ethics, specifically regarding treatment for hepatitis C (HCV). The impact of this expensive treatment has been a challenge in balancing the cost considerations to insurance companies, and federal programs like Medicare and Medicaid, and the ethics of treating a disease that can be cured, resulting in the prevention of infection in others. Today there is a very effective but very expensive treatment for HCV, called sofosbuvir, that has a cure rate greater than 90%, but is priced at approximately $84,000 per treatment, which is roughly $1,000 per pill (Liao & Fischer, 2017). Liao and Fischer noted that similar treatments are cheaper in other settings (e.g., $50,000 to $60,000 in the United Kingdom) and that Medicaid beneficiaries include both low socioeconomic groups and individuals who are more likely to have HCV compared to the US population. This has, predictably, put significant demands on the state budgets associated with Medicaid. But the demand has differed from state to state, with more than 6% in some states and less than 0.5% in others (Liao & Fischer, 2017). One of the strategies to reduce costs has been to use coverage restrictions such as substance abuse history, HIV treatment status, and sometimes demonstrated substance abstinence over time. Their results suggested that not all types of strict restrictions reduced costs, but strict abstinence components were associated with a significant 1.03% decrease in Medicaid drug spending. This combination of medical, budgetary, and other preferences raises significant ethical and public health concerns in determining who will receive treatment and who will not qualify. Once again the pharmacoeconomic analysis is balanced by many other considerations.

In summary, pharmacists with a pharmacoeconomic background are creating a contribution to public health that will continue to grow as drug therapy becomes more complicated and interdisciplinary teams of health care providers become more essential. One of a pharmacist's contributions can be the awareness of pharmacoeconomic issues in areas of public health. When this is coupled with a sophisticated understanding of how medications work and how the health care system's forces operate, the opportunities for the pharmacy to make important contributions to health seem limitless.

References

Bootman, J. L., Townsend, R. J., & McGhan, W. F. (2005). *Principles of pharmacoeconomics* (3rd ed.). Cincinnati, OH: Harvey Whitney Book Company.

Chan, M. (2017). Zika: We must be ready for the long haul. [Press release]. Geneva: World Health Organization. Retrieved from http://www.who.int/mediacentre/commentaries/2017/zika-long-haul/en/

Centers for Medicare & Medicaid Services (2016). *National health expenditure data*. Baltimore, MD: U.S. Department of Health and Human Services. Retrieved from https://www.cms.gov/Research-Statistics-Data-and-Systems/Statistics-Trends-and-Reports/NationalHealthExpendData/Downloads/highlights.pdf

Globe, A. E. & May, M. B. (2017). Rising cost of cancer pharmaceuticals: Cost issues and interventions to control costs. *Pharmacotherapy*, 37(1): 85–93. doi:10.1002/phar.1867

Greer, S. L., & Singer, P. M. (2016). The United States confronts Ebola: suasion, executive action and fragmentation. *Health Economics, Policy, and Law*, 12(1), 81–104. doi:10.1017/s1744133116000244

Griggs, S. K., Coleman, C. I., Park, T., & Schafermeyer, K. W. (2017). Pharmacoeconomics. In K. S. Plake, K. W. Schafermeyer, & R. L. McCarthy (Eds.), *Introduction to health care delivery: A primer for pharmacists* (6th ed., pp. 451–481). Burlington, MA: Jones and Bartlett Learning.

Hughes, D., Charles, J., Dawoud, D., Edwards, R. T., Holmes, E., Jones, C., . . . Yeo, S. T. (2016). Conducting economic evaluations alongside randomised trials: Current methodological issues and novel approaches. *Pharmacoeconomics, 34*(5), 447–461. doi:10.1007/s40273-015-0371-y

Husereau, D., Drummond, M., Petrou, S., Carswell, C., Moher, D., Greenberg, D., . . . Loder, E. (2013). Consolidated Health Economic Evaluation Reporting Standards (CHEERS) statement. *Pharmacoeconomics, 31*(5), 361–367.

Liao, J. M., & Fischer M. A. (2017). Restrictions of hepatitis C treatment for substance-using Medicaid patients: Cost versus ethics. *American Journal of Public Health, 107*(6), 893–899. doi:10.2105/AJPH.2017.303748

McConnell, K. J., Guzman, O. E., Pherwani, N., Spencer, D. D., Van Cura, J. D., & Shea, K. M. (2017). Operational and clinical strategies to address drug cost containment in the acute care setting. *Pharmacotherapy, 37*(1), 25–35. doi:10.1002/phar.1858

Petrou, S., & Gray, A. (2011). Economic evaluation alongside randomised controlled trials: Design, conduct, analysis, and reporting. *BMJ, 342*, d1548. doi:10.1136/bmj.d1548

Petrou, S., Rivero-Arias, O., Dakin, H., Longworth, L., Oppe, M., Froud, R., & Gray, A. (2015). The MAPS Reporting Statement for studies mapping onto generic preference-based outcome measures: Explanation and elaboration. *Pharmacoeconomics, 33*(10), 993–1011. doi:10.1007/s40273-015-0312-9

QunitilesIMS. (2015). *Global medicines use in 2020: Outlook and implications.* Parsippany, NJ: Author. Retrieved from http://www.imshealth.com:90/en/thought-leadership/quintilesims-institute/reports/global-medicines-use-in-2020#ims-form

QuintilesIMS. (2016, April 16). IMS health study: U.S. drug spending growth reaches 8.5 percent in 2015 (Press release). Parsippany, NJ: Author. Retrieved http://www.imshealth.com/en/about-us/news/ims-health-study-us-drug-spending-growth-reaches-8.5-percent-in-2015

Rascati, K. (2014). *Essentials of pharmacoeconomics* (2nd ed.). Baltimore, MD: Lippincott Williams & Wilkins.

Shaw, J. W. (2011). Use of patient versus population preferences in economic evaluations of health care interventions. *Clinical Therapeutics, 33*(7), 898–900. doi:10.1016/j.clinthera.2011.06.009

Shaw, J. W. & Delate, T. (2008). Pharmacoeconomics, In B. L. Levin, P. D. Hurd, & A. Hanson (Eds.), *Introduction to public health in pharmacy* (pp. 227–246). Sudbury, MA: Jones and Bartlett.

Thorn, J. C., Noble, S. M., & Hollingworth, W. (2014). Methodological developments in randomized controlled trial-based economic evaluations. *Expert Review of Pharmacoeconomics & Outcomes Research, 14*(6), 843–856. doi:10.1586/14737167.2014.953934

Townsend, R. J. (1986). Post marketing drug research and development: An industry clinical pharmacist's perspective. *American Journal of Pharmacy Education, 50*, 480–482.

12

Evidence-Based Practice and Public Health

PATRICK J. BRYANT, PETER D. HURD, AND ARDIS HANSON

The Oxford English Dictionary (2017, para. 1) defines evidence as "the available body of facts or information indicating whether a belief or proposition is true or valid." We use evidence-based approaches every day in medicine and public health for problem-solving and for decision-making. However, the most difficult step of evidence-based medicine (EBM) and evidence-based public health (EBPH) is to link the evidence with current clinical knowledge and experience. Although both EBM and EBPH emphasize proof of efficacy, EBPH also must have evidence of protective efficacy and effectiveness before an agency or organization launches a control or eradication program (Jenicek, 1997). This is critical since any population-based health programming, including health promotion and disease prevention, should prove themselves beneficial (Jenicek, 1997, p. 193).

The evidence-based process is the framework for this chapter. In this chapter, we examine relevant background issues, including concepts underlying EBM, EBPH, and definitions of evidence; describe key analytic tools to enhance the adoption of evidence-based decision-making; and finish with challenges and opportunities for implementation in public health practice.

Evidence-Based Medicine: A Brief History

In the 1970s, faculty at the McMaster Medical School in Canada were in the process of developing a clinical learning strategy they called "evidence-based medicine" (Evidence-Based Medicine Working Group, 1992). Concurrently, Archibald Cochrane and David Sackett were working on the tenets of evidence-based medicine. Cochrane's (1972) *Effectiveness and Efficiency: Random Reflections on Health Services,* was influential in promoting evidence-based clinical practice, calling for relevant, valid research conducted in a systematic fashion. He promoted the use of cumulative evidence (i.e., systematic reviews), and today, the Cochrane name stands for explicit quality criteria for the appraisal of published research. Sackett, a clinical epidemiologist, who was significantly influenced by the importance of a well-documented clinical trial, turned his attention to evaluating clinical research for evidence of best clinical practices (Sackett, 2015). Working with colleagues, Sackett et al. (1996, p. 71) defined EBM as "the conscientious and judicious use of current best evidence in making decisions about the care of individual patients." They further defined the practice of EBM as "integrating individual clinical expertise with the best available external clinical evidence from systematic research . . . especially from patient centered clinical research" (Sackett et al., 1996, pp. 71–72).

Today, thanks to the pioneering efforts of Cochrane, Sackett, and others, we have international registries of randomized and quasi-randomized controlled trials, centers for evidence-based medicine across the world, stringent protocols for the systematic review of the literature, and evolving clinical learning strategies to improve patient care and outcomes.

Prior to the establishment of these evidence-grounded processes, medicine primarily was practiced using a "sage" model, which put the clinician's clinical experience and judgment in the center of making decisions involving patients. However, studies show that relying on clinical experience and/or judgment to make a clinical decision tends to overestimate efficacy and underestimate safety risks associated with therapy (Balogh, Miller, & Ball, 2015; Cook, Guyatt, Laupacis, & Sackett, 1992; Institute of Medicine, 2009, 2013; Kohn, Corrigan, & Donaldson, 2000). Hence, many medical errors occur under conditions of uncertainty, when data is ambiguous and judgmental heuristics and biases come into play.

Interestingly, many health care professionals did not accept the EBM process when it was first proposed. Only relatively recently has EBM been accepted more completely. The influence of managed care on the way physicians make decisions and practice medicine these days has played a part in the acceptance of EBM principles. However, although EBM is used to compile practice guidelines that determine the norm for how diseases should be treated, few guidelines lead to consistent changes in provider behavior, especially with the persistence of the "autonomous medical decision maker" model (Timmermans & Mauck, 2005, p. 26). On the other hand, advances in implementation science provide insight into the adoption of new ways of working and have increased the acceptance of EBM (Rapport et al., 2017; Sedlar, Bruns, Walker, Kerns, & Negrete, 2017).

The emphasis on established patient-centered scientific evidence requires health care professionals to evaluate the literature systematically to establish the quality of the study design, the conduct of the trial, and the significance of the study. We discuss best practices and reviewing the literature in detail in the section on key analytic tools.

Evidence-Based Public Health: A Brief History

Evidence-based public health (EBPH) has been defined as "the development, implementation, and evaluation of effective programs and policies in public health through application of principles of scientific reasoning, including systematic uses of data and information systems, and appropriate use of program planning models" (Brownson, Gurney, & Land, 1999, p. 87). This definition emphasizes the importance of empirical reasoning in appraising and interpreting evidence derived from the use of specific public health models, studies, and data.

Key components of EBPH include making decisions using the best available scientific evidence, systematically using data and information systems, applying program planning frameworks, engaging stakeholders and the community in decision-making, conducting sound evaluation, and disseminating lessons learned (Brownson, Fielding, & Maylahn, 2009). Further, the eight core domains and 26 competencies for EBPH are likely to improve decision-making in public health practice to better address agency-level conditions and practices (Brownson et al., 2009). This is a critical component when we are examining interventions from a population or public health perspective.

There are many issues when evaluating the effectiveness of public health programs. Consider the following prevention programs, one in California, and one in Missouri. The California Tobacco Control Program determined increased tobacco taxes and a successful media campaign led to a drop in the sale of cigarettes and a decrease in smoking (Brownson et al., 1999). The drop in both sales of cigarettes and in smoking (for 1988–1993) was double the expected rate based on the previous sales/smoking trend (for 1974–1987) and substantiated the success of the program.

The Missouri Take a Seat, Please! (TASP) Program, designed to decrease motor vehicle injuries and deaths among children, attempted to increase compliance with Missouri's child restraint legislation. Volunteers sent business-reply postcards to the Missouri Department of Health to "report" drivers who were ignoring the law. Those drivers then received information about the importance of using child safety seats. Two years later, TASP was evaluated. Although Missouri discontinued the program due to lack of effectiveness, other states adopted similar programs, with little supporting evidence (Brownson et al., 1999). Decades later, universal implementation of proper child restraint use in cars is still problematic (Sauber-Schatz, Thomas, & Cook, 2015). These two examples highlight both the need for EBPH and the reality that many public health education programs could benefit from an EBPH approach.

One of the challenges in EBPH is finding and assessing the evidence. Brownson et al. (1999, 2003) suggest two categories of evidence: Type 1 and Type 2. Type 1 evidence examines risk-disease relations (i.e., the magnitude, severity, and preventability of identified public health problems). Type 2 evidence examines the relative effectiveness of specific interventions designed to address an identified public health problem. Rychetnik, Hawe, Waters, Barratt, and Frommer (2004) suggest a third type of evidence, Type 3, which highlights implementation of the intervention, including design, contextual circumstances of the implementation environment, and the reception of the implementation by its stakeholders/patients. Clearly, the descriptive and/or qualitative information gathered in Type 3 evidence would complement the more quantitative data gathered in Type 1 and 2 evidence. It would also complete the snapshot as to identifying a problem that needs to be solved, what should be done to solve the problem, and how the solution should be implemented.

Public health approaches also typically include a needs assessment of a community sometimes coupled with an economic analysis comparing the costs, benefits, and effectiveness of interventions. Ideally, stakeholders also assess the project during and after implementation using formative and summative evaluations. Yet, from a practical viewpoint, a project may address a new public health problem, but stakeholders need to use the best *available* evidence rather than the *perfect* set of information.

Comparing EBM and EBPH

While both EBM and EBPH are based on the use of the best evidence to inform decisions, the two approaches differ in important ways. Perhaps the most fundamental difference is the EBPH focus on groups of people in a community and the EBM responsibility for individual patient care. EBPH will be planning community interventions and EBM will be writing a patient's prescription. Public health places a greater emphasis on health promotion and disease prevention for communities, while EBM focuses on the treatment plan for a patient, which may include recommendations to help prevent further disease ("take this medication for your blood pressure") and promote health ("exercise more"). EBM has more of a diagnosis imperative ("does the patient have Zika?") while EBPH focuses on surveillance and protection components ("what evidence is available regarding where the Zika virus is currently causing disease; what can the community do to minimize this risk?"). EBM includes randomized controlled trials (RCTs) more often than for EBPH, where epidemiological research and quasi-experimental approaches are more commonly used.

Another key differentiating characteristic between EBPH and EBM is the type of trials used to develop the evidence for decision-making purposes. With EBPH, large observational epidemiologic-type trials with many variables and confounders are used to study a population and gain insights into that population's health issues. The randomized clinical trial, which represents a relatively smaller trial size due to expense and inclusion/exclusion criteria used to limit the number of variables and confounding factors, is the "holy grail" for EBM. Since pharmaceutical companies generate and support much of the clinical research, government agencies, such as the Food and Drug Administration in the United States or the Medicines and Healthcare Products Regulatory Agency in the United Kingdom, have strict guidelines on the conduct of these studies, often in concert with other federal or national funding agencies.

RCTs are explanatory trials conducted in ideal conditions with carefully chosen groups to determine the *efficacy* of a specific drug or intervention. To be clinically meaningful, results must be relevant to specific patient populations in specific settings. Efficacy studies generally are conducted in large tertiary-care referral health centers, which mean more innovative technologies and available specialty providers. Subjects typically live near to these facilities, are often better educated, and have better insurance coverage. These carefully constructed trials of a potential new medication can be fundamental in showing that the compound does make a difference (efficacy). However, this difference is demonstrated under carefully controlled conditions and with patients who may not have complicating environmental or medical factors.

The design of an RCT shows the efficacy of a drug in ideal conditions with carefully chosen groups, including a comparison group. When these carefully constructed trials of a potential new medication are conducted, they can be fundamental in showing that the compound itself makes a difference, not some other variable. However, this difference is demonstrated under carefully controlled conditions and with patients who may not have complicating environmental or medical factors.

Effectiveness trials are pragmatic trials, which measure the degree of beneficial effect of drugs or other behavioral interventions. These trials occur in "real-world" clinical settings, affected by geography (urban vs. rural) and/or health care systems (neighborhood clinic vs. hospital, Medicaid vs. private payer). Hence, hypotheses and study designs of an effectiveness trial are formulated based on conditions of routine clinical practice and on outcomes essential for clinical decisions. Unlike medicine, which uses the efficacy of an RCT (effects of treatment) as its gold standard, public health interventions are judged more frequently on their effectiveness. Does the drug work in the "real world" of patients with multiple disease states, genetic differences, who have poor adherence to treatment, or who take multiple medications? Again, moving between EBM and EBPH can be critical for optimum health care but should be done cautiously.

Comparing EBM of Individuals and Populations

EBM principles can be used to make clinical decisions for an individual patient and/or a specific patient population, such as a state Medicaid population (Bryant

& Pace, 2009). With individual patient clinical decisions, the practitioner has the advantage of having the medical and medication history of the patient. For this reason, health care providers can consider a more aggressive approach to therapy. Not only do providers know specifics about *this* patient, such as allergies, previously failed therapies, comorbid disease state/disorders, but they also know whether the current decision is the final attempt to help the patient.

When entire patient populations are involved in the decision-making process, providers generally do not have this type of detailed information generally for each of the patients. In the case of a state Medicaid population, for example, aggregate data would be easily available as to frequency and instance of treatment for particular disorders. For this reason, a more cautious or conservative approach to making the clinical decision is appropriate. In both situations, the same evidence-based process is utilized; however, at the point of making the actual decision based on the evidence, the clinician should take into consideration the individual patient versus an entire patient population as the target for the therapeutic decision.

Comparing EBPH to Individuals and Populations

Epidemiology is a central component in most public health programs. Applying this group-focused approach to a patient-care setting has been called clinical epidemiology (Sackett, Haynes, Guyatt, & Tugwell, 1991), blending more of the science approach to clinical medicine. Terms, such as "relative risk reduction" and "number needed to treat," use evidence to help decide what the best therapy might be for a patient.

In a similar way, pharmacoeconomic analysis, also used in EBPH, analyzes the cost-effectiveness of treatments and the "quality-adjusted life years" that are associated with different interventions, medication therapy, or preventive approaches to improve patient outcomes. Health care providers use these data (based on groups of individuals) to make individual patient treatment decisions. Although moving between EBM and EBPH can be critical for optimum health care, such moves should be done cautiously, using a standardized framework for selection of best practices to facilitate optimal utilization of evidence-based practice.

Evidence-Based Decision-Making

To help explain the importance of EBPH, one might start by exploring some of the ways by which individuals make decisions. Different decision-making strategies and approaches have both strengths and drawbacks; hence, each strategy or approach needs consideration before adoption. While one hopes individuals make decisions in the best possible way, human nature often plays a role that can confound the process. Decisions are subjective; they often have an emotional component (e.g., "we are in love," "I believe in this treatment," "they feel very strongly about this decision"). This emotional energy often drives researchers to find a cure to a disease. In today's health environment, however, the focus has shifted to an evidence-based framework.

Evidence-based decision-making is both a product and a process for making decisions about a program, practice, or policy. A group uses the best available research evidence, practice (experiential) evidence, and relevant contextual evidence as it works through the decision-making process. Evidence-based decision-making requires participants to gather evidence, interpret the evidence, and apply what they have learned from the evidence. This requires drawing upon stakeholder knowledge and expertise and using evidence that is replicable, credible, verifiable, and observable. It also requires a process to address the underlying subjective responses humans have, individually and as a group, regardless of how objective they try to be.

To explore this emotional component and learn ways of using an awareness of one's emotional response in working effectively with others, Bradberry and Greaves (2009) developed "Emotional Intelligence 2.0," an effective way to develop personal competence through self-awareness and self-management and then social competence through social awareness and relationship management. These skills can be crucial for those implementing and using evidence-based decision-making in the application of EBPH by reducing the subjective-only component in favor of established research and published findings. Being objective is a challenge and a central component of EBPH.

While not seen as "emotional" choices, health care professionals often base clinical or health decisions on experience, perhaps related to a "gut feeling" or a similarity with other cases or events. A complex, iterative, and collaborative activity, the decision-making process takes time and occurs within the context of an identified health problem and system. The goal is to reduce uncertainty, narrow down possibilities, and develop a more precise understanding of the health problem under review. Hence, finding a pattern or comparing to a prototype case can be a very effective way of making an initial decision, especially for those with a strong background in critical areas.

Unfortunately, research suggests that physicians providing health care to adults will follow literature-recommended approaches about half the time (McGlynn et al., 2003). Those practitioners who feel they can judge the level of adherence to a prescribed drug or procedure often are wrong when reviewing the actual data. Again, basing judgments on appropriate data can lead to decisions that are more effective.

Similarly, a straightforward logical approach would seem to lead to an unbiased decision; however, that assumes the information available is relatively complete and correct. Research can be following a logical pathway or testing a logical hypothesis only to find that the data do not support the "logical" approach because other factors have not been considered, or sometimes even discovered. This can be the beginning of a great discovery, but it also helps illustrate the challenges of decision-making.

Epidemiology, one of the foundational disciplines in public health, generally brings a macro-centered perspective for decision-making. However, clinical epidemiology shifted its focus from a community setting approach to focusing on groups of patients and individual patients in clinical settings in the 1960s (Feinstein, 1985). Using the clinical epidemiologic approach, Sackett and colleagues (1991) examined different strategies of clinical diagnosis that illustrate different ways of thinking in a clinical setting. The intent was to improve the credibility and validity of the RCT for both groups of patients and individual patients, determine the benefit of the medication or intervention, and improve compliance with best standards of care.

Combining good evidence-based information with good clinical judgment takes skill, knowledge, and years of experience. Using an EBM process, pharmacists can answer clinical questions more accurately and determine if one medication is more suitable than another and address alternative or behavioral approaches to care.

Steps in the EBM Process for Pharmacy

Although several EBM processes are in current use, these processes tend to be complex, labor intensive, and time consuming, and they differ primarily in rigor. In an attempt to develop an EBM process for the busy clinician, faculty at the University of Missouri–Kansas City School of Pharmacy developed a process that has been used over the past 20 years to teach PharmD students who then apply the process to their practice following graduation (Bryant & Pace, 2009). This EBM process involves five steps: (1) define the question; (2) retrieve pertinent literature, (3) critically evaluate this literature, (4) categorize the quality of the literature, and (5) develop a conclusion/recommendation. To minimize complexity and assist users in incorporating the process into their decision-making process, we offer "10 Major Considerations" as a tool for critically evaluating the literature. The 10 considerations look at the strength and limitations of a number of variables. These variables include the power of the study, the appropriateness of the dosage/treatment/regimen; if the length of the study shows effect; if the inclusion and exclusion criteria are adequate; if the study blinded; if randomization similar across study groups; if the appropriate statistical tests are used; if the measures used have validity and reliability; and whether the results support the conclusions of the authors (Bryant & Pace, 2009).

The 10 Major Considerations assist in determining how well the researcher conducted and documented the study. If any one of these considerations is not present or present but not done appropriately, the study is potentially flawed. In most cases, the user will need to identify how this flaw could have affected the results before judging the usefulness of the article. In addition, a categorization of quality, modified from the Cook et al. (1992) Levels of Evidence rating system, is applied to the study that is based primarily on study design. This is similar to the many levels of evidence models that emphasize increasing rigor and quality of evidence, starting with the lowest level of evidence (5), generally interventional or observational studies with no randomization or control group, moving up to the highest level of evidence (1), interventional studies with randomized control groups, with power requirements met. In between, levels 3 and 4 are observational, with level 3 comprising nonrandomized prospective cohorts and level 4 comprised of nonrandomized retrospective cohorts. Level 2 is also comprised of randomized control groups; however, in these interventional studies, power requirements are not met.

To determine overall quality of a study, the user combines the results of the categorization step (study design) and how the study was conducted (10 Major Considerations). Once the quality of the study or studies is determined, it is possible to formulate an evidence-based conclusion and/or recommendation.

Along with the recommendation, researchers develop a series of justification statements to support the conclusion/recommendation. These justification statements should cover efficacy, safety, cost, and other considerations such as route and frequency of therapy obtained from the article(s) evaluated. The supportive relationship between the justification statements and the recommendation statement centers upon efficacy, safety, cost, and other considerations. As mentioned in an earlier section of this chapter, the user needs to take into consideration whether this is a conclusion/recommendation for an individual patient (more aggressive) or a patient population (more conservative) clinical decision and modify the recommendation and justification statements accordingly.

Standard of Care and Clinical Practice Guidelines

Standard of care, a complex concept that has evolved over time, is currently defined as "that which a minimally competent physician in the same field would do under similar circumstances" (Moffett & Moore, 2011, p. 111). The decision of *Hall v. Hilbun* (1985), cited by Moffett and Moore (2011), among others, held physicians accountable to a competence-based national standard of care and a limited role of local custom. In brief, that means national standards are used to judge a doctor's duty of care to a patient, with respect to cognizance of what facilities are available locally. This is an important distinction when we look at the ongoing development of evidence-based care. Today, we can understand the standard of care more fully by examining the development of *clinical practice guidelines* that describe how to diagnosis and treat a particular disease state or disorder.

In 1990, the Institute of Medicine (IOM) defined clinical practice guidelines as "systematically developed statements to assist practitioner and patient decisions about appropriate health care for specific clinical circumstances" (Field, Lohr, & Committee to Advise the Public Health Service on Clinical Practice Guidelines, 1990). Twenty years later, the IOM redefined clinical practice guidelines as "statements that include recommendations intended to optimize patient care that are informed by a systematic review of evidence and an assessment of the benefit and harms of alternative care options" (Graham, Mancher, Wolman, Greenfield, & Steinberg, 2011). This was a major reworking of the 1990 IOM definition to distinguish clearly the differences between a clinical practice guideline and other expert or evidentiary texts, such as consensus statements, expert bodies, and other types of appropriate use criteria.

Examples of clinical practice guidelines are available from many agencies and professional associations from across the world. The World Health Organization (WHO; 2014, 2017) has a protocol for the development of its global clinical practice guidelines that incorporates equity, human rights, gender, and social determinants.

The U.S. Agency for Healthcare Research and Quality's (AHRQ; 2017) National Guideline Clearinghouse™ (NGC) is a publicly accessible database of evidence-based clinical guidelines from a variety of partners. The Institute for Clinical Systems Improvement, for example, a partnership of more than 50 medical groups and hospitals, has disseminated 152 evidence-based guidelines and protocols through the NGC.

Not only does the NGC provide summaries by clinical specialty, but guideline syntheses provide comparison discussions on selected guidelines and expert commentaries offer discussions on issues of importance to evidence-based practice, such as measure development and implementation concerns. AHRQ's Clinical Guidelines and Recommendations site also provides the *Guide to Clinical Preventive Services 2014*, which includes the recent U.S. Preventive Services Task Force recommendations on screening, counseling, and preventive medication topics in a variety of formats (AHRQ, 2014).

Evidence-based practice standards rely upon standard nomenclature, crosswalks between disparate terminologies across disciplines, and interoperability. All NGC summaries follow the NGC Template of Guideline Attributes, associated Glossaries, and Classification Scheme (AHRQ, 2016). These include controlled vocabularies from the U.S. National Library of Medicine's Medical Subject Headings and Unified Medical Language System, ECRI Institute's Universal Medical Device Nomenclature System, the International Classification of Diseases, and the U.S. Health Care Financing Administration Common Procedure Coding System to classify disease, treatment, and intervention concepts.

Clinical practice guidelines have also evolved over time, having initially been compiled by a consensus process among a group of experts in the area (Burgers,

Grol, Klazinga, Makela, & Zaat, 2003). The application of EBM principles has greatly increased the scientific validity of clinical practice guidelines by providing a systematic process of integrating the results from clinical trials with the clinical judgment/experience of these experts developing the document.

Standard of care and, more importantly, *minimal standard of care* are used in medical malpractice cases, and physicians are held to these standards by managed care and insurance providers (Boyd et al., 2005; Moffett & Moore, 2011). Often new information from clinical trials is created faster than the clinical practice guidelines are updated, and therefore the date of last revision should be checked (Shekelle et al., 2001). This requires the end users to update the clinical practice guidelines as needed since recommendations can change based on recent new studies. For this reason, it is imperative that practitioners and researchers use a systematic EBM process, such as the one described in this chapter, to assure a specific guideline is current as needed between formal revisions.

Other Evidence to Decision Analytic Tools

The need to assemble and systematically review the abundance of evidence on the effects of health care has led to the development of a number of evidence-synthesis strategies, based on the level of evidence, with their own vocabularies. The WHO (2014), for example, defines the quality of the evidence as the "extent to which one can be confident that an estimate of the effect or association is correct" in its evidence to decision (EtD) clinical framework for RCTs. The European Observatory on Health Systems and Policies uses health technology assessment to examine "the medical, organizational, economic and societal consequences of implementing health technologies or interventions within the health system" (Velasco-Garrido & Busse, 2005, p. 2) as does the U.S. National Library of Medicine's National Information Center on Health Services Research and Health Care Technology.

The Cochrane Collaboration is a nongovernmental organization that is truly international, with over 37,000 Cochrane collaborators from more than 130 countries. The Cochrane Library, part of the Cochrane Collaboration, contains the Cochrane Database of Systematic Reviews (CDSR), the Cochrane Central Register of Controlled Trials (CENTRAL), and the Cochrane Methodology Register (CMR). The CDSR contains all the Cochrane Reviews (approximately 9,800 systematic reviews) and review protocols prepared by the Cochrane Review Groups. The CENTRAL has more than 1 million registered trials, and the CMR has more than 15,700 trial methods. All of these reviews and protocols are peer-reviewed and prepared according to one of two stringent guidelines: the *Cochrane Handbook for Systematic Reviews of Interventions* or the *Cochrane Handbook for Diagnostic Test*

Accuracy (DTA) Reviews (Cochrane Screening and Diagnostic Tests Methods Group, 2017; Higgins & Green, 2011).

Other databases, such as PROSPERO (UK), an international database of prospectively registered systematic reviews, use the Cochrane guidelines in their trials registry for health and social sciences research where there is a health-related outcome care (e.g., social welfare, public health, education, crime, justice, and international development).

In addition to the Cochrane guidelines, there is the Grading of Recommendations Assessment, Development and Evaluation (GRADE) methodology (Guyatt et al., 2011; Guyatt et al., 2008; Mustafa et al., 2013). The GRADE approach attempts to separate the quality of evidence from the strength of the recommendations. This is an important distinction in that, although the quality of evidence influences the strength of a recommendation, it is important to determine the magnitude of the benefits and harms to public health (Davoli et al., 2015). Similar to the PICO model for clinical questions, the GRADE approach examines the relevant setting, as well as the population, intervention, comparator, and outcomes. These evidence-oriented organizations and their guidelines are representative of many other organizations also concerned with building a strong EtD knowledge base; hence there is a strong focus on the hierarchy of research designs (level of evidence) and the quality of the research execution.

However, there are a number of experimental and quasi-experimental studies that are used in addition to RCTs. Comparative effectiveness research studies and patient-centered outcomes studies, for example, systematically compare existing health care interventions to determine which provide the greatest benefits for which patients and are used increasingly in EtD. When building the evidence base for a particular medication or intervention, consistency in the syntheses of the studies is critical. Hence all syntheses begin with a formal protocol.

The *protocol* describes how the existing studies are found (the search strategies and eligibility criteria), how data from the selected studies will be extracted for analysis, how useful the studies are in answering the review question, and how the overall measure of effectiveness is determined. The protocol also describes the analytical approach used to calculate pooled prevalence estimates and discusses the use of meta-regression to assess how the studies' characteristics influence the prevalence estimates.

The *systematic review* summarizes the results of available controlled trials and provides a high level of evidence on the effectiveness of identified health care interventions. By explicitly stating a priori hypotheses and methods, without advance knowledge of results, systematic review protocols help minimize bias.

Meta-analyses are specific methodologic and statistical technique for combining quantitative data from RCTs. To minimize confounding variable bias, meta-analyses should be conducted with high methodological quality homogenous studies (Level

I or II) or evidence randomized studies. What is critical for these types of evidence-based syntheses and studies is that researchers clearly and thoroughly *document and report* the planned review methods, outcomes, and analyses. Complete transparency of the conduct of experimental research, systematic reviews, and meta-analyses permits reproducibility and improves fidelity of its conclusions.

Since the selective reporting of outcomes may bias the evidence base for clinical decision-making and policy, transparency is essential when documenting therapeutic efficacy. To facilitate the completeness and transparent reporting of trials and aid their critical appraisal and interpretation, there are a number of reporting guidelines used that help determine how well designed and executed the trials are, such as CONSORT, PRISMA, and methodologies, such as Statistical Analyses and Methods in the Published Literature (SAMPL).

The "CONsolidated Standards Of Reporting Trials" (CONSORT) Statement is an evidence-based minimum set of 25 recommendations with a checklist and flow diagram for reporting RCTs and their abstracts (CONSORT Group, 2017) as well as new guidelines for pilot and feasibility studies (Eldridge et al., 2016).

The Preferred Reporting Items for Systematic Reviews and Meta-analyses (PRISMA) guidelines emphasize that systematic reviews and meta-analyses are iterative processes, conducting research and reporting research are intertwined yet distinct concepts, risk of bias is addressed at the study level and the outcome level, and reporting biases are critical (Moher, Liberati, Tetzlaff, Altman, & PRISMA Group, 2009). Similar to the CONSORT statement, the PRISMA statement consists of a 27-item checklist and a four-phase flow diagram to aid in the reporting of systematic reviews and meta-analyses of RCTs and evaluations of interventions. More recently, the PRISMA-P (for protocols) 2015 documents the 17 items considered to be the minimum required components of a systematic review or meta-analysis protocol (Shamseer et al., 2015).

SAMPL addresses long-standing, widespread, and potentially serious statistical concerns in the biomedical literature with general principles for reporting statistical results (numbers and descriptive statistics); risk, rates, and ratios; hypotheses tests; association, correlation, and regression analyses; survival (time-to-event) analyses; and Bayesian analyses (Lang & Altman, 2015).

There are numerous other standards, such as Strengthening the Reporting of Observational Studies in Epidemiology (STROBE) Statement and the CARE Guidelines: Consensus-based Clinical Case Reporting Guideline Development. These reporting guidelines and many other quantitative and qualitative reporting standards can be found on the EQUATOR (Enhancing the Quality and Transparency Of health Research) Network site. In addition to the reporting guidelines and checklists, the site also features a simple flow chart to determine the most appropriate checklist and reporting guideline (UK EQUATOR Centre, 2013). Using that flowchart, an online EQUATOR wizard, developed in collaboration with Penelope Research, is available that checks uploaded manuscripts for completeness, data, ethics and permissions, statistics, citations and references, tables and figures, scientific reporting, and registry information for clinical trials (Penelope Research, 2017).

Journals, such as *BMC*, and editorial consortia, such as ICMJE, have adopted specific reporting guidelines for use in manuscript submissions, have established clinical trial registration policies, and are adding tools like PENELOPE to improve the rigor of reporting and improve the quality of manuscript submissions.

Implications for Public Health and Pharmacy Practice

Much like in EBM, which combines individual clinical experience with the best clinical evidence, those working in public health will benefit from a similar combination of experience and evidence. While some of the data may differ in methods of collection, data analysis, and focus, the process can lead to better health outcomes. Rather than making decisions about individual patients, however, EBPH is concerned with programs and policies that impact groups of people and populations.

Finding the best available evidence, as described in the EBM sections, is similar in EBPH. Perhaps in public health, review articles of the relevant scientific literature would be one of the most objective bodies of evidence (Brownson et al., 2009), and other searches of scientific literature would look at both journal articles and surveillance data from sources such as the Centers for Disease Control and Prevention or public health agencies (health data and prevalence information). Community need assessments and interactions would also be important but are more subjective, as would be personal experiences. Each of these types of evidence would be important in EBPH.

To illustrate the value of review articles, an evidence-based review by Marcum, Hanlon, and Murray (2017) is helpful. Their study looked at RCTs with the goal of determining if interventions to improve medication adherence also improved health outcomes. They looked at articles using older individuals listed in searches of three databases, including MEDLINE. They found 12 studies, which were listed in their references and could be reviewed by a researcher, which would be especially useful if one of the projects or interventions was similar to the one that other researchers wanted to implement. They concluded that patient-centered and multidisciplinary interventions were worthy of testing further to determine the degree of impact on health outcomes.

For public health professionals working on similar problems, this work would be invaluable to support patient-centered and multidisciplinary approaches. Further, the study designs could help in the development of similar interventions because they would provide evidence of successful implementations.

Brownson et al. (1999) provide a very useful framework for applying evidence-based decision-making to public health. As in many problem-solving models, the first stage is the development of a statement of the issue. While this sounds straightforward, one of the common mistakes in problem-solving is to inaccurately define the problem at the start. Stage 2 is to assess the scientific literature to determine what is already known (the EBM guidelines will help assess the strength of the individual articles). Stage 3 looks for descriptive studies and data that would complement the first two stages; factors like age and gender may already be available, but additional data collection may also be important in this stage. Stage 4 involves the development of program or policy options; what might work based on the evidence, and what choices might need to be made. Stage 5 is the development of an action plan, including objectives that are linked to desired outcomes and will be measured in the plan. Stage 6 is the evaluation of the program. This stage should include the dissemination of the information in some way so that others can benefit from the efforts and results of the project. In addition, lessons learned can be used to adjust the next iteration of the program to increase effectiveness in the future.

To facilitate connections between public health and health care providers, all groups benefit from common communications and thought processes. With the continued adoption of the EBM approach in health care, those working in public health need to share this way of thinking and this commitment to using current evidence in the decision-making process. The EBPH process will also lead to interventions based on evidence of what has (or has not) worked in the past, more cost-effective programs, and ideally better health outcomes for populations.

References

Agency for Healthcare Research and Quality. (2014, May). *The guide to clinical preventive services 2014: Recommendations of the U.S. Preventive Services Task Force*. Washington, DC: Retrieved from https://www.ahrq.gov/sites/default/files/publications/files/cpsguide.pdf

Agency for Healthcare Research and Quality. (2016, July 15). NGC template of guideline attributes. Washington, DC: Author. Retrieved from (https://www.guideline.gov/help-and-about/summaries/template-of-guideline-attributes)

Agency for Healthcare Research and Quality. (2017). National Guideline Clearinghouse. Rockville, MD: Author. Retrieved from https://www.guideline.gov/

Balogh, E. P., Miller, B. T., & Ball, J. R. (2015). *Improving diagnosis in health care*. Washington, DC: National Academies Press.

Boyd, C. M., Darer, J., Boult, C., Fried, L. P., Boult, L., & Wu, A. W. (2005). Clinical practice guidelines and quality of care for older patients with multiple comorbid diseases: Implications for pay for performance. *JAMA, 294*(6), 716–724. doi:10.1001/jama.294.6.716

Bradberry, T., & Greaves, J. (2009). *Emotional Intelligence 2.0: The world's most popular emotional intelligence test*. San Diego, CA: TalentSmart.

Brownson, R. C., Baker, E. A., Leet, T. L., & Gillespie, K. N. (2003). *Evidence-based public health*. New York: Oxford University Press.

Brownson, R. C., Fielding, J. E., & Maylahn, C. M. (2009). Evidence-based public health: A fundamental concept for public health practice. *Annual Review of Public Health, 30*, 175–201. doi:10.1146/annurev.publhealth.031308.100134

Brownson, R. C., Gurney, J. G., & Land, G. H. (1999). Evidence-based decision making in public health. *Journal of Public Health Management & Practice, 5*(5), 86–97.

Bryant, P. J., & Pace, H. A. (2009). *The pharmacist's guide to evidence-based medicine for clinical decision making.* Bethesda, MD: American Society of Health-System Pharmacists.

Burgers, J. S., Grol, R., Klazinga, N. S., Makela, M., & Zaat, J. (2003). Towards evidence-based clinical practice: An international survey of 18 clinical guideline programs. *International Journal for Quality in Health Care, 15*(1), 31–45.

Cochrane, A. L. (1972). *Effectiveness and efficiency: Random reflections on health services.* London: Nuffield Provincial Hospitals Trust.

Cochrane Screening and Diagnostic Tests Methods Group. (2017). *Cochrane handbook for diagnostic test accuracy reviews.* London: Author. Retrieved from http://methods.cochrane.org/sdt/handbook-dta-reviews

Consolidated Standards of Reporting Trials Group. (2017). CONSORT 2010. London: Author. Retrieved from http://www.consort-statement.org/consort-2010

Cook, D. J., Guyatt, G. H., Laupacis, A., & Sackett, D. L. (1992). Rules of evidence and clinical recommendations on the use of antithrombotic agents. *Chest, 102*(4 Suppl.), 305s–311s.

Davoli, M., Amato, L., Clark, N., Farrell, M., Hickman, M., Hill, S., . . . Schunemann, H. J. (2015). The role of Cochrane reviews in informing international guidelines: A case study of using the Grading of Recommendations, Assessment, Development and Evaluation system to develop World Health Organization guidelines for the psychosocially assisted pharmacological treatment of opioid dependence. *Addiction, 110*(6), 891–898. doi:10.1111/add.12788

Eldridge, S. M., Chan, C. L., Campbell, M. J., Bond, C. M., Hopewell, S., Thabane, L., & Lancaster, G. A. (2016). CONSORT 2010 statement: Extension to randomised pilot and feasibility trials. *Pilot and Feasibility Studies, 2*, 64. doi:10.1186/s40814-016-0105-8

Evidence-Based Medicine Working Group. (1992). Evidence-based medicine: A new approach to teaching the practice of medicine. *JAMA, 268*(17), 2420–2425. doi:10.1001/jama.1992.03490170092032

Feinstein, A. R. (1985). *Clinical epidemiology: The architecture of clinical research.* Philadelphia, PA: W. B. Saunders.

Field, M. J., Lohr, K. N., & Committee to Advise the Public Health Service on Clinical Practice Guidelines. (1990). *Clinical practice guidelines: Directions of a new program.* Washington, DC: National Academy Press. Retrieved from https://www.nap.edu/catalog/1626/clinical-practice-guidelines-directions-for-a-new-program

Graham, R., Mancher, M., Wolman, D. M., Greenfield, S., & Steinberg, E. (Eds.). (2011). *Clinical practice guidelines we can trust.* Washington DC: National Academies Press. Retrieved from https://www.nap.edu/catalog/13058/clinical-practice-guidelines-we-can-trust.

Guyatt, G. H., Oxman, A. D., Akl, E. A., Kunz, R., Vist, G., Brozek, J., . . . Schunemann, H. J. (2011). GRADE guidelines: 1. Introduction—GRADE evidence profiles and summary of findings tables. *Journal of Clinical Epidemiology, 64*(4), 383–394. doi:10.1016/j.jclinepi.2010.04.026

Guyatt, G. H., Oxman, A. D., Vist, G. E., Kunz, R., Falck-Ytter, Y., Alonso-Coello, P., & Schunemann, H. J. (2008). GRADE: An emerging consensus on rating quality of evidence and strength of recommendations. *BMJ, 336*(7650), 924–926. doi:10.1136/bmj.39489.470347.AD

Hall v. Hilbun, No. 466 So.2d 856 (Supreme Court of Mississippi 1985).

Higgins, J. P. T., & Green, S. (2011, March). *Cochrane handbook for systematic reviews of interventions, 5.1.0.* London: Cochrane Collaboration. Retrieved from http://handbook.cochrane.org/

Institute of Medicine. (2009). *Transforming clinical research in the United States: Challenges and opportunities: Workshop summary.* Washington, DC: National Academies Press.

Institute of Medicine. (2013). *Best care at lower cost: The path to continuously learning health care in America.* Washington, DC: National Academies Press.

Jenicek, M. (1997). Epidemiology, evidenced-based medicine, and evidence-based public health. *Journal of Epidemiology, 7*(4), 187–197.

Kohn, L. T., Corrigan, J. M., & Donaldson, M. S. (Eds.). (2000). *To err is human: Building a safer health system*. Washington, DC: National Academies Press.

Lang, T. A., & Altman, D. G. (2015). Basic statistical reporting for articles published in biomedical journals: The "Statistical Analyses and Methods in the Published Literature" or the SAMPL guidelines. *International Journal of Nursing Studies, 52*(1), 5–9. doi:10.1016/j.ijnurstu.2014.09.006

Marcum, Z. A., Hanlon, J. T., & Murray, M. D. (2017). Improving medication adherence and health outcomes in older adults: An evidence-based review of randomized controlled trials. *Drugs and Aging, 34*(3), 191–201. doi:10.1007/s40266-016-0433-7

McGlynn, E. A., Asch, S. M., Adams, J., Keesey, J., Hicks, J., DeCristofaro, A., & Kerr, E. A. (2003). The quality of health care delivered to adults in the United States. *New England Journal of Medicine, 348*(26), 2635–2645. doi:10.1056/NEJMsa022615

Moffett, P., & Moore, G. (2011). The standard of care: Legal history and definitions: The bad and good news. *Western Journal of Emergency Medicine, 12*(1), 109–112.

Moher, D., Liberati, A., Tetzlaff, J., Altman, D. G., & the PRISMA Group. (2009). Preferred reporting items for systematic reviews and meta-analyses: The PRISMA statement. *Journal of Clinical Epidemiology, 62*(10), 1006–1012. doi:10.1016/j.jclinepi.2009.06.005

Mustafa, R. A., Santesso, N., Brozek, J., Akl, E. A., Walter, S. D., Norman, G., . . . Schunemann, H. J. (2013). The GRADE approach is reproducible in assessing the quality of evidence of quantitative evidence syntheses. *Journal of Clinical Epidemiology, 66*(7), 736–742; quiz, 742. doi:10.1016/j.jclinepi.2013.02.004

Oxford English Dictionary. (2017). Evidence. [Web Page]. Retrieved from https://en.oxforddictionaries.com/definition/evidence

Penelope Research. (2017). Have you remembered everything? [Online tool]. London: Author. Retrieved from https://www.penelope.ai/equatorwizard/

Rapport, F., Clay-Williams, R., Churruca, K., Shih, P., Hogden, A., & Braithwaite, J. (2017). The struggle of translating science into action: Foundational concepts of implementation science. *Journal of Evaluation in Clinical Practice*. Advance online publication. doi:10.1111/jep.12741

Rychetnik, L., Hawe, P., Waters, E., Barratt, A., & Frommer, M. (2004). A glossary for evidence based public health. *Journal of Epidemiology & Community Health, 58*(7), 538–545. doi:10.1136/jech.2003.011585

Sackett, D. L. (2015). Why did the randomized clinical trial become the primary focus of my career? *Value in Health, 18*(5), 550–552. doi:10.1016/j.jval.2015.04.001

Sackett, D. L., Haynes, R. B., Guyatt, G. H., & Tugwell, P. (1991). *Clinical epidemiology: A basic science for clinical medicine* (2nd ed.). Boston: Little, Brown.

Sackett, D. L., Rosenberg, W. M., Gray, J. A., Haynes, R. B., & Richardson, W. S. (1996). Evidence based medicine: What it is and what it isn't. *BMJ, 312*(7023), 71–72.

Sauber-Schatz, E. K., Thomas, A. M., & Cook, L. J. (2015). Motor vehicle crashes, medical outcomes, and hospital charges among children aged 1–12 years—crash outcome data evaluation system, 11 states, 2005–2008. *MMWR Surveillance Summaries, 64*(8), 1–32. doi:10.15585/mmwr.ss6408a1

Sedlar, G., Bruns, E. J., Walker, S. C., Kerns, S. E., & Negrete, A. (2017). Developing a quality assurance system for multiple evidence based practices in a statewide service improvement initiative. *Administration and Policy in Mental Health, 44*(1), 29–41. doi:10.1007/s10488-015-0663-8

Shamseer, L., Moher, D., Clarke, M., Ghersi, D., Liberati, A., Petticrew, M., . . . Stewart, L. A. (2015). Preferred Reporting Items for Systematic Review and Meta-Analysis Protocols (PRISMA-P) 2015: Elaboration and explanation. *BMJ, 350*, g7647. doi:10.1136/bmj.g7647

Shekelle, P. G., Ortiz, E., Rhodes, S., Morton, S. C., Eccles, M. P., Grimshaw, J. M., & Woolf, S. H. (2001). Validity of the Agency for Healthcare Research and Quality clinical practice guidelines: How quickly do guidelines become outdated? *JAMA, 286*(12), 1461–1467.

Stevenson, A. (Ed.). (2010). *Oxford dictionary of English* (3rd ed.). Oxford: Oxford University Press.

Timmermans, S., & Mauck, A. (2005). The promises and pitfalls of evidence-based medicine. *Health Affairs, 24*(1), 18–28. doi:10.1377/hlthaff.24.1.18

UK EQUATOR Centre. (2013). *EQUATOR Reporting Guideline Decision Tree: Which guidelines are relevant to my work?* Oxford: Author. Retrieved from http://www.equator-network.org/wp-content/uploads/2013/11/20160301-RG-Decision-Tree-used-for-EQUATOR-wizard-vn-1.pdf

Velasco-Garrido, M., & Busse, R. (2005). *Health technology assessment: An introduction to objectives, role of evidence, and structure in Europe.* Brussels, Belgium: WHO European Centre for Health Policy. Retrieved from http://www.euro.who.int/__data/assets/pdf_file/0018/90432/E87866.pdf

World Health Organization. (2014). *WHO handbook for guideline development.* Geneva: Author. Retrieved from http://www.who.int/publications/guidelines/handbook_2nd_ed.pdf?ua=1

World Health Organization. (2017). WHO guidelines approved by the Guidelines Review Committee. Geneva: Author. Retrieved from http://www.who.int/publications/guidelines/en/

13

Informatics

ARDIS HANSON, BRUCE LUBOTSKY LEVIN, AND AIMON MIRANDA

Introduction

Informatics, as an academic discipline, involves the practice and theory of information processing, systems engineering, and classification research and is related to the study and practice of creating, storing, finding, manipulating, sharing, and communicating information. Using theoretical frameworks and practical theory from computation, communication, and cognition, we suggest informatics is how we transform data and information to create a body of knowledge that can answer the questions we ask about populations, geographic areas, disease surveillance, and much more.

Informatics is not new. The early 1990s saw the development of electronic office management software that could address computerized medication administration records, implement pharmacotherapy standards, and document pharmacist activities (Canaday & Yarborough, 1994; Cherici & Remillard, 1993; Teich, Spurr, Schmiz, O'Connell, & Thomas, 1995; Zimmerman, Smolarek, & Stevenson, 1995). Sujansky (1998) wrote of the need for decision support tools embedded in the electronic health record to make it more than just a paper analog, as well as the use of bibliographic retrieval systems, such as PubMed, to facilitate clinical decision-making. Today, informatics hardware and software handles decision support functions, as well as in-house administrative tasks, such as billing and scheduling, and many managed care functions, such as certifications, authorizations, treatment plans, medication evaluation forms, treatment summary forms, and outcome assessments. To do so, informatics utilizes data, contextualizes information, and builds a body of knowledge.

If the primary focus of an information system is a measurement or a personal characteristic of an individual, then we are talking about *data. Information* is data placed within a specific context (after analysis). Information applied within specific rules or guidelines is a *body of knowledge* or, in a shortened form, knowledge.

Take for example the emergence of vital statistics (birth and death records) in the United States in the early 20th century. We took discrete data at the local and state levels of government and examined it in light of the effects of three public health activities—(a) immunization, (b) sanitation, and (c) nutrition—on the health of individuals and communities. The information we gleaned from viewing data in this way led to the control of infectious diseases in the United States.

Public health practice has three core functions: (a) the identification or assessment of public health problems; (b) policy development (education, partnerships, and regulation); and (c) provision of necessary services (enforcement, linkages, workforce, evaluation, and research). We suggest the essential component in each of the three public health core functions is the availability and quality of data and information to create an accurate and complete body of knowledge. However, data comes in many formats—textual, visual, geospatial, and numeric—and levels, including primary or secondary data. Textual data are reports, best practice guidelines, and state or federal regulations. Visual data may be excerpts of larger numeric or geospatial datasets. Geospatial and numeric data form the basis for statistical data.

Given the amount and types of data collected by public and private organizations, as well as by local, city, county, state, and national agencies, for various purposes, information systems remain disparate in their structure and function. Hence there is a significant need to develop high-quality data standards that provide the basis for uniform, comparable, and good-quality information on populations, disorders, and services that address the dual needs of pharmacy and public health.

International Perspective: WHO

At an international level, the World Health Organization (WHO) Programme for International Drug Monitoring is an excellent example of an integrated public health pharmacy informatics solution. Created in 1961 as a response to the global outcry about thalidomide, over 130 countries are part of the WHO's pharmacovigilance program (WHO, 2016b). The WHO Collaborating Centre for International Drug Monitoring is the Uppsala Monitoring Centre (UMC), located in Uppsala, Sweden. The UMC screens for and analyzes international adverse-reaction data, provides current awareness services to keep health professionals up to date on the state of the science and tools, and provides technical assistance and training to establish and run national pharmacovigilance programs and UMC tools (UMC, 2000).

The UMC has created a number of tools using the WHO Global Database of Individual Case Safety Reports (ICSR). VigiBase® contains data on more than 10 million ICSRs submitted from over 100 countries since 1968 and includes conventional medicines, traditional medicines, and biological medicines (e.g., vaccines) (Viklund & Biiriell, 2015). VigiBase uses the *WHO Drug Dictionary* and the medical terminology classifications from WHO-Adverse Drug Reaction Terminologoy (ART), the International Classification of Diseases (ICD), and the Medical Dictionary for Regulatory Activities (MedDRA) to provide standardized and/or crosswalked nomenclature and ontologies.

Standardized Nomenclature

The importance of standardized and/or crosswalked nomenclature and ontologies is critical, especially when working with specialized vocabularies across multiple language groups, medical models, and/or cultural frames, at the global, national, and state levels. The *WHO Drug Dictionary Enhanced*, for example, is the world's most comprehensive source of pharmaceutical and medicinal product information. Although most of the entries are prescription-only products, the *Drug Dictionary Enhanced* also includes over-the-counter drugs and products, pharmacist-dispensed preparations, biotech and blood products, diagnostic substances, and contrast media. There is also an expanded version of the *Drug Dictionary Enhanced*, which includes the *WHO Herbal Dictionary*. Herbal medicines and traditional/complementary medical practices are used extensively across the globe (WHO, 2013); approximately 75% of the global population uses herbs for basic health care needs (Pan et al., 2014).

The WHO-ART is used for coding clinical information related to adverse drug reactions. It is a four-level hierarchical terminology, which begins at the body system/organ level classes used by drug regulatory agencies and pharmaceutical manufacturers.

Used in epidemiology, health management, and quality and clinical settings, the ICD is the standard global diagnostic tool (WHO, 2016a). Its diagnostic classes are used as a standard for vital statistics entries, reimbursement and resource allocation, and storage and retrieval queries for administrative data analysis and quality reviews. Translated into 43 languages, the ICD is used by all European Union (EU) member states, and most of the member states use the ICD to report mortality data.

Created by the International Council for Harmonisation of Technical Requirements for Registration of Pharmaceuticals for Human Use (2013), MedDRA standardizes the sharing of regulatory information for medical products used by humans. MedDRA covers data on pharmaceuticals, biologics, vaccines, and drug-device combination products from the clinical phase 1 to marketed product phase IV. Used by regulatory agencies, public health officials, medical researchers, and the drug industry, MedDRA's multiaxial hierarchical classification system allows signal detection and/or monitoring of clinical syndromes when symptoms encompass numerous systems or organs.

Other Tools

Other tools include CemFlow, a prototype data monitoring tool to analyze anti-malarial treatment data from cohort event monitoring programs developed for use in Nigeria and Tanzania Suku (Suku et al., 2015), and PaniFlow, developed for the Swiss medicines agency Swissmedic to monitor adverse events following administration of drugs and vaccines against the influenza A (H1N1) pandemic (Viklund & Biiriell, 2015). In addition to these tools specifically developed for WHO and UMC staff collaborators, there is VigiAccess™, a publicly accessible interface to VigiBase˚. Users can find information about possible side effects of medication, gain a more global understanding of the effects of drugs on people, and learn more about drug safety (Uppsala Monitoring Centre, 2015).

Regional Perspective: SemanticHEALTH

In 2008, the WHO conducted the Public Health Informatics Key Informant Survey, which became the basis for a EU project. The 28 member states of the EU, which vary widely in size, wealth, and political systems, began the SemanticHEALTH project, which addresses sematic interoperability in health systems in the EU.

Overall interoperability is defined as

> the ability, facilitated by ICT applications and systems, to exchange, understand and act on citizens/patients and other health-related information and knowledge among linguistically and culturally disparate health professionals, patients and other actors and organizations within and across health system jurisdictions in a collaborative manner. (Stroetmann et al., 2009, p. 10)

Sematic interoperability (SIOp) therefore identifies best practices in the coding, transmission, and use of meaning of health information between patients, providers, and institutions and in research and training across local, regional, and national borders. To do this, SIOp examines three key components: who delivers and receives health care (actors), how health care is delivered (processes), and the relationship of the actors and processes within the context of existing national health policy frameworks (laws, regulations, stakeholders) and infrastructures (institutional, technological, and service systems).

Semantic HEALTH emphasizes the importance of standardization in clinical data to ensure semantic interoperability. It identified as key the following three items: (a) generic reference models for clinical data from international standards organizations, (b) agreed-upon clinical data structure definitions, and (c) clinical terminology systems, such as Logical Observation Identifiers Names and

Codes (LOINC) and Systematized Nomenclature of Medicine—Clinical Terms (SNOMED CT).

The generic reference models were ISO/EN 13606 Part 1, openEHR, and HL7 Clinical Document Architecture. A reference model is an abstract framework or domain-specific ontology, which consists of an interlinked set of clearly defined concepts, objects, and relationships. Reference models can create standards for software or for a health record. Reference models also can help establish clear communication, such as "this" = "that," if one is working across different terminologies or languages. They help clinical specialists define the semantics of clinical information systems or transmission protocols for online health exchanges. All three create archetypes, (e.g., machine-readable specifications of how to store patient data), which are then used to provide true analytic functions, such as decision support, and allow complex queries. The ISO/EN 13606 Part 1 standard defines a means by which computer systems can exchange health care records with each other (Austin, Sun, Hassan, & Kalra, 2013) while Part 2 defines how archetypes should be formally represented (Tapuria, Kalra, & Kobayashi, 2013). Similarly, the openEHR Foundation publishes specifications for building "clinical models," or archetypes.

Health Level Seven (HL7) refers to a set of international standards for the transfer of clinical and administrative data between software applications used by various healthcare providers (Hanson & Levin, 2013). HL7 is one of several American National Standards Institute–accredited standards developing organizations (SDOs). Since the HL7 SDO develops standards for interoperability across platforms and data, this enhances the ability to share data, reduce ambiguity, improve care, and optimize workflow (Dolin, Rogers, & Jaffe, 2015). The HL7 is one of the standards used by the U.S. National Health Information Infrastructure (NHII).

National Perspective: CDC, Informatics, and Surveillance

The NHII was a health care standardization initiative to develop an interoperable, health information technology (HIT) system for the United States. The NHII report addressed three dimensions of health information: personal health, the health care provider, and population health (National Committee on Vital Health Statistics, 2001). Today, the NHII is called the Nationwide Health Information Network (NwHIN), sponsored by the Office of the National Coordinator for Health Information Technology. The NwHIN focuses on standards, services, and policies that enable secure health information exchange over the Internet (Office of the National Coordinator, 2013).

Perhaps the best-known public health organization in the United States working in informatics is the U.S. Centers for Disease Control and Prevention (CDC). The CDC's Division of Health Informatics and Surveillance provides access to a number of public health information and surveillance systems of interest in public health pharmacy. The National Syndromic Surveillance Program uses almost "real-time" prediagnostic data to detect and identify unusual disease or hazardous event activities for further investigation or response. The BioSense application is an electronic health information system with standardized tools and procedures to facilitate the collection, sharing, and analyzing of health data.

Take the case of mosquito-borne viruses, an increasing public health concern in the subtropical continental United States and in Puerto Rico. In 2010, the CDC identified an increase in the number of persons seeking care at Veterans Administration facilities who showed dengue-like signs and symptoms (Schirmer et al., 2013). The dengue virus is a leading cause of illness and death in the tropics and subtropics. In 2014, in Florida, the CDC confirmed 24 cases of dengue fever and 18 cases of a new mosquito-transmitted virus called chikungunya. To date, the presence of the chikungunya virus is confirmed in 44 countries in the Americas, with over 1 million suspected cases (Sharp et al., 2014).

The CDC National Notifiable Diseases Surveillance System Modernization Initiative (NNDSS NMI; 2014) is a surveillance system for the collection, analysis, and sharing of health data. The NNDSS NMI is standardizing the nation's health data and exchange systems. Two components of the NMI that are of especial interest to individuals working in public health/pharmacy are the development of new HL7 Message Mapping Guides (MMGs) and the CDC Message Validation, Processing, and Provisioning System (MVPS). The MMGs provide a structure for case notifications to the U.S. Public Health Information Network, using messaging standards and specifications, vocabulary standards and value sets, and business rules (CDC, 2012). Each MMG is designed for a specific disease event. The MVPS receives, processes, and manages the data for all nationally notifiable diseases based on HL7 standards (CDC, 2014). Since the MVPS is compliant with the HL7 standards, the amount of data that can be processed and the increased granularity of the data that can be processed should enhance the CDC's ability to surveil, identify, and respond to disease and/or hazardous events.

The CDC's Electronic Laboratory Reporting (ELR) is another public health priority. Clinical laboratory test results that are not uniformly coded or documented in a standardized manner across multiple standards are problematic. Part of the Centers for Medicare & Medicaid Services' Medicare and Medicaid Programs Electronic Health Records Incentive Program (Lamb et al., 2015), the intent of the ELR is to encourage professionals and providers participating in Medicare and Medicaid to adopt, implement, and sustain use of certified electronic health records (EHR) technology in the delivery of care.

Although many ELR and EHR systems uniformly code to the International Classification of Diseases, 9th revision Clinical Modification: Current Procedural Terminology and National Drug Codes, few ELR systems consistently use LOINC, which is used by the U.S. Food and Drug Administration (U.S. FDA) and the

Clinical Data Interchange Standards Consortium (Hanson & Levin, 2013). The CDC incorporated LOINC into its Reportable Condition Mapping Tool (RCMT). The RCMT, also HL7 compliant, maps between reportable conditions, their associated LOINC laboratory tests, and SNOMED CT. SNOMED CT addresses clinical findings, symptoms, diagnoses, procedures, body structures, organisms and other etiologies, substances, pharmaceuticals, devices, and specimen. More importantly, SNOMED CT crosswalks to other international standards and classifications, which is an important consideration for an increasingly global health perspective (McBride, Lawley, Leroux, & Gibson, 2012). Consider that even English changes as one moves across English-speaking countries. There are guides to understand medical terminology in every country. Consider health care provided in Australia and New Zealand. Not only do these guides provide Australian terminology and sociocultural perspectives common in the Australian health care environment (Walker, Wood, & Nicol, 2012), but they also provide frameworks for standard naming conventions and terminology to accurately describe medications.

Pharmacy Practice

Technology to support pharmacy practice is not new. The use of technology in pharmacy in the United States dates back to the 1970s and possibly earlier. In 1992, an expert conference arranged by U.S. Pharmacopeia predicted that, by 2020, the future of pharmacy practice would be affected by three factors: movement from a local to a global market, achieving cost-effectiveness in health care, and benefits from information technology (Bezold, Halperin, & Eng, 1993). More than 20 years later, another international study on pharmacy practice found that the vision for community pharmacy would have a strong patient care orientation and equally strong support from technology, including through work optimization, online documentation and follow-up, access to evidence-based practice and decision-making, shared patient data, and e-prescribing (Westerling, Haikala, & Airaksinen, 2011). These predictions and visions have come true. These did not only affect community pharmacy but almost all areas of pharmacy such as institutional, ambulatory care, and hospitals. There has even been the rapid development of an area of pharmacy informatics to meet major national and international needs and goals. Technology continues to affect many aspect of public health pharmacy, such as mobile health (m-health), electronic health records, and e-prescribing.

M-HEALTH

M-health uses mobile technologies as tools and platforms for health research and health care delivery (Fogarty International Center, 2016). This is a broad area that can include the most commonly used item such as smartphones (i.e., iPhone,

Android) and tablets (i.e., iPad, Surface) to the more advanced items such as wireless medical devices (i.e., blood pressure cuffs, glucometers) via Bluetooth, medical mobile applications (apps), and sensors linked to pacemakers. Different platforms of social media (i.e., Twitter, Instagram) and simple short messaging services can be utilized in m-health and have been to achieve different outcomes. Currently there is limited literature related to m-health as compared to other areas of pharmacy informatics, but the existing literature has been positive.

Text messaging, an early form of m-health, can be used to facilitate behavior change and improve health (Clauson, Elrod, Fox, Hajar, & Dzenowagis, 2013). A systematic review found text messaging to be effective in terms of addressing diabetes self-management, weight loss, physical activity, smoking cessation, and medication adherence (Hall, Cole-Lewis, & Bernhardt, 2015). Especially promising is its accessibility in developing nations as mobile phones rather than other health infrastructures reach further into developing countries for education and awareness, remote data collection and monitoring, communication and training, and epidemic tracking (Vital Wave Consulting, 2009). In South Africa, text messaging has been used in campaigns to build awareness of HIV/AIDs, leading to an increase in contact with helplines and HIV self-testing for Project Masiluleke (PopTech, 2016). Text messaging has experienced rapid growth due to its ease of use and accessibility, but related research is still limited and is difficult to interpret due to heterogeneity of health conditions and patient populations.

Mobile medical applications, or apps, can be used in several different ways. There has been substantial growth of mobile applications with certain apps targeted for patient use or clinician use. They can be used by clinicians to help increase access to clinical information for point-of-care by allowing access to drug information references and clinical practice guidelines. This can help with workflow and increase productivity and patient quality of care. For patients, there are apps that promote patient engagement through education, data collection, and feedback. There are also apps that can be used to help improve medication adherence that can be recommended for patient use (Dayer, Heldenbrand, Anderson, Gubbins, & Martin, 2013). Although readily available and easy to use, there are issues with mobile app development. There is a lack of evidence-based information or accuracy as most apps available often lack medical references or medical professional input (Ferrero, Morrell, & Burkhart, 2013; Mosa, Yoo, & Sheets, 2012; Wolf et al., 2013). Currently, the U.S. FDA (2015) only regulates a subset of apps that meet the definition of "device" and that "are intended to be used as an accessory to a regulated medical device" or "transform a mobile platform into a regulated medical device.". As the number of apps and popularity continues to grow, there may be future oversight needed to help regulate these apps.

Mobile technology has undergone rapid advances in the past several years with smartphones and tablets, as these devices have become a societal mainstay and their use has increased in clinical care due to the amalgamation of different functions that can used (Aungst, Miranda, & Serag-Bolos, 2015). These devices can be used to serve simpler functions for pharmacist as clinical references, ordering processing, communication, patient engagement, and documentation. Some mobile technology devices are much more advanced and are geared toward consumer use, such as wearable devices (i.e. Fitbit, Misfit Shine) that allow users to track certain biometrics such as steps, calories burned, sleep, and heart rate. Other mobile technology devices that are not wearables and available to consumers can be used to collect data such as blood pressure, blood glucose, and electrocardiograms on patients (i.e., iHealth iglucometer, Withings blood pressure cuff, and AliveCor). Many organizations are recognizing the potential benefits of incorporating such technology into practice, but the overarching issue is training health care professionals to be ready to integrate such devices into their workflow and practice (Miranda, Serag-Bolos, Aungst, & Chowdhury, 2016).

M-health is a rapidly growing area that is gaining much interest. Its major strengths are its scalability, increased reach to populations, and integrative data collection. These technologies are making the concept of telemedicine more robust. While this area seems promising, many barriers still exist, such as the need for additional research, the idea that technology changes quickly, and the integration of such technologies. Although data collection is also a strength, it can be seen as a weakness as well as there is the concept of data overload and the need to manage large enough amounts of data to make it clinically useful.

ELECTRONIC MEDICAL RECORDS, ELECTRONIC HEALTH RECORDS, AND PERSONAL HEALTH RECORDS

Electronic medical records (EMRs) are electronic records of health-related information on an individual that can be created, gathered, managed, and consulted by authorized clinicians and staff within one health care organization (National Alliance for Health Information Technology, 2008). EMRs are not synonymous with EHRs, which aggregate all of the data being generated by individual EMRs. Personal health records (PHRs) contain the same type of information as EHRs, such as diagnoses, medications, immunizations, family medical histories, and provider contact information, but they are designed to be set up, accessed, and managed by patients (HealthIT.gov, 2015).

Implementation of EMRs hold the promise of improved patient care, reducing medical errors, and coordinated care (DesRoches, Painter, & Jha, 2015). EMRs have several features that assist with pharmacy practice such as documentation of clinical services and patient care, medication lists, and allergy documentation and as a means of conducting clinical research. Incentives from the Health Information Technology Act of 2009 have drastically increased the adoption rate of certified EHRs. The increased use of EHRs makes it possible to capture massive amounts of clinical data that can be used in areas of data mining and data application and integration (Ross, Wei, & Ohno-Machado, 2014). Through data mining and applying predictive analytics and decision support, adverse drug events have been detected through utilizations of EHRs (Chazard, Ficheur, Bernonville, Luyckx, & Beuscart, 2011; Ji et al., 2011). This process is not proactive nor expeditious and can be used to augment the current process (Coloma, Trifiro, Patadia, & Sturkenboom, 2013).

A component of EMRs are clinical decision support (CDS) tools. CDS provides clinicians, patients, or individuals with knowledge and person-specific or population-specific information, intelligently filtered or presented at appropriate times, to foster better health processes, better individual care, and better population health (Osheroff et al., 2007). These tools have become very helpful in practice as a means to assist with clinical care, preventative care, diagnosis, and follow-up. For preventative care, they have been used to provide reminders for vaccinations and screenings. A meta-analysis found that computerized reminders increased preventative practices when these reminders were used (Shea, DuMouchel, & Bahamonde, 1996). Such practices are often missed when there are other issues that need to be addressed during the patient visit.

Although EMRs have become the center of clinical practice in a very short matter of time, there are still significant efforts being made to create a fully functioning interopertability model of health information exchange across the United States. EHRs could be used to bridge a gap between public health practice and clinical medicine. EHRs could support public health surveillance by designing standard computer algorithms to identify cases that meet surveillance case definitions and present them to public health agencies or facilitate surveillance for common chronic disease states by providing additional information on clinical parameters and risk factors (Birkhead, Klompas, & Shah, 2015).

PHRs are a relatively new area that is meant to improve patient engagement and encourage family health management. Currently, there are two types of PHR: (a) standalone/web-based and (b) incorporated/tethered (Pushpangadan & Seckman, 2015). Standalone/web-based PHRs can be printed, downloaded, or accessed via smartphones or tablets. Incorporated/tethered PHRs, also known as patient portals, are connected to EHRs, which are usually associated with a health care institution or insurance company (George & Hopla, 2015). There are several consumer concerns regarding its use, privacy, and security of these systems, leading to a slow adaption of PHRs (Pushpangadan & Seckman, 2015). This may change as time progresses due to millennials and baby boomers wanting online access to their health information through the use of patient portals.

TO ERR IS HUMAN: ADDRESSING MEDICATION ERRORS THROUGH TECHNOLOGY

One of the best-known instances of the use of technology to improve pharmacy practice came about with the Institute of Medicine's (IOM) publication of *To Err is Human: Building a Safer Health System* (Kohn, Corrigan, & Donaldson, 2000), which addressed the increased mortality and morbidity in American hospitals due to medication errors. Three main causes of medication errors are similar-sounding drug names (e.g., Celexa for depression and Celebrex for arthritis), illegible physician handwriting, and the continued expansion of the drug universe, that is, the number of new drugs and the number of prescriptions filled annually.

The IOM report recommended a number of changes, such as workplace changes to improve medication safety practices, standardization of terminology, minimizing data handoffs, and creating protocols and checklists. A year later, a second IOM (2011) report, *Crossing the Quality Chasm: A New Health System for the 21st Century*, called for the automation of patient health records, which could be integrated with computerized prescriber-order-entry (CPOE) systems, drug distribution systems, and medication administration systems.

By 2003, the Medicare Prescription Drug, Improvement, and Modernization Act required that Part D plans support an "electronic prescription program" (Bell & Friedman, 2005). By 2005, Medicare had issued a number of technical standards for these systems. However, subparts of existing standards that were used rarely, such as the fill status notification feature of the NCPDP SCRIPT standard, needed to be tested. Other possible standards were identified, such as RxNorm, created by the National Library of Medicine, which creates crosswalks across similar generic and brand-name drugs to their active ingredients, components, and dose forms (Hanson & Levin, 2013).

REENGINEERING VERSUS AUTOMATION

Automating patient records and CPOE systems present an interesting example of the use of reengineering and automation in patient care and pharmacy services. Re-engineering is determining how a system performs and deciding how to change the system to make it perform more effectively. Automation is the act of replacing human work with work done by machines. So, when we talk of re-engineering, the topic under discussion can range from re-engineering pharmacy layout to become more productive to re-engineering the medication error-reporting process to re-engineering biosimilar drugs. However, re-engineering and automation are not always distinct form the other. Automation of a workflow process is a key component for many re-engineering initiatives.

Automation Issues for Formularies

Automation and re-engineering can play an important role in addressing formulary management. Traditionally, a formulary was a collection of formulas used to compound and test medication. Today, a formulary is an authoritative list of prescription drugs and drug products available to enrollees approved for use by a hospital, health system provider, or a state/national health service. Basic information in a formulary database generally includes the names of the discrete therapeutic entities and commercially packaged drug products, a unique identifier (e.g., a National Drug Code, the names of the drugs contained in a drug product, administration protocol, side effects, contraindications, strength and dosage range, and price).

A national formulary contains a list of medicines approved for prescription throughout the country. According to the WHO (2015), over 156 countries now have national lists of essential medicines, with separate lists for adults and for children. Two examples of national formularies are the U.S. Centers for Medicare and Medicaid Services and the British National Formulary managed by the National Health Service.

Automated pharmacy systems and pharmacy information system formularies need automatic and synchronous updates to ensure accuracy across related purchasing, inventory, and dispensing systems. However, there are a number of problems related to formulary interoperability, including formulary-database synchronization and syntactic and sematic interoperability (McManus et al., 2012).

In a study on two American Society of Health-System Pharmacists Section of Pharmacy Informatics and Technology webinars, participants voiced their frustration with the lack of synchronization among their formularies, the EMR, and "downstream" systems (Volpe et al., 2014). The inability to synchronize formularies with CPOE, e-prescribing systems, inventory and purchasing systems, automated dispensing cabinets, and unit dose robots, to name just a few, means pharmacists spend a significant amount of time doing manual entry and maintenance across numerous systems. Seventy-eight percent of participants did manual entry; almost half of participants reported spending 10 or more hours a week to keep the formulary data updated, and 51% reported they managed between five to nine online systems to maintain current and updated formulary data (Volpe et al., 2014).

Why are these issues problematic? Brookins et al. (2011) argue that manual synchronization is a major challenge for formularies. Manual entry increases risk of data-entry error, is labor and personnel-intensive, may not reflect actual time-dependent product or activity changes, and result in less accuracy for downstream automated systems. Further, with the increased reliance on robotics and compounding devices, new data requirements will emerge specific to these new tools and applications to ensure patient safety, reduce prescribing error, and manage costs. Working with large, distributed, aggregated data sets also presents a significant challenge for integrated HIT and health information exchange systems, especially in the normalization of formulary data collected over time or across institutions (Wynden et al., 2011). Such data is reused in clinical translational research, administrative data/service utilization review across health systems, or comparative effectiveness reviews.

Challenges in Re-engineering
Re-engineering procedures and processes is much more than figuring out how to improve a process. The success of re-engineering often depends on a number of

factors: financial, workforce, strategic, cultural, structural, technological, and security. Financial factors, such as the cost of implementing HIT systems and potential liabilities in implementation and maintenance of HIT systems, often limit the use of these systems. Existing IT workforce may not be able to address the added complexity of implementing and integrating HIT systems. Organizations may not have incorporated HIT into their long-range strategic or operational plans, which would affect all of the factors named previously. Workplace culture may not be primed to adapt successfully to new ways of working in addition to new technology. Structurally, technology, as in hardware, is inherently problematic, with interoperability and cross-platform migration issues to address. Operating new technologies is a major technological challenge. The more complex the HIT, the less likely intuitive "click here" buttons or easy-to-use "plug and play" modules will be available. It is difficult for users to change roles or workflow processes, especially with new systems to learn and use.

Finally, security in HIT and health service delivery in the United States focuses on privacy and confidentiality framed by the Health Insurance Portability and Accountability Act (HIPAA) standards. However, since federal HIPAA legislation may be preempted by more rigorous state standards, there are hindrances to interstate flow of patient information that cannot be easily resolved.

PHARMACOVIGILANCE

Pharmacovigilance, defined as the detection, assessment, and prevention of long- and short-term adverse effects of medicines, is part of postmarketing product surveillance, which tracks drugs, appliances, and devices postrelease to the public. Pharmacovigilance is very important from a global perspective. There may be significant differences in the occurrence and frequency of adverse drug reactions and drug-related problems between countries and within regions within countries. This may be due to many factors, such as pharmaceutical quality and composition of locally produced pharmaceutical products or the use of nonorthodox drugs (e.g., traditional or indigenous remedies). Additional factors also include access to and distribution of drugs, drug use (e.g., indications, dose, availability), and sociocultural factors, such as genetics, diet, and traditions.

An interesting study on the use of VigiBase˚ was the identification of substandard medicines. Substandard medicines have the potential to pose a significant threat to patient safety and community health. In 2008, the CDC began an investigation of rapid-onset, acute, and severe adverse drug reactions (ADRs) to injected heparin sodium; many of the ADRs had been fatal (Blossom et al., 2008). In addition to the U.S. cluster, countries in the EU and Asia reported ADRs with heparin products from different manufacturers. It was determined that a heparin supply in China had been contaminated with a semisynthetic oversulfated chondroitin sulfate and distributed (Liu, Zhang, & Linhardt, 2009). However, this ADR emphasized the complexity of monitoring and analyzing polydispersed, polycomponent, polypharmacologic agents (Liu et al., 2009).

In 2011, the UMC developed a novel algorithm for VigiBase to identify reporting patterns that may indicate substandard medicines (Juhlin et al., 2015). The algorithm was successful in identifying historical clusters; however, the researchers concluded there needed to be additional data reported at the national level and processes created to allow the algorithm to be truly useful. Additional data needed include detailed information on the product and its distribution channels, samples of suspected products for analysis, and laboratory capacity to analyze suspected samples at the national level (Juhlin et al., 2015).

Implications for Public Health and Pharmacy Practice

There are a number of challenges when we examine public health pharmacy informatics, such as integrating surveillance systems, improving data mining, enhancing online analytical processing, standardizing public health vocabulary and classification systems, addressing emerging automated coding systems and legacy systems, and workforce development. These are in addition to other technological solutions in the workday of a pharmacist.

Accurate transmission, encryption, reception, and storage of client information and public health data are critical to ensure appropriate treatment decisions. However, existing legislation and professional rules of conduct often hinder implementation of informatics projects and programs. As legislation plays "catch up" with the advances in technology, there is great uncertainty about the application of existing legislation to HIT and health information exchange, what actions constitute statutory violations, or what actions create litigation risks. There is no easy solution, as shown by the number of case law decisions dealing with antitrust concerns, fraud and abuse, malpractice, state licensing and credentialing, and anti-kickback laws.

One of the areas for which informatics looks promising in pharmacy practice is the management of vulnerable older inpatients on high-risk medication or polypharmeutical regimens. Another area is identifying discrepancies in EMRs through pharmacist medication reconciliation. A third area is continuity of care in transitional care settings, as patients are shifted from one health care setting or service to another.

However, there are also a number of concerns as public health pharmacy continues to rely on technology. One major challenge is integrating patient care services into current and emerging business models. Some pharmacists may decide to base their practice on dispensing and sales; others may focus on services provision. Each of these has different implications for public health pharmacy practice.

References

Aungst, T. D., Miranda, A. C., & Serag-Bolos, E. S. (2015). How mobile devices are changing pharmacy practice. *American Journal of Health-System Pharmacy, 72*(6), 494–500. doi:10.2146/ajhp140139

Austin, T., Sun, S., Hassan, T., & Kalra, D. (2013). Evaluation of ISO EN 13606 as a result of its implementation in XML. *Health Informatics Journal, 19*(4), 264–280. doi:10.1177/1460458212473993

Bell, D. S., & Friedman, M. A. (2005). E-prescribing and the Medicare Modernization Act of 2003. *Health Affairs, 24*(5), 1159–1169. doi:10.1377/hlthaff.24.5.1159

Bezold, C., Halperin, J. A., & Eng, J. L. (1993). *2020 visions: Health care information standards and technologies.* Rockville, MD: U.S. Pharmacopeial Convention.

Birkhead, G. S., Klompas, M., & Shah, N. R. (2015). Uses of electronic health records for public health surveillance to advance public health. *Annual Review of Public Health, 36*, 345–359. doi:10.1146/annurev-publhealth-031914-122747

Blossom, D. B., Kallen, A. J., Patel, P. R., Elward, A., Robinson, L., Gao, G., . . . Sasisekharan, R. (2008). Outbreak of adverse reactions associated with contaminated heparin. *New England Journal of Medicine, 359*(25), 2674–2684. doi:10.1056/NEJMoa0806450

Brookins, L., Burnette, R., De la Torre, C., Dumitru, D., McManus, R. B., Urbanski, C. J., . . . Tribble, D. A. (2011). Formulary and database synchronization. *American Journal of Health-System Pharmacy, 68*(3), 204, 206. doi:10.2146/ajhp100354

Canaday, B. R., & Yarborough, P. C. (1994). Documenting pharmaceutical care: Creating a standard. *Annals of Pharmacotherapy, 28*(11), 1292–1296.

Centers for Disease Control & Prevention. (2012, February). *Public Health Information Network (PHIN) National Notifiable Diseases Surveillance System (NNDSS) case notification certification process.* Atlanta, GA: Author.

Centers for Disease Control & Prevention. (2014, December 22). *National Notifiable Diseases Surveillance System Modernization Initiative: Questions & answers.* Atlanta, GA: U.S. Department of Health and Human Services, Public Health Service, Centers for Disease Control and Prevention.

Chazard, E., Ficheur, G., Bernonville, S., Luyckx, M., & Beuscart, R. (2011). Data mining to generate adverse drive events detection rules. *IEEE Transactions in Information Technology in Biomedicine, 16*(6), 823–830.

Cherici, C. A., & Remillard, P. (1993). Implementation of a computerized medication administration record. *Hospital Pharmarcy, 28*(3), 193–195, 198–200, 201–195.

Clauson, K. A., Elrod, S., Fox, B. I., Hajar, Z., & Dzenowagis, J. H. (2013). Opportunities for pharmacists in mobile health. *American Journal of Health-System Pharmacy, 70*(15), 1348–1352.

Coloma, P. M., Trifiro, G., Patadia, V., & Sturkenboom, M. (2013). Postmarketing safety surveillance: Where does signal detection using electronic healthcare records fit into the big picture? *Drug Safety, 36*(3), 183–197. doi:10.1007/s40264-013-0018-x

Dayer, L., Heldenbrand, S., Anderson, P., Gubbins, P. O., & Martin, B. C. (2013). Smartphone medication adherence apps: Potential benefits to patients and providers. *Journal of the American Pharmacists Association, 53*(2), 172–181. doi:10.1331/JAPhA.2013.12202

DesRoches, C., Painter, M. W., & Jha, A. K. (2015). *Health information technology in the United States, 2015: Transition to a Post-HITECH world.* Princeton, NJ: Robert Wood Johnson Foundation.

Dolin, R. H., Rogers, B., & Jaffe, C. (2015). Health level seven interoperability strategy: Big data, incrementally structured. *Methods of Information in Medicine, 54*(1), 75–82. doi:10.3414/me14-01-0030

Ferrero, N. A., Morrell, D. S., & Burkhart, C. N. (2013). Skin scan: A demonstration of the need for FDA regulation of medical apps on iPhone. *Journal of the American Academy of Dermatology, 68*(3), 515–516. doi:10.1016/j.jaad.2012.10.045

Fogarty International Center. (2016). Mobile health (mHealth) information and resources. Bethesda, MD: National Institute of Health. Retrieved from http://www.fic.nih.gov/RESEARCHTOPICS/Pages/MobileHealth.aspx

George, T., P., & Hopla, D. L. (2015). Advantages of personal health records. *Nursing Critical Care, 10*(6), 10–12.

Hall, A. K., Cole-Lewis, H., & Bernhardt, J. M. (2015). Mobile text messaging for health: A systematic review of reviews. *Annual Review of Public Health, 36,* 393–415. doi:10.1146/annurev-publhealth-031914-122855

Hanson, A., & Levin, B. L. (2013). *Mental health informatics.* New York: Oxford University Press.

HealthIT.gov. (2015, November 2). What are the differences between electronic medical records, electronic health records, and personal health records? Washington, DC: Office of the National Coordinator for Health Information Technology. Retrieved from https://www.healthit.gov/providers-professionals/faqs/what-are-differences-between-electronic-medical-records-electronic

International Council for Harmonisation of Technical Requirements for Registration of Pharmaceuticals for Human Use. (2013). *Understanding MedDRA: The medical dictionary for regulatory activities.* McLean, VA: Author.

Institute of Medicine. (2001). *Crossing the quality chasm: A new health system for the 21st century.* Washington, DC: National Academy Press.

Ji, Y., Ying, H., Dews, P., Mansour, A., Tran, J., Miller, R. E., & Massanari, R. M. (2011). A potential causal association mining algorithm for screening adverse drug reactions in postmarketing surveillance. *IEEE Transactions on Information Technology in Biomedicine, 15*(3), 428–437. doi:10.1109/titb.2011.2131669

Juhlin, K., Karimi, G., Ander, M., Camilli, S., Dheda, M., Har, T. S., . . . Noren, G. N. (2015). Using VigiBase to identify substandard medicines: Detection capacity and key prerequisites. *Drug Safety, 38*(4), 373–382. doi:10.1007/s40264-015-0271-2

Kohn, L. T., Corrigan, J. M., & Donaldson, M. S. (Eds.). (2000). *To err is human: Building a safer health system.* Washington, DC: National Academies Press.

Lamb, E., Satre, J., Hurd-Kundeti, G., Liscek, B., Hall, C. J., Pinner, R. W., . . . Smith, K. (2015). Update on progress in electronic reporting of laboratory results to public health agencies—United States, 2014. *MMWR Morbidity & Mortality Weekly Report, 64*(12), 328–330.

Liu, H., Zhang, Z., & Linhardt, R. J. (2009). Lessons learned from the contamination of heparin. *Natural Product Reports, 26*(3), 313–321. doi:10.1039/b819896a

McBride, S. J., Lawley, M. J., Leroux, H., & Gibson, S. (2012). Using Australian Medicines Terminology (AMT) and SNOMED CT-AU to better support clinical research. *Studies in Health Technology and Informatics, 178,* 144–149.

McManus, R., Nemec, E. C., Ferer, D.S., Gumpper, K.F., Volpe G., Giacomelli B., et al. (2012). Suggested definitions for informatics terms: Interfacing, integration, and interoperability. *American Journal of Health-System Pharmacy, 69*(13), 1163–1165.

Miranda, A. C., Serag-Bolos, E. S., Aungst, T. D., & Chowdhury, R. (2016). A mobile health technology workshop to evaluate available technologies and their potential use in pharmacy practice. *BMJ Simulation and Technology Enhanced Learning.* doi:10.1136/bmjstel-2015-000067

Mosa, A. S., Yoo, I., & Sheets, L. (2012). A systematic review of healthcare applications for smartphones. *BMC Medical Informatics and Decision Making, 12,* 67. doi:10.1186/1472-6947-12-67

National Alliance for Health Information Technology. (2008, April). *Defining key health information technology terms: Report to the Office of the National Coordinator for Health Information Technology.* Washington, DC: U.S. Department of health & Human Services.

National Committee on Vital Health Statistics. (2001). *Information for health: A strategy for building the National Health Information Infrastructure: Report and recommendations.* Washington, DC: U.S. Department of Health and Human Services, Office of Disease Prevention and Health Promotion, Office of Public Health and Science; National Center for Health Statistics, Centers for Disease Control and Prevention.

Office of the National Coordinator for Health Information Technology. (2013). Nationwide Health Information Network. Washington, DC: Author. Retrieved from https://www.healthit.gov/policy-researchers-implementers/nationwide-health-information-network-nwhin

Osheroff, J. A., Teich, J. M., Middleton, B., Steen, E. B., Wright, A., & Detmer, D. E. (2007). A roadmap for national action on clinical decision support. *Journal of the American Medical Informatics Association, 14*(2), 141–145. doi:10.1197/jamia.M2334

Pan, S. Y., Litscher, G., Gao, S. H., Zhou, S. F., Yu, Z. L., Chen, H. Q., ... Ko, K. M. (2014). Historical perspective of traditional indigenous medical practices: The current renaissance and conservation of herbal resources. *Evidence-Based Complementary and Alternative Medicine, 2014,* 525340. doi:10.1155/2014/525340

PopTech. (2016). Project Masiluleke: A breakthrough approach to reversing HIV and TB in South Africa and beyond. Camden, ME: Author. Retrieved from http://www.poptech.org/project_m

Pushpangadan, S., & Seckman, C. (2015). Consumer perspective on personal health records: A review of the literature. *Online Journal of Nursing Informatics, 19*(1). Retrieved from http://www.himss.org/ResourceLibrary/GenResourceDetail.aspx?ItemNumber=39756

Ross, M. K., Wei, W., & Ohno-Machado, L. (2014). "Big data" and the electronic health record. *Yearbook of Medical Informatics, 9,* 97–104. doi:10.15265/iy-2014-0003

Schirmer, P. L., Lucero-Obusan, C. A., Benoit, S. R., Santiago, L. M., Stanek, D., Dey, A., ... Holodniy, M. (2013). Dengue surveillance in Veterans Affairs healthcare facilities, 2007–2010. *PLoS Neglected Tropical Diseases, 7*(3), e2040. doi:10.1371/journal.pntd.0002040

Sharp, T. M., Roth, N. M., Torres, J., Ryff, K. R., Perez Rodriguez, N. M., Mercado, C., ... Garcia, B. R. (2014). Chikungunya cases identified through passive surveillance and household investigations—Puerto Rico, May 5–August 12, 2014. *MMWR Morbidity & Mortality Weekly Report, 63*(48), 1121–1128. http://www.cdc.gov/mmwr/pdf/wk/mm6348.pdf

Shea, S., DuMouchel, W., & Bahamonde, L. (1996). A meta-analysis of 16 randomized controlled trials to evaluate computer-based clinical reminder systems for preventive care in the ambulatory setting. *Journal of the American Medical Informatics Association, 3*(6), 399–409.

Stroetmann, V. N., Kalra, D., Lewalle, P., Rodrigues, J. M., Stroetmann, K. A., Surjan, G., ... Zanstra, P. E. (2009). *Semantic interoperability for better health and safer healthcare: Research and deployment roadmap for Europe.* Luxembourg: Office for Official Publications of the European Communities.

Sujansky, W. V. (1998). The benefits and challenges of an electronic medical record: Much more than a "word-processed" patient chart. *Western Journal of Medicine, 169*(3), 176–183. http://www.ncbi.nlm.nih.gov/pmc/articles/PMC1305206/pdf/westjmed00324-0050.pdf

Suku, C. K., Hill, G., Sabblah, G., Darko, M., Muthuri, G., Abwao, E., ... Pal, S. N. (2015). Experiences and lessons from implementing cohort event monitoring programmes for antimalarials in four African countries: Results of a questionnaire-based survey. *Drug Safety, 38*(11), 1115–1126. doi:10.1007/s40264-015-0331-7

Tapuria, A., Kalra, D., & Kobayashi, S. (2013). Contribution of clinical archetypes, and the challenges, towards achieving semantic interoperability for EHRs. *Healthcare Informatics Research, 19*(4), 286–292. doi:10.4258/hir.2013.19.4.286

Teich, J. M., Spurr, C. D., Schmiz, J. L., O'Connell, E. M., & Thomas, D. (1995). Enhancement of clinician workflow with computer order entry. *Proceedings of the Annual Symposium of Computer Applications in Medical Care, 1995,* 459–463.

U.S. Food and Drug Administration. (2015, September 22). Mobile medical applications. Silver Spring, MD: U.S. Department of Health and Human Services. Retrieved from http://www.fda.gov/MedicalDevices/DigitalHealth/MobileMedicalApplications/default.htm#b

Uppsala Monitoring Centre. (2000). *Safety monitoring of medicinal products: Guidelines for setting up and running a pharmacovigilance centre.* Uppsala, Sweden: Author.

Uppsala Monitoring Centre. (2015). *VigiAccess™.* Uppsala, Sweden: Author.

Viklund, A., & Biiriell, C. (2015, July). *VigiBase scales new heights* (Uppsala Reports, 70). Uppsala, Sweden: Uppsala Monitoring Centre.

Vital Wave Consulting. (2009). *mHealth for development: The opportunity of mobile technology for healthcare in the developing world.* Washington, DC.; Berkshire, UK: UN Foundation; Vodafone Foundation Partnership.

Volpe, G., Nickman, N. A., Bussard, W. E., Giacomelli, B., Ferer, D. S., Urbanski, C., & Brookins, L. (2014). Automation and improved technology to promote database synchronization *American Journal of Health-System Pharmacy, 71*(8), 675–678. doi:10.2146/ajhp130286

Walker, S., Wood, M., & Nicol, J. (2012). *Mastering medical terminology Australia and New Zealand.* Chatswood, NSW: Elsevier Australia.

Westerling, A. M., Haikala, V., & Airaksinen, M. (2011). The role of information technology in the development of community pharmacy services: Visions and strategic views of international experts. *Research in Social & Administrative Pharmacy, 7*(4), 430–437. doi:10.1016/j.sapharm.2010.09.004

Wolf, J. A., Moreau, J. F., Akilov, O., Patton, T., English, J. C. 3rd, Ho, J., & Ferris, L. K. (2013). Diagnostic inaccuracy of smartphone applications for melanoma detection. *JAMA Dermatology, 149*(4), 422–426. doi:10.1001/jamadermatol.2013.2382

World Health Organization. (2013, December). *WHO traditional medicine strategy: 2014–2023.* Geneva: Author.

World Health Organization. (2015). WHO model lists of essential medicines. Geneva: Author. Retrieved from http://www.who.int/medicines/publications/essentialmedicines/en/

World Health Organization. (2016a). *International statistical classification of diseases and related health problems.* Geneva: Author.

World Health Organization. (2016b). Pharmacovigilance. Geneva: Author. Retrieved from http://www.who.int/medicines/areas/quality_safety/safety_efficacy/pharmvigi/en/

Wynden, R., Anderson, N., Casale, M., Lakshminarayanan, P., Anderson, K., Prosser, J., . . . Weiner, M. (2011). Using RxNorm for cross-institutional formulary data normalization within a distributed grid-computing environment. *AMIA Annual Symposium Proceedings, 2011,* 1559–1563.

Zimmerman, C. R., Smolarek, R. T., & Stevenson, J. G. (1995). A computerized system to improve documentation and reporting of pharmacists' clinical interventions, cost savings, and workload activities. *Pharmacotherapy, 15*(2), 220–227. http://onlinelibrary.wiley.com/doi/10.1002/j.1875-9114.1995.tb04357.x/abstract

14

Emergency Preparedness

PETER D. HURD, STEPHENIE LUKAS, AND ARDIS HANSON

While this chapter focuses on the US health care systems and emergency preparedness within its borders, other chapters in this book have highlighted public health emergencies in other parts of the world, ranging from tuberculosis, polio, measles, tobacco, and Ebola to the earthquake in Haiti. However, other manmade events affect public health and result in great suffering to countries. One such public health emergency/disaster was the 1994 genocide in Rwanda, which took place during the Rwandan Civil War (1990–1994) against ethnic Tutsis and moderate Hutus. This led to the deaths of 1 million people and the displacement of millions more (Binagwaho et al., 2014; Centers for Disease Control and Prevention [CDC], 1996; Hintjens, 1999).

From a public health perspective, this was on overwhelming catastrophe: bodies to be buried, endemic rape and violence against women and girls, the spread of HIV/AIDS, and a very slow response from outside countries (Dabelstein, 1996; Mandelbaum-Schmid, 2004; Verwimp, 2004). Refugee camps led to dysentery, dehydration, and cholera (CDC, 1996). The lack of food, potable water, and health infrastructure contributed to the spread of disease and rising death rates. The public health needs included such basics as clean water and safe food, access to health care and mental health care, housing, and care for orphaned children. More than 20 years later, there remain a number of postconflict and generational trauma that still require intervention, such as mental illnesses, the lack of adequate housing, refugee repatriation, care for orphaned children, violence perpetration, alcohol use, infectious disease transmission and treatment, and at-risk behaviors (Caserta, Pirttila-Backman, & Punamaki, 2016; Chaudhury et al., 2016; Neugebauer et al., 2016; Rubanzana, Hedt-Gauthier, Ntaganira, & Freeman, 2015). The Rwandan tragedy helps emphasize that public health's role has expanded to include working through war, crisis, and violence (Willis & Levy, 2000). However, today, pharmacy also has a large role to play within US borders.

Basic Terminology and Concepts

When people think of emergency preparedness, they often consider it in the context of some disaster. The Federal Emergency Management Agency (FEMA, 1996, p. GLO-1) defines disaster as "an occurrence of a natural catastrophe, technological accident, or human-caused event that has resulted in severe property damage, deaths, and/or multiple injuries." This is similar to how "emergency" is defined: "Any occasion or instance, such as a hurricane, tornado, storm, flood, tidal wave, tsunami, earthquake, volcanic eruption, landslide, mudslide, snowstorm, fire, explosion, nuclear accident, or any other natural or man-made catastrophe, that warrants action to save lives and to protect property, public health, and safety" (FEMA, 1996, p. GLO-2). From a public health perspective, we define emergencies by their causes, precipitating events, and health consequences, whose scale, timing, or unpredictability could overwhelm routine capabilities. The definition also aligns with FEMA's (1996) all-hazards approach to preparedness used within the United States as well as other health care and government responders (Joint Commission, 2016; Office of Public Health Preparedness and Response, 2013).

Most people consider an epidemic or a pandemic a public health emergency. An epidemic is the occurrence of more cases of a disease than would be expected in a local community during a given time period. A pandemic is when an epidemic becomes very widespread and affects a whole region, a continent, or the world, such as avian flu or AIDS. However, a natural disaster, that is, a natural event with catastrophic consequences (e.g., hurricane, flood, or earthquake), also may have public health consequences (e.g., sanitation, water, decreased access to medication and health care), which may set the stage for somatic and/or psychiatric diseases. Preparing for these types of events requires numerous types of responses at multiple perspectives. Hence the public health viewpoint addresses each level of response (local, state, regional, national, international) and across numerous stakeholders.

Since disasters are difficult to predict or control, planning for them is critical so responders can implement carefully made plans with very little delay when they occur. In the United States, emergency preparedness is designed to help communities prepare for both natural events and manmade events (Office of Public Health Preparedness and Response, 2013). The CDC's Office of Public Health Preparedness and Response (2013) defines category types by five major categories (see Figure 14-1). However, it is easy to see how these categories may overlap when looking at disasters.

Epidemic disease has a strong patient-care focus and a close relationship to health care needs and is "biological," which would include pandemics, such as bubonic plague, HIV/AIDS, and Ebola. Manmade disasters include both accidental and intentional disasters. These would include a forest fire started by a careless

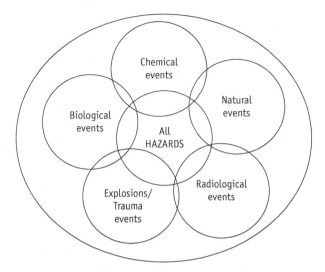

Figure 14-1. CDC All Hazards Model.

camper, the meltdown of the Fukashima or Chernobyl nuclear plants, or terror-ist events, which can come in many forms. Terrorist events are biologically based, such as an anthrax release; others are conventional explosions, such as a car bomb. Nuclear terrorism would include a dirty bomb that spreads radiation; chemical terrorism may include poisonous gas or nerve gas. Whether natural, manmade, or terrorist, these types of disaster events all have profound impacts on the public health system.

Some disasters/emergencies are fundamentally health emergencies; in oth-ers, health is just one of many facets affected. Following the 2005 hurricane sea-son in Louisiana, individuals living in housing provided by FEMA faced numerous problems. In addition to a lack of shelter, safe drinking water, electricity, and food, individuals also lacked access to prescription medications and to appropriate care, exacerbating previous and immediate mental health problems (Abramson & Garfield, 2006). Typical reactions included fear of another attack or of expo-sure, grief over the loss of others, confusion and disorientation in the immediate aftermath, and depression as a reaction to the devastation or loss. Hence current thinking on disaster preparedness uses a socioecological framework that addresses housing stability, economic stability, physical health, mental health, and social role adaptation (Abramson, Stehling-Ariza, Park, Walsh, & Culp, 2010). Therefore, when planning a pharmacy response to a disaster, pharmacists need to address the psychological needs, somatic needs, and basic survival needs of the affected popu-lation to increase community resilience and pharmacist response (Arya, Medina, Scaccia, Mathew, & Starr, 2016).

Key Components of the Emergency Preparedness and Response System

The Robert T. Stafford Disaster Relief and Emergency Assistant Act (42 U.S.C. §§ 5121-5207 §401) allows the president to formally declare a region or area as an emergency or disaster event. The Act requires the governor of an affected state or territory to ask the president to make a formal declaration. Once an emergency or disaster is declared, local, state, and federal agencies (private and public) work together to respond quickly. However, emergency powers, responders, and resources vary widely across levels and locations. At the national level, the National Preparedness System describes how the federal government organizes and responds to natural disasters, terrorist attacks, and other catastrophic events as well as provides guidance for community response.

The National Preparedness System and Goal

Presidential Policy Directive 8: National Preparedness calls for national preparedness to be based on core capabilities aimed at "strengthening the security and resilience of the United States through systematic preparation for the threats that pose the greatest risk to the security of the Nation, including acts of terrorism, cyberattacks, pandemics and catastrophic natural disasters" (Obama, 2011). A national preparedness goal and a national preparedness system allows the United States to track capacity and improve capability to prevent, protect against, mitigate the effects of, respond to, and recover from such events. Further, all affected stakeholders (e.g., individuals; families; communities; the private and nonprofit sectors; faith-based organizations; and local, state, tribal, territorial, and federal governments) are engaged in planning, preparedness, and response (U.S. Department of Homeland Security [USDHS], 2016e).

The National Preparedness Goal defines three key themes, five frameworks, and 32 core capabilities needed for the US response to emergencies and disasters. The themes are (a) Engaged Partnership with the Whole Community; (b) Scalability, Flexibility, and Adaptability in Implementation; and (c) Integration among the Frameworks (USDHS, 2015). The National Preparedness System describes the processes used to build, sustain, and deliver core functions and activities necessary to achieve the goal of a secure and resilient nation. Comprised of five individual frameworks (mission areas), the National Planning Frameworks address prevention, protection, mitigation, response, and recovery (USDHS, 2015) (see Table 14-1).

Table 14-1 Capabilities by Mission Area

Prevention	Protection	Mitigation	Response	Recovery
Planning				
Public Information and Warning				
Operational Coordination				
Intelligence and Information Sharing		Community Resilience	Infrastructure Systems	Economic Recovery
Interdiction and Disruption		Long-term Vulnerability Reduction	Critical Transportation	Health and Social Services
Screening, Search, and Detection		Risk and Disaster Resilience Assessment	Environmental Response/Health and Safety	Housing
Forensics and Attribution	Access Control and Identity Verification	Threats and Hazards identification	Fatality Management Services	Natural and Cultural Resources.
	Cybersecurity		Fire Management and Suppression	
	Physical Protective Measures		Logistics and Supply Chain Management	
	Risk Management for Protection Programs and Activities		Mass Care Services	
	Supply Chain integrity and Security		Mass Search and Rescue Operations	
			On-scene Security, Protection, and Law Enforcement	
			Operational Communications	
			Public Health Healthcare, and Emergency Medical Services	
			Situational Assessment	

THE NATIONAL PREVENTION FRAMEWORK

To combat the most dangerous potential bioterrorism agents (e.g., anthrax micro-organisms, cultures of viral encephalitis, and toxic chemicals introduced in foods and water) requires forethought and planning. Hence, the Prevention Framework includes those actions necessary to avoid, prevent, or stop an act of imminent terrorism (threatened or actual) (USDHS, 2016e). As shown in Table 14-1, the seven Prevention core capabilities are Planning; Public Information and Warning; Operational Coordination; Intelligence and Information Sharing; Interdiction and Disruption; Screening, Search, and Detection; and Forensics and Attribution.

THE NATIONAL PROTECTION FRAMEWORK

This Framework focuses on key roles and responsibilities, creating stronger coordinated operational structures that will synchronize community and government stakeholders across the Prevention, Mitigation, Response, and Recovery mission areas (USDHS, 2016d). Sharing the first six core capabilities as the Prevention Framework, Protection adds Physical Protective Measures; Risk Management for Protection Programs and Activities; Screening, Search, and Detection; and Supply Chain Integrity and Security. Stakeholders include but are not limited to operations centers; law enforcement task forces; critical infrastructure partnerships; governance boards; regional consortiums; information sharing mechanisms/consortia; health surveillance networks; and public–private partnership organizations at local, state, regional, and national levels.

THE NATIONAL MITIGATION FRAMEWORK

The Mitigation Framework seeks to reduce the loss of life and property and the impact of disasters/emergencies by fostering a culture of preparedness centered on risk and resilience and emphasizing continuity of operations planning (USDHS, 2016b). In addition to Planning, Public Information and Warning, Operational Coordination, the Mitigation Framework addresses Community Resilience, Long-Term Vulnerability Reduction, Risk and Disaster Resilience Assessment, and Threats and Hazards Identification.

THE NATIONAL RESPONSE FRAMEWORK

The Response Framework describes how the federal government organizes and responds to disasters, public health emergencies, and other catastrophic events within a community response framework. Key concepts for response are scalability, flexibility, and adaptability, as there is no "one-size-fits-all" model for emergency/disaster responses. Of its 15 core capabilities, 11 are unique to its mission: Critical

Transportation; Environmental Response/Health and Safety; Fatality Management Services; Fire Management and Suppression; Infrastructure Systems, Logistics and Supply Chain Management; Mass Care Services; Mass Search and Rescue Operations; On-Scene Security, Protection, and Law Enforcement; Operational Communications; Public Health, Health Care, and Emergency Medical Services; and Situational Assessment (USDHS, 2016e).

THE NATIONAL DISASTER RECOVERY FRAMEWORK

One of the predominant themes surrounding disaster recovery is the concept of resilience, defined by the National Preparedness Goal as "the ability to adapt to changing conditions and withstand and rapidly recover from disruption due to emergencies" (USDHS, 2015, p. A-2). Hence the unique areas of focus for the National Disaster Recovery Framework (NDRF) are Economic Recovery, Health (somatic and behavioral) and Social Services, Housing, Infrastructure Systems, and Natural and Cultural Resources. Hence recovery must be prepared to handle series of interdependent, concurrent, and cascading activities that must address the immediate incident, as well as short-term, intermediate, and long-term effects, needs, and consequences. The Recovery Continuum espoused by the NDRF highlights the reality that "preparedness, response, and recovery are not and cannot be separate and sequential efforts" (USDHS, 2016a, p. 5). The ability to manage recovery effectively begins with predisaster preparedness and requires support and resources focused on recovery at the immediate onset of an incident. It is a series of interdependent, concurrent activities that occur across the short, intermediate, and long term.

THE NATIONAL INCIDENT MANAGEMENT SYSTEM

In 2003, Homeland Security Presidential Directive-5, Management of Domestic Incidents, called for the creation of "a single, comprehensive approach to domestic incident management" (Bush, 2003). This resulted in the creation of the National Incident Management System (NIMS) (USDHS, 2008). While the NRF provides the structure and mechanisms for national level policy to address emergency response, NIMS provides the template for incident management at local, state, regional, and national levels. Since NIMS is based on the concept that all incidents begin and end locally, command remains with state and local authorities and the ability of responders is enhanced by establishing standard procedures and terminology. A common operating picture, for example, offers a standard overview of an incident, compiling data from multiple sources, thus ensuring all responders have a shared understanding and awareness of incident status and information when conducting operations.

The Incident Command Structure (ICS) in NIMS has become the standard for emergency management across the United States. The ICS integrates procedures, personnel, facilities, equipment, and communications into a common organizational structure from the initial occurrence of the event to its conclusion. It specifically addresses Preparedness, Communications and Information Management, Resource Management, Command and Management, and Ongoing Management and Maintenance (USDHS, 2008). Currently undergoing review, the NIMS should be in its updated, second edition by the end of 2017.

In addition to these national response functions, there are a number of other agencies engaged in emergency preparedness in the United States. At the federal level, the list is quite extensive.

The Department of Health and Human Services (DHHS) Secretary of Health and Human Services directs all DHHS emergency response activities. The Office of Assistant Secretary for Health also coordinates emergency activities and monitors progress. The Office of the Assistant Secretary for Public Health Emergency Preparedness coordinates DHHS response activities with other federal departments and agencies. The National Vaccine Program Office coordinates and monitors pandemic preparedness and response plans and activities. The Office of the General Counsel advises on legal and regulatory issues that emerge before, during, or after emergency response activities. The Office of the Assistant Secretary of Public Affairs develops communications plans and disseminates emergency information. The Office of Global Health Affairs oversees interactions with other governments, international organizations, and nongovernmental organizations related to emergency preparedness. The Food and Drug Administration regulates and licenses vaccines and antiviral agents. The National Institutes of Health conducts and supports biomedical research. The Health Resources and Services Administration coordinates emergency preparedness planning for hospital and health care surge capacity. The DHS has overall authority for emergency response activities. The Department of Defense and Department of Veterans Affairs also provides surge capacity of medical equipment, materials, and personnel. The Department of Agriculture conducts surveillance for infectious diseases in domestic animals. The Department of Energy and the Department of Transportation maintain critical infrastructure during emergencies and disasters.

Each department has numerous divisions and units under it. In addition, each state and territory has its own government infrastructure to address emergency preparedness; this does not even address other private- or public-sector organizations that participate in emergency preparedness, planning, mitigation, response, and recovery. Here we examine three more closely: the CDC, FEMA, and the Hospital Preparedness Program.

Centers for Disease Control and Prevention

Founded in 1946, the CDC is one of the 13 major operating components of the DHHS (see chapter 2 for a fuller discussion on the CDC as a federal agency). The

CDC is one of the key components of the federal government when looking for guidance about health care needs in an emergency.

The Public Health Emergency Response Guide for State, Local, and Tribal Public Health Directors Version 2.0 (CDC, 2011) provides information about the public health response in the first 24 hours following a disaster. One component of the information is communications, but other pieces include determining the extent of the problem, such as safe water, transportation, and services access; developing and implementing a plan; and including the many agencies that will respond and provide assistance. Even in the first 24 hours, the response needs vary between the immediate needs (0–2 hours) and the extended phase (12–24 hours). This awareness and response to the changing nature of the needs of the community is very important (Hurd & Mount, 2008).

The CDC Emergency Operations Center uses an Incident Management System to respond to emergencies. This system outlines roles and responsibilities ahead of time; essentially the response plan is in place before the actual emergency is identified (Redd & Frieden, 2017). The CDC uses three levels of CDC response, with Level 1 being a full 24/7 CDC response, the highest level. Examples of past Level 1 responses include Hurricane Katrina in 2005, the 2009 H1N1 influenza outbreak, the 2014 Ebola outbreak, and the 2016 Zika virus (ZIKV) outbreak (Office of the Assistant Secretary for Preparedness and Response [ASPR], 2016).

The emergence of ZIKV in the southeastern United States is an example of the CDC's role in planning for new health events (Hennessey, Fischer, & Staples, 2016). Transmitted by mosquitos to humans, ZIKV has a devastating effect on the developing babies of women who are pregnant, leading to babies who are born with microcephaly (an underdeveloped head) or other serious birth defects (Sampathkumar & Sanchez, 2016). After ZIKV was determined a "Public Health Emergency of international concern" by the World Health Organization, the CDC began emergency countermeasures (Imperato, 2016).

The CDC received $350 million in funding under the Zika Response and Preparedness Act of 2016 (Pub. L. 114–223). By the end of 2016, it had funded a number of initiatives (CDC, 2016). It had distributed $25 million in funding to 53 state, city, and territorial health department in areas at risk for outbreaks of ZIKV based on the risk of local transmission as determined by the estimated range of the two Aedes mosquito species known to transmit ZIKV in the United States (specifically, *Aedes aegypti* and *Aedes albopictus*). Florida and Texas received the largest share, approximately $5 million; other locations included New York City and Puerto Rico.

The act also funded emergency preparedness and response ZIKV activities in 21 jurisdictions at the greatest risk of ZIKV infections, added epidemiologic and birth defects surveillance and investigation, improved mosquito control and monitoring, and strengthened laboratory capacity; it also developed the US Zika Pregnancy Registry to monitor pregnant women with ZIKV and the health and developmental outcomes of children affected by ZIKV. Clearly, ZIKV is a global threat, especially in warmer areas with a mosquito population that can transmit the virus (Imperato, 2016).

Another CDC initiative was the Preparedness and Emergency Response Learning Centers (PERLCs) to continue public health workforce preparedness development. Fourteen PERLCs, located within accredited schools of public health, support organizational and community readiness locally, regionally, or nationally through technical consultation aligned with national preparedness competency frameworks and public health preparedness capabilities (Richmond, Sobelson, & Cioffi, 2014).

Federal Emergency Management Agency

In 1979, Executive Order 12127 created FEMA by merging six federal administrations and programs (FEMA, 2008). In 2003, FEMA and 22 other federal agencies became part of the new USDHS. Dedicated to rapid response to manmade and natural disasters, FEMA provides financial assistance to individuals and governments to rebuild homes, businesses, and public facilities; trains firefighters and emergency medical professionals; and funds emergency planning throughout the United States.

In September 2011, FEMA implemented its "Whole Community" approach to emergency management. The "Whole Community" is FEMA's approach to increase community resilience (FEMA, 2011). Private and nonprofit, the general public, and local, tribal, state, territorial, and federal government partners are participants (Sobelson, Wigington, Harp, & Bronson, 2015).

FEMA asked the CDC Foundation (2013) to evaluate promising programs across the nation to determine how such examples understand community complexity; how these programs recognize the actual needs and collective capabilities of the community; and how they foster, build, and maintain relationships with community leaders and multiorganizational partnerships. The Foundation also examined how these programs leveraged and strengthened the community's social infrastructure, networks, and assets. These and other questions became the basis of a joint FEMA/CDC curriculum designed to teach others how to engage the "whole community."

Hospital Preparedness Program

Also a part of the DHHS, the ASPR helps hospitals and other parts of the health care system prepare for emergencies. This federal program coordinates emergency preparedness and encourages cooperation of providers even though they might normally be competitors. Through coalitions that include health care providers, public health organizations, and other responders, ASPR facilitates collaboration within a community to enable the health care system to continue to function despite the surge in demand during an emergency.

As a part of developing this collaboration, ASPR facilitates drills that simulate an overwhelming need for a community. In its National Guidance for Healthcare System Preparedness report (Office of the Assistant Secretary for Preparedness and Response, 2012), "Capability 14: Responder Safety and Health" (pp. 46–48) specifically addresses pharmaceutical protections, needs assessments, cache management and protection, and medical countermeasure dispensing. In the 2017–2022 Health Care Preparedness and Response Capabilities report, ASPR identifies pharmacy as a key health care function (Office of the Assistant Secretary for Preparedness and Response, 2016, p. 33).

Pharmacists' Role in the National Response Frameworks

Pharmacists play an integral role in prevention by using a public health surveillance model to monitor increases in prescription medications commonly prescribed for potential bioterrorism agents. This prevention strategy has been used successfully in many countries, including the United States and Japan (Ijuin, Kusu, Matsuda, & Hayashi, 2006).

Pharmacists can also assist in the rapid selection of patient-appropriate prophylactic antimicrobials to address possible exposure to bioterrorist agents (Montello, Ostroff, Frank, Haffer, & Rogers, 2002; Veltri, Yaghdjian, Morgan-Joseph, Prlesi, & Rudnick, 2012).

Pharmacists perform credible risk assessments and ensure regulatory compliance for critical medical countermeasures against potential threats from natural, chemical, biological, radiological, or nuclear events (Bhavsar, Kim, & Yu, 2010). They can provide valuable insights as consultants for statewide bioterrorism and emergency preparedness (Feret & Bratberg, 2012; Zod, Fick-Osborne, & Peters, 2014). Just from these examples, we can see the roles pharmacists play in planning, public information and warning, operational coordination, health services, and infrastructure systems

PLANS AND PLANNING

The pharmacist's contribution to emergency preparedness has been recognized by the federal government since at least the 1960s (Cohen, 2003). Indeed, pharmacists have been a key source of public health information and response in their communities whenever they help others. The American Pharmacists Association has a long history of concern for public health in general and for pharmacists who are involved in emergency readiness. It has provided a variety of options for the pharmacist, including training in administering vaccinations, smoking cessation, and disaster preparedness, to name a few. Other pharmacy organizations, such as the American

Society of Health-Systems Pharmacists (Eppert & Reznek, 2011), have made similar contributions. However, most authors are careful to choose inclusive terminology, such as "health care providers" or "first responders," in recognition of the many types of professionals who will find themselves as central decision-makers in health care emergencies (Hurd & Mount, 2008).

From a public health pharmacy point of view, pharmacy also needs to be aware of the changing needs following the crisis. Immediate needs might include first aid and related supplies. One of the immediate concerns is securing the pharmacy's medication supply so that the public, hopefully, has a safe and secure source of medications in the immediate future and remains safe from any kind of drug misuse or abuse. Providing medications related to the crisis or emergency medications would follow. For a damaged pharmacy, a more delayed response is a temporary structure (such as a trailer or bus) to serve as the pharmacy until the bricks-and-mortar structure is repaired.

Community preparedness includes coordinated plans, strategies to treat or quarantine, communications between various health providers and service groups, and supplies that would be needed (from drugs to chemical protection suits to radiation monitors). For example, stockpiling ciprofloxacin, which is a treatment for anthrax, has become more important as a result of the contamination of mail and postal facilities (Leitenberg, 2005).

The NIMS Incident Command Structure includes subcomponents at the state and local level, including the response from pharmacists and pharmacies. Pharmacists' involvement includes preventing disease (e.g., through vaccinations, including tetanus), preventing injury, and decreasing the exposure to environmental hazards such as unsafe water, sanitation problems, and mold clean-up. Emergency medication and pharmacy dispensing, of course, is another part of this response.

In his history of emergency medical services in the United States, Shah (2006) found much of the early emphasis was on transportation needs, especially related to traumatic injuries and cardiovascular disease. The focus on accidents and heart attacks also led to an increase in the medical technology available to those who were first responders. The provision of these services used a decentralized government approach, emphasizing local control more than national rules and regulations. With this background, coordinating emergency medical services for large disasters becomes very challenging. Along a similar line of thought, the public health data that might be very useful to set boundaries on a particular disaster or to detect a common problem are difficult to collect and compile.

Disaster plans are part of the accreditation requirements for hospitals and other health care organizations through the Joint Commission on Accreditation of Healthcare Organizations (Joint Commission, 2006, 2016). After the September 11 terrorist attack on the United States in 2001, the National Hospital Ambulatory Medical Care Survey surveyed approximately 500 non-federal hospitals in the United States regarding the level of their preparedness in the event of terrorism

(Niska & Burt, 2005). Almost all hospitals (97.3%) had plans for natural disasters, and most hospitals (75% or higher) had plans for chemical, biological, explosive, or nuclear/radiological events. In addition to plans, hospitals had included training of their personnel and drills to practice the institution's response. In many cases, hospitals collaborated with other groups in these drills or simulations, and most of the plans included contact with public health departments.

Since then, hospitals have made great strides in preparing for disasters and large numbers of injured people. The hospital planning and response to the Boston Marathon bombings in 2013 provide insights into the steps that hospitals have taken to prepare for mass casualty incidents (Gates et al., 2014). A joint USDHS and FEMA (2014) report describes the coordinated response of first responders and hospitals, the communications between providers, the exercises and planning that occurred prior to the event, and the effectiveness of triaged care.

A state-level after-action review of the Boston Marathon bombing, coordinated by a multidisciplinary, multijurisdictional project management team of key responders, found a number of best practices already in place provided the supports necessary to triage and transport the injured quickly from the scene of the incident to trauma centers for care (Project Management Team, 2014). These included the all-hazards medical system put in place on Marathon Day; hospitals scheduling fewer surgeries and other medical appointments on race day, which allowed their respective departments to be ready to handle a surge; and the establishment of a multiagency coordination center (MACC). The MACC played an integral role coordinating with the Unified Command Center in response to the bombings as did member participation in multijurisdictional exercises to handle a surge (mass casualty) event.

However, preparedness means eternal vigilance, as situations change rapidly and it can be difficult to envision best-response practice to scenarios. We can learn from the experiences of other countries. Similar to the United States, Israeli emergency personnel, health care providers, and medical facilities operate under national policies based on an "all hazards" approach (Adini & Peleg, 2013). Reviewing the preparedness of US hospitals through an Israeli lens, a number of security recommendations were recommended (Golabek-Goldman, 2016). These included conducting more frequent and realistic lockdown exercises; adding permanent emergency signage; enhancing security perimeter protocols; in-depth training to increase an institution's defense against primary and secondary attacks; and better coordination with local, state, and national law enforcement (e.g., the police and sheriff departments, National Guard) and other outside security agencies (Golabek-Goldman, 2016).

In addition, compulsory emergency response training for all medical institutions and first responders and regular exercises for all acute care facilities responding to mass-casualty incidents are central to ensure accurate and appropriate responses

(Adini & Peleg, 2013). These recommendations would apply to public health facilities and personnel as well as pharmacist networks.

PERSONNEL

While health professionals, such as pharmacists, are an essential part of a response to disaster, they are often represent the second wave of response, helping those individuals brought to the hospital or clinic for care. The first professional people to respond often include law enforcement personnel, firefighters, paramedics, and security personnel. Public safety personnel and public works personnel are also involved. With more time, state emergency management offices, the Red Cross, local government, and community groups have time to respond. Other groups, such as not-for-profit organizations and offices of the federal government, also may respond, depending on the nature of the disaster. The list goes on to include volunteers, church groups, specialized response people (e.g., trained dog handlers or scuba divers), and service organizations.

SUPPLIES (PHYSICAL RESOURCES)

The Public Health Security and Bioterrorism Preparedness Act of 2002 directs the Secretary of the USDHHS to maintain a Strategic National Stockpile (SNS) whose statutory mission is to provide for the emergency health security of the United States in the event of a bioterrorist attack or other public health emergency. The act also specifically includes provisions for stockpile management and security requirements.

At the national level, stockpiling drugs and vaccines is an important step in the planned response to a threat, but it is a step that is less appropriate for state, city, or local government. Coordinating the use of materials in the SNS with individuals at a specific site is often quite challenging. One example is delivering drugs to an emergency pharmacy operation. What paperwork is appropriate? How is security assured? How do federal, state, and local laws apply to the distribution of these products?

The CDC's SNS is the nation's largest supply of antibiotics, chemical antidotes, antitoxins, vaccines, antiviral drugs, and other medical material for use in a serious public health emergency when local supplies are exhausted (Board on Health Sciences Policy, 2016). Since the 2001 anthrax attacks, the CDC has responded to three major public health emergencies using the SNS: (a) the 2009–2010 H1N1 influenza pandemic, (b) the 2014–2016 Ebola epidemic in West Africa, and (c) the current ZIKV epidemic (Redd & Frieden, 2017).

The SNS handles medical countermeasure (MCMs) requests from state, local, tribal, territorial, and national responders. The development of federal medical stations and the Cities Readiness Initiative (Jones, Neff, Ely, & Parker, 2012) established protocols to disperse MCMs to people within less than 48 hours after a decision to dispense, using multiple points of dispensing and rapid dispensing processes. In addition, the SNS also provides supplemental funds to stockpile pandemic influenza MCMs and personal protective equipment.

Established in 2006 as a partner with the SNS, the Public Health Emergency Medical Countermeasures Enterprise develops strategic plans on MCM prioritization and the use of MCMs against chemical, biological, radiological, nuclear, and explosive (CBRNE) threats and emerging infectious diseases, including influenza. In addition, the joint National Science and Technology Council and Committee on Homeland and National Security Subcommittee on Standards (2011) established a working document to develop a national strategy to create CBRNE equipment standards by 2020 that will include evaluating equipment, interoperability, training of users, standard vocabulary, and standard operating procedures for response.

PREPARATION: DRILLS AND EXERCISES

One of the changes in public health preparedness in the recent past has been the efforts to assess preparedness for public health emergencies like bioterrorism, with the lessons learned extending to preparedness for other crises (Katz, Staiti, & McKenzie, 2006). Drills range from part-day local drills to multiday national events (e.g., TOPOFF exercises using the top officials in multistate events). Some of these drills are in the field, using a community or a stadium, and some are tabletop activities with less realistic simulations.

Preparation also can be assessed by examining the response to real crises, such as the 2004–2005 flu vaccine shortage, that would be similar to problems that resulted from a bioterrorism event like anthrax. Public health emergencies, such as the Midwest blackout in 2003, have provided valuable real-life situations that help evaluate both the regional and national response.

One of our major challenges is the inadequate surge capacity in responding to a crisis, especially in the areas of staff, materials, structure, and system (Katz et al., 2006). To scale up operations to handle these surges, emergency agencies require access to resources in larger than normal quantities and specialized equipment or personnel. Local workforces (public health and emergency responders), hospital staff and bed space, and stockpiled resources often are inadequate for a major crisis. Electric companies that send repair teams across the country to deal with a regional power outage provide one example of the kind of response that is necessary when the available resources at the local level cannot possibly meet the demand caused by a crisis. The sudden need for many buses to evacuate individuals without transportation, the elderly, or handicapped people from New Orleans is another example of a surge demand that required coordinated effort.

Especially in the hospital setting and to a lesser extent in community settings, pharmacists have a rather direct involvement in dealing with hazardous materials, such as disposing of dangerous drugs, preparing chemotherapy under a hood, dealing with sharps (used syringes), and disposing of tubing and containers that cannot be used again. These skills and training can be especially useful in disaster situations, both from a knowledge/advice perspective and from a hands-on service angle (Cohen, 2003).

Reviewing the literature on infectious diseases likely to be used in a bioterrorist attack, pharmacists can make recommendations regarding diagnosis, therapy, and prevention through such means as vaccination. Terriff, Schwartz, and Lomaestro (2003) provide an example of this kind of endeavor. In the response to a biological threat or disaster, pharmacy personnel are needed in the hospital setting to provide treatment, in the pharmacy to provide medication, and potentially in the pharmacy and other clinics to provide vaccinations.

How a public health service (PHS) team responded to Hurricane Katrina by setting up a facility to meet the needs of low-acuity hospitalized patients provides key insights into the type of challenges that are faced in responding to an emergency. In a study by Velazquez et al. (2006), the PHS team of 70 officers included eight pharmacists. One of the first requirements was to establish a secure space for the pharmacy. Although they were on a naval air base, where security already was provided, they needed to find a safe place for medications and controlled substances. A locked, caged area in the airplane hangar that housed the hospital was the best choice available. When the pharmacy received pharmaceutical supplies from the SNS, these supplies did not include many of the drugs needed for an emergency of this size, such as insulin and tetanus toxoid vaccines.

The team also received an order of controlled medications through an umbrella Drug Enforcement Administration number, solving some of the problems of acquiring these types of medications. They established a way to order drugs from a national wholesaler, again helping to stock the pharmacy. Establishing Internet access, policies and procedures for drug distribution, and medication security at nursing stations added to the work of setting up this pharmacy. With a limited supply of medications, policies needed to be established about the amount of drug to be distributed to a patient at any one time (Velazquez et al., 2006).

Basic equipment, such as shelving, refrigerators, furniture, photocopiers, and word-processing equipment, had to be found or purchased (Velazquez et al., 2006). Non-pharmacy staff were constantly updated on the drugs that were available in the pharmacy through photocopies of updated word-processed documents. Further, upon patient discharge, all the medical information that had been reconstructed from the patient and the care of the patient needed to be provided to his or her relocation provider. Many creative responses were needed; backpacks filled with emergency supplies and equipment became "crash carts" for those with cardiac emergencies in the facility; patients who could administer their own medications were allowed to do this, with labeled bags tied to their beds (Velazquez et al., 2006). One can only imagine the hard work, cooperation, and creativity that were a necessary part of this effort. Reading the description provided by these pharmacists is instructional and inspiring; realizing that others were providing similarly valiant assistance throughout the region can be overwhelming.

Disaster situations have great moments of altruism, but they also have many self-centered behaviors. For example, during the anthrax scare, when individuals were exposed to anthrax via letters that had been sent through the postal system, the demand for ciprofloxacin (an antibiotic that is prescribed for anthrax) increased drastically. People were stockpiling the drug for future anthrax exposures. Some pharmacies had trouble keeping the drug in stock. Those who might need the drug faced the possibility of not being able to find a source of supply in a major crisis. Those planning responses to this kind of disaster need to include plans to deal with this kind of individual behavior early in the crisis.

In a disaster, the collection of information and the coordination of the use of that information can be a crucial part of an effective response. If it is a biological threat, pharmacists can play a key role because of their knowledge of drugs and diseases. The choice of drug, administration, storage, delivery, and sources of supply are all key pieces of information that others might not have. Other information may help estimate the extent of the potential threat, the number of cases, the timing of the disease in the population, and the necessary preventive actions.

After a disaster, many individuals have refill difficulties. With no phones, no pharmacist, and potentially no pharmacy building, it would be difficult to determine if the individual was in a pharmacy network or if there was a record of the prescription, or to call the old pharmacy to verify information. A pharmacist's natural response would be to contact his or her own state board to ask for guidance on how to help these individuals. A state board with no plan or no broad-based communication will likely be overwhelmed with calls asking very similar questions. Sometimes the prescription container might be available to document the prescription, but that is not the same as a prescription. An urgent care center or physician visit would be required. In any event, records that include the basic information needed by the pharmacy should be kept.

Pharmacists and other health professionals can be trained to detect early signs of disease that might indicate a bioterrorist attack. In addition, pharmacy drug records have the potential, in an aggregate format, to help identify the location and extent of a public health problem through the prescription and/or over-the-counter drug sale changes. Public health surveillance has begun to include nontraditional warnings, including the sale of pharmaceutical products that are unusual in a particular region, in the detection of a bioterrorist attack and other health crises (Turnock, 2012).

In a 2004 survey of pharmacy practice in ambulatory care settings, pharmacist involvement in emergency preparedness was greater than 50% of all respondents and over 90% in such specific areas as involvement in emergency preparedness within the organization (Knapp, Okamoto, & Black, 2005). Emergency preparedness was a topic surveyed for the first time in this longitudinal project, as an emerging area of pharmacist activity along with medication management services, indigent care programs, and others. Claver et al. (2012) emphasize general and mental health status and services use, patient tracking, evacuation, and disaster planning/prepa ration. Noe and Smith (2013) recommend pharmacists have a manual for disaster preparedness that addresses applicable pharmacy regulations, risk assessment, and public needs during a disaster that focus on the response of the pharmacy to the community.

Sometimes the effects of a tragedy are long term and yet have application to pharmacy. For example, Wu et al. (2006) reported an increase in smoking by high school students after the September 11, 2001, attack on the World Trade Center. The authors pointed out the need for targeted substance-use interventions following disasters. Bass et al. (2016) reported the need for trauma-informed interventions for survivors of torture and related trauma in Kurdistan and Iraq. Potentially, this type of follow-up intervention, whether for smoking, posttraumatic stress disorder, or some other area, offers a real opportunity for pharmacists to continue to support their communities in the long-term response to a tragedy.

Implications for Pharmacists and Pharmacy Practice

The areas of emergency preparedness that would benefit from pharmacy involvement are significant. For example, pharmacists with knowledge of burn care can assist in providing optimum care, getting patients ready to leave hospital care, recommending the most recent products, and providing valuable information to other health care providers. Pharmacists with a knowledge of dangerous chemicals can help in identifying the hazardous substances involved and the recommended treatment. Some pharmacies have programs to notify patients prior to an emergency to pick up their refills in advance of a possible disaster.

The implications, however, can also be more fundamental. Boards of pharmacy may not be ready to deal with disasters/emergencies within their states. Professional boards are encouraged to have existing statutory or regulatory language to address practice issues during a disaster before a disaster occurs; hence model acts can help to standardize language, operational practice, reciprocal licensing, and so on across states to expedite response and mitigation. After Hurricane Katrina, the National Association of Boards of Pharmacy developed a Model Pharmacy Act, containing eight Rules for Public Health Emergencies. In 2015, Ford, Trent, and Wickizer (2016) reviewed state statutes, rules, and regulations to determine if any of the eight

Rules for Public Health Emergencies from the National Association of Boards of Pharmacy Model Pharmacy Act were incorporated into existing documentation.

Twenty states had adopted no Rules for Public Health Emergencies (Ford et al., 2016). Rule 2, addressing policies and procedures for reporting disasters, was the most adopted rule. Although 10 states had addressed emergency refill dispensing in some way, emergency refill quantities differed between the states that had established this guideline (Ford et al., 2016). While state boards of pharmacy can and indeed have adopted emergency rules to deal with a disaster, the ideal plan would be to have this in place prior to an event so the response can be immediate and planned for by pharmacies. For example, hurricanes normally are anticipated events and allow time for health care providers, including pharmacies, to put plans in place prior to the event. Indeed, Ford et al.'s research suggested that the southeastern states were better prepared to deal with disasters (e.g., refills, emergency licenses for out-of-state pharmacists, and the use of pharmacies outside the immediate area).

Pharmacist work in disaster preparedness has taken many focuses. Efforts have been made to help prepare community pharmacists for disasters by developing a disaster preparedness manual (Noe & Smith, 2013). Cohen (2003) gives a detailed example of how a health-system pharmacy team might be organized in order to respond to terrorism attacks. Other researchers have developed a classification scheme for pharmacy personnel to identify essential actions that would ensure an effective emergency response (Alkhalili, Ma, & Grenier, 2017).

The American Association of Colleges of Pharmacy has produced a white paper on public health and the CAPE 2013 Educational Outcomes, which cover numerous ways to include public health in both introductory and advanced practice experiences, focusing mostly on providing patient/population care but including disaster preparedness (Covvey et al., 2016).

Another project describes emergency preparedness modules used in an Introductory Pharmacy Practice Experience (Hannings, von Waldner, McEwen, & White, 2016). These simulations included triage of injured patients, transport decisions, simulated injuries, and a mass-dispensing simulation. Students were evaluated on the accuracy of their performances and provided feedback about their experiences. Exposing students to these less than traditional pharmacy roles can help prepare them for real emergencies, both small and regional.

These types of educational projects put disaster/emergency preparedness in perspective for a pharmacy education program. Disaster preparedness correctly is considered a nontraditional role and is one that requires specialized training. Much of public health pharmacy has focused on disease prevention and health promotion.

Pharmacists, and pharmacy students, normally have a limited exposure to the principles and structures of emergency management necessary to help coordinate effective and rapid responses. Finding ways to weave these components of public health into a curriculum can be challenging but can also help pharmacy build on a strong foundation of patient and population care. Finding ways to communicate pharmacists' capabilities and training to others will also be a challenge for the profession.

References

Abramson, D. M., & Garfield, R. (2006). *On the edge: Children and families displaced by Hurricanes Katrina and Rita face a looming medical and mental health crisis.* New York: National Center for Disaster Preparedness, Mailman School of Public Health, Columbia University and Operation Assist.

Abramson, D. M., Stehling-Ariza, T., Park, Y. S., Walsh, L., & Culp, D. (2010). Measuring individual disaster recovery: A socioecological framework. *Disaster Medicine and Public Health Preparedness, 4*(Suppl. 1), S46–S54. doi:10.1001/dmp.2010.14

Adini, B., & Peleg, K. (2013). On constant alert: Lessons to be learned from Israel's emergency response to mass-casualty terrorism incidents. *Health Affairs, 32*(12), 2179–2185. doi:10.1377/hlthaff.2013.0956

Alkhalili, M., Ma, J., & Grenier, S. (2017). Defining roles for pharmacy personnel in disaster response and emergency preparedness. *Disaster Medicine and Public Health Preparedness.* Advance online publication. doi:10.1017/dmp.2016.172

Arya, V., Medina, E., Scaccia, A., Mathew, C., & Starr, D. (2016). Impact of Hurricane Sandy on community pharmacies in severely affected areas of New York City: A qualitative assessment. *American Journal of Disaster Medicine, 11*(1), 21–30. doi:10.5055/ajdm.2016.0221

Bass, J., Murray, S. M., Mohammed, T. A., Bunn, M., Gorman, W., Ahmed, A. M., . . . Bolton, P. (2016). A randomized controlled trial of a trauma-informed support, skills, and psychoeducation intervention for survivors of torture and related trauma in Kurdistan, Northern Iraq. *Global Health, Science and Practice, 4*(3), 452–466. doi:10.9745/ghsp-d-16-00017

Bhavsar, T. R., Kim, H. J., & Yu, Y. (2010). Roles and contributions of pharmacists in regulatory affairs at the Centers for Disease Control and Prevention for public health emergency preparedness and response. *Journal of the American Pharmacists Association, 50*(2), 165–168.

Binagwaho, A., Farmer, P. E., Nsanzimana, S., Karema, C., Gasana, M., de Dieu Ngirabega, J., . . . Drobac, P. C. (2014). Rwanda 20 years on: Investing in life. *The Lancet, 384*(9940), 371–375. doi:10.1016/s0140-6736(14)60574-2

Board on Health Sciences Policy. (2016). *The nation's medical countermeasure stockpile: Opportunities to improve the efficiency, effectiveness, and sustainability of the CDC Strategic National Stockpile: Workshop summary.* Washington, DC: National Academies Press.

Bush, G. W. (2003, February 28). Homeland Security presidential directive (HSPD)-5: Management of domestic incidents. Retrieved from https://www.gpo.gov/fdsys/pkg/PPP-2003-book1/pdf/PPP-2003-book1-doc-pg229.pdf

Caserta, T. A., Pirttila-Backman, A. M., & Punamaki, R. L. (2016). Stigma, marginalization and psychosocial well-being of orphans in Rwanda: Exploring the mediation role of social support. *AIDS Care, 28*(6), 736–744. doi:10.1080/09540121.2016.1147012

Centers for Disease Control and Prevention. (1996). Morbidity and mortality surveillance in Rwandan refugees: Burundi and Zaire, 1994. *MMWR: Morbidity and Mortality Weekly Report, 45*(5), 104–107.

Centers for Disease Control and Prevention. (2011). *Public health emergency response guide for state, local, and tribal public health directors—version 2.0.* Atlanta, GA: Author.

Centers for Disease Control and Prevention. (2016, December 22). CDC awards nearly $184 million to continue the fight against Zika [Press release]. Retrieved from https://www.cdc.gov/media/releases/2016/p1222-zika-funding.html

Chaudhury, S., Brown, F. L., Kirk, C. M., Mukunzi, S., Nyirandagijimana, B., Mukandanga, J., . . . Betancourt, T. S. (2016). Exploring the potential of a family-based prevention intervention to reduce alcohol use and violence within HIV-affected families in Rwanda. *AIDS Care, 28*(Suppl. 2), 118–129. doi:10.1080/09540121.2016.1176686

Claver, M., Friedman, D., Dobalian, A., Ricci, K., & Horn Mallers, M. (2012). The role of Veterans Affairs in emergency management: A systematic literature review. *PLoS Currents, 4,* 1–14. doi:10.1371/198d344bc40a75f927c9bc5024279815

Cohen, V. (2003). Organization of a health-system pharmacy team to respond to episodes of terrorism. *American Journal of Health-System Pharmacy, 60*(12), 1257–1263.

Covvey, J. R., Conry, J. M., Bullock, K. C., DiPietro, N. A., Goad, J., Golchin, N., . . . Patterson-Browning, B. (2016). *Public health and the CAPE 2013 educational outcomes: Inclusion, pedagogical considerations and assessment.* Alexandria, VA: American Association of Colleges of Pharmacy.

Dabelstein, N. (1996). Evaluating the international humanitarian system: Rationale, process and management of the joint evaluation of the international response to the Rwanda genocide. *Disasters, 20*(4), 286–294.

Eppert, H. D., & Reznek, A. J. (2011). ASHP guidelines on emergency medicine pharmacist services. *American Journal of Health-System Pharmacy, 68*(23), e81–e95. doi:10.2146/sp110020e

Federal Emergency Management Agency. (1996). Guide for all-hazards emergency operations planning. Washington, DC: Author. Retrieved from http://www.fema.gov/pdf/plan/slg101.pdf.

Federal Emergency Management Agency. (2008, July). FEMA: Prepared. Responsive. Committed FEMA B-653. Washington, DC: Author.

Federal Emergency Management Agency. (December, 2011). A Whole Community Approach to Emergency Management: Principles, Themes, and Pathways for Action. Washington, DC: Author. Retrieved from https://www.fema.gov/media-library-data/20130726-1813-25045-0649/whole_community_dec2011__2_.pdf.

Feret, B., & Bratberg, J. (2012). A ten-year experience of a pharmacist consulting team for statewide bioterrorism and emergency preparedness. *Medicine and Health, Rhode Island, 95*(9), 279–280.

Ford, H., Trent, S., & Wickizer, S. (2016). An assessment of state board of pharmacy legal documents for public health emergency preparedness. *American Journal of Pharmaceutical Education, 80*(2), 20. doi:10.5688/ajpe80220

Gates, J. D., Arabian, S., Biddinger, P., Blansfield, J., Burke, P., Chung, S., . . . Yaffe, M. B. (2014). The initial response to the Boston Marathon bombing: Lessons learned to prepare for the next disaster. *Annals of Surgery, 260*(6), 960–966. doi:10.1097/sla.0000000000000914

Golabek-Goldman, M. (2016). Adequacy of US hospital security preparedness for mass casualty incidents: Critical lessons from the Israeli Experience. *Journal of Public Health Management and Practice, 22*(1), 68–80. doi:10.1097/phh.0000000000000298

Hannings, A. N., von Waldner, T., McEwen, D. W., & White, C. A. (2016). Assessment of emergency preparedness modules in introductory pharmacy practice experiences. *American Journal of Pharmaceutical Education, 80*(2), 23. doi:10.5688/ajpe80223

Hennessey, M., Fischer, M., & Staples, J. E. (2016). Zika virus spreads to new areas: Region of the Americas, May 2015–January 2016. *MMWR: Morbidity and Mortality Weekly Report, 65*(3), 55–58. doi:10.15585/mmwr.mm6503e1

Hintjens, H. M. (1999). Explaining the 1994 genocide in Rwanda. *Journal of Modern African Studies, 37*(2), 241–287.

Hurd, P. D., & Mount, J. K. (2008). Health emergency preparedness and response. In B. L. Levin, P. D. Hurd, & A. Hanson (Eds.), *Introduction to public health in pharmacy* (pp. 321–336). Sudbury, MA: Jones and Bartlett.

Ijuin, K., Kusu, F., Matsuda, R., & Hayashi, Y. (2006). Method for detecting health injury from prescriptions at a pharmacy. *Yakugaku Zasshi: Journal of the Pharmaceutical Society of Japan, 126*(4), 283–287. doi:10.1248/yakushi.126.283

Imperato, P. J. (2016). The convergence of a virus, mosquitoes, and human travel in globalizing the Zika epidemic. *Journal of Community Health, 41*(3), 674–679. doi:10.1007/s10900-016-0177-7

Joint Commission. (2006). *Surge hospitals: Providing safe care in emergencies.* Oakbrook, IL: Author.

Joint Commission. (2016). *Emergency management in health care: An all-hazards approach* (3rd ed.). Oakbrook, IL: Author.

Jones, J. R., Neff, L. J., Ely, E. K., & Parker, A. M. (2012). Results of medical countermeasure drills among 72 cities readiness initiative metropolitan statistical areas, 2008–2009. *Disaster Medicine and Public Health Preparedness, 6*(4), 357–362. doi:10.1001/dmp.2012.68

Katz, A., Staiti, A. B., & McKenzie, K. L. (2006). Preparing for the unknown, responding to the known: Communities and public health preparedness. *Health Affairs, 25*(4), 946–957. doi:10.1377/hlthaff.25.4.946

Knapp, K. K., Okamoto, M. P., & Black, B. L. (2005). ASHP survey of ambulatory care pharmacy practice in health systems—2004. *American Journal of Health-System Pharmacy, 62*(3), 274–284.

Leitenberg, M. (2005). *Assessing the biological weapons and bioterrorism threat* (Strategic Studies Institute series). Carlisle, PA: Strategic Studies Institute.

Mandelbaum-Schmid, J. (2004). Rwandan genocide survivors in need of HIV treatment. *Bulletin of the World Health Organization, 82*(6), 472.

Montello, M. J., Ostroff, C., Frank, E. C., Haffer, A. S., & Rogers, J. R. (2002). 2001 anthrax crisis in Washington, D.C.: Pharmacists' role in screening patients and selecting prophylaxis. *American Journal of Health-System Pharmacy, 59*(12), 1193–1199.

National Science and Technology Council and Committee on Homeland and National Security Subcommittee on Standards. (2011, May). *A national strategy for CBRNE standards.* Washington, DC: Author.

Neugebauer, R., Forde, A., Fodor, K. E., Fisher, P. W., Turner, J. B., Stehling-Ariza, T., & Yamabe, S. (2016). Are children or adolescents more at risk for posttraumatic stress reactions following exposure to violence? Evidence from post-genocide Rwanda. *Journal of Nervous and Mental Disease.* Advance online publication. doi:10.1097/nmd.0000000000000582

Niska, R. W., & Burt, C. W. (2005). Bioterrorism and mass casualty preparedness in hospitals: United States, 2003. *Advanced Data, 364,* 1–14.

Noe, B., & Smith, A. (2013). Development of a community pharmacy disaster preparedness manual. *Journal of the American Pharmacists Association, 53*(4), 432–437. doi:10.1331/JAPhA.2013.12115

Obama, B. (2011). Presidential policy directive/PPD-8: National preparedness. Retrieved from http://www.dhs.gov/presidential-policy-directive-8-national-preparedness

Office of Public Health Preparedness and Response. (2013). *The all-hazards preparedness guide.* Atlanta, GA: Centers for Disease Control and Prevention.

Office of the Assistant Secretary for Preparedness and Response. (2012, January). *The healthcare preparedness capabilities: National guidance for healthcare system preparedness.* Washington, DC: Author.

Office of the Assistant Secretary for Preparedness and Response. (2016, November). *2017–2022 health care preparedness and response capabilities* Washington, DC: Author. Retrieved from http://www.phe.gov/Preparedness/planning/hpp/reports/Documents/2017-2022-healthcare-pr-capablities.pdf

Project Management Team. (2014, December). *After action report for the response to the 2013 Boston Marathon bombings.* Boston: Author.

Redd, S. C., & Frieden, T. R. (2017). CDC's evolving approach to emergency response. *Health Security, 15*(1), 41–52. doi:10.1089/hs.2017.0006

Richmond, A. L., Sobelson, R. K., & Cioffi, J. P. (2014). Preparedness and emergency response learning centers: Supporting the workforce for national health security. *Journal of Public Health Management and Practice, 20*(Suppl. 5), S7–S16. doi:10.1097/phh.0000000000000107

Rubanzana, W., Hedt-Gauthier, B. L., Ntaganira, J., & Freeman, M. D. (2015). Exposure to genocide as a risk factor for homicide perpetration in Rwanda: A population-based case-control study. *Journal of Interpersonal Violence.* doi:10.1177/0886260515619749

Sampathkumar, P., & Sanchez, J. L. (2016). Zika virus in the Americas: A review for clinicians. *Mayo Clinic Proceedings, 91*(4), 514–521. doi:10.1016/j.mayocp.2016.02.017

Shah, M. N. (2006). The formation of the emergency medical services system. *American Journal of Public Health, 96*(3), 414–423. doi:10.2105/AJPH.2004.048793

Sobelson, R. K., Wigington, C. J., Harp, V., & Bronson, B. B. (2015). A whole community approach to emergency management: Strategies and best practices of seven community programs. *Journal of Emergency Management, 13*(4), 349–357. doi:10.5055/jem.2015.0247

Terriff, C. M., Schwartz, M. D., & Lomaestro, B. M. (2003). Bioterrorism: Pivotal clinical issues. Consensus review of the Society of Infectious Diseases Pharmacists. *Pharmacotherapy, 23*(3), 274–290. doi:10.1592/phco.23.3.274.32097

Turnock, B. J. (2012). Public health emergency preparedness and response. In *Public health: What it is and how it works* (pp. 423–484). Sudbury, MA: Jones and Bartlett.

U.S. Department of Homeland Security. (2008, December). *National Incident Management System.* Washington, DC: Author.

U.S. Department of Homeland Security. (2015, September). *National Preparedness Goal* (2nd ed.). Washington, DC: Author.

U.S. Department of Homeland Security. (2016a, June). *National Disaster Recovery Framework* (2nd ed.). Washington, DC: Author.

U.S. Department of Homeland Security. (2016b). *National Mitigation Framework* Washington, DC: Author.

U.S. Department of Homeland Security. (2016c, June). *National Prevention Framework* (2nd ed.). Washington, DC: Author.

U.S. Department of Homeland Security. (2016d, June). *National Protection Framework.* Washington, DC: Author.

U.S. Department of Homeland Security. (2016e, June). *National Response Framework* (3rd ed.). Washington, DC: Author.

U.S. Department of Homeland Security, & Federal Emergency Management Agency. (2014). *Boston Marathon bombings: Hospital readiness and response* (Lessons Learned). Washington, DC: Author.

Velazquez, L., Dallas, S., Rose, L., Evans, K. S., Saville, R., Wang, J., . . . Bona, J. D. (2006). A PHS pharmacist team's response to Hurricane Katrina. *American Journal of Health-System Pharmacy, 63*(14), 1332–1335. doi:10.2146/ajhp060020

Veltri, K., Yaghdjian, V., Morgan-Joseph, T., Prlesi, L., & Rudnick, E. (2012). Hospital emergency preparedness: Push-POD operation and pharmacists as immunizers. *Journal of the American Pharmacists Association, 52*(1), 81–85. doi:10.1331/JAPhA.2012.11191

Verwimp, P. (2004). Death and survival during the 1994 genocide in Rwanda. *Population Studies, 58*(2), 233–245. doi:10.1080/0032472042000224422

Willis, B. M., & Levy, B. S. (2000). Recognizing the public health impact of genocide. *JAMA, 284*(5), 612–614. doi:10.1001/jama.284.5.612

Wu, P., Duarte, C. S., Mandell, D. J., Fan, B., Liu, X., Fuller, C. J., . . . Hoven, C. W. (2006). Exposure to the World Trade Center attack and the use of cigarettes and alcohol among New York City public high-school students. *American Journal of Public Health, 96*(5), 804–807. doi:10.2105/ajph.2004.058925

Zod, R., Fick-Osborne, R., & Peters, E. B. (2014). A functional needs approach to emergency planning. *Disaster Medicine and Public Health Preparedness, 8*(4), 301–309. doi:10.1017/dmp.2014.57

15

Education and Training

ANGELA S. GARCIA, DANIEL FORRISTER,

KRYSTAL BULLERS, AND PETER D. HURD

History of Public Health Training in Pharmacy Education

The first mention of public health in the pharmacy curriculum was in 1932 in the fourth edition of *The Pharmaceutical Syllabus*, a work used by the American Council on Pharmaceutical Education (ACPE) to guide accreditation decisions (Gibson, 1972). While the health literature recognized the unique position held by pharmacists to interact with the community, public health was not emphasized in curricular requirements in the United States until the inception of the *Healthy People* program in 1979 (Babb & Babb, 2003; Calis et al., 2004; Lenz, Monaghan, & Hetterman, 2007). More recently, the Association for Prevention Teaching and Research formed the interprofessional Healthy People Curriculum Task Force (2015) to ensure that core competencies were included in each of the health professions training curricula that would prepare future health professionals to understand the principles of population health and generally improve health outcomes at the individual, clinical, and community levels.

This growing focus on training pharmacists in public health has influenced each iteration of the Center for the Advancement of Pharmaceutical Education (CAPE) Educational Outcomes produced by the American Association of Colleges of Pharmacy (AACP). Each CAPE Educational Outcomes document since 1998 has included recommendations regarding population-based health improvement, wellness, and disease prevention (AACP, 1998, 2004, 2013). As a result, the ACPE now requires that schools and colleges conferring a doctor of pharmacy (PharmD) degree not only inform candidates about public health programs but also provide opportunities to participate in public health focused skills, such as immunization delivery (ACPE, 2015).

Training and Certification in Public Health

Formal and informal certification and training are available in public health through-out the field of pharmacy. Opportunities to gain public health knowledge and skills are available at all levels within the pharmacy profession, from pharmacy technician certification to doctoral and postgraduate studies.

PHARMACY TECHNICIAN

The first level of formal certification available in the field of pharmacy in the United States is that of pharmacy technician. While some states require a high school diploma and on-the-job training, most states require certification either through completing a postsecondary degree program, passing an exam, or both (Anderson, Draime, & Anderson, 2016; Bureau of Labor Statistics, 2015b). The American Society of Health-System Pharmacists (ASHP) has developed public health objec-tives for pharmacy technician training that include a grasp of the concepts of well-ness promotion and disease prevention, such as health screenings and substance abuse, as well as an understanding of the circumstances that influence health (ASHP, 2015).

DOCTOR OF PHARMACY

The required entry-level degree for a pharmacist is a PharmD. This program requires four academic years of education (although this may be compressed into three cal-endar years) and, while most PharmD candidates enter the program with an average of three years of postsecondary education, students able to meet the program pre-requisites may enter with just a high school diploma. The National Association of Boards of Pharmacy (NABP) requires candidates to have a PharmD from an ACPE-accredited institution to sit for the North American Pharmacist Licensure Exam (NAPLEX). This represents a change from the previous requirements for a five-year bachelor's degree in pharmacy after the NABP deemed more hands-on clinical practice experience was necessary. Passing both the NAPLEX and the Multistate Pharmacy Jurisprudence Examination, in addition to state-specific requirements, such as completing a set number of hours of internship under a licensed pharma-cist, are required prerequisites to state licensure to practice pharmacy in that state (Bureau of Labor Statistics, 2015a). Pharmacists must renew their license at regular intervals as determined by the state issuing the license.

Students pursuing a PharmD can expect to encounter public health throughout the didactic and experiential portions of their degree. The ACPE (2015) requires the curricula to include "exploration of population health management strate-gies, national and community-based public health programs, and implementation of activities that advance public health and wellness, as well as provide an avenue through which student earn certificates in immunization delivery and other public health-focused skills" (p. 23).

The latest ACPE 2016 standards incorporates an additional obligation for institutions to administer the NABP's Pharmacy Curriculum Outcomes Assessment® (PCOA®) to assess student proficiency as they complete the didactic portion of their education and prepare to begin the final phase of Advanced Pharmacy Practice Experiences (ACPE, 2015). The social/behavioral/administration sciences section (3.0) of the PCOA® represents 22% of the exam and measures students' understanding of public health and wellness, specifically in the areas of promoting health, preventing both chronic and infectious disease, and recognizing the various factors that affect public health and individual medical care (NAPB, 2016a). This section also measures student comprehension of how health care is delivered in the United States as compared to other industrialized countries.

The 2015 NABP survey of US schools and colleges of pharmacy ranked student competencies in order of importance to the overall curricula based on the number of contact or credit hours, which in turn is the basis of how the test is apportioned (NABP, 2016b). In the survey, schools ranked "health care delivery systems and public health" 11th out of 30 areas of competencies. "Disease prevention and population health" and "population-based care and pharmacoepidemiology" ranked in the bottom third at 21st and 26th place, respectively.

While the ACPE requires accredited institutions to ensure that pharmacy students achieve competencies in public health, the method is left up to the institution. Schools may elect to achieve this through a stand-alone course on public health or to incorporate public health topics into other courses as appropriate (Naughton, Friesner, Scott, Miller, & Albano, 2010). Topics most often cited in the literature were motivational interviewing, behavior modification, particularly with regard to smoking cessation, and educational strategies for prevention and management of chronic diseases (Woodard, McKennon, Danielson, Knuth, & Odegard, 2016).

Methodologies for teaching public health during the first portion of most pharmacy curricula is done through both didactic and active learning activities, such as case studies, problem-based learning, oral presentations, journal club presentations, in-class simulations, and tabletop exercises or opportunities to give educational presentations to specific groups or to participate in wellness centers, free clinics, or medical missions (Bailey & DiPietro Mager, 2016; Dennis et al., 2016; O'Neil & Berdine, 2007; Whitley, 2012). The final year of the PharmD gives students the most cited opportunities to incorporate public health into practice, with hands-on experience of conducting health screenings, providing immunizations, and chronic care counseling (Dennis et al., 2016; Patterson, 2008).

Two areas of public health that seems to be underrepresented in pharmacy curricula at present are emergency preparedness and global health (Accreditation Council for Pharmacy Education, 2015; AACP, 2013; Woodard et al., 2016). Not only are pharmacists in communities and hospitals well positioned to respond to natural disasters, but they are also likely to become aware of potential infectious disease outbreaks. Pharmacists are often included in disaster response preparations and response, yet the necessary skills may not be taught in many schools and colleges of pharmacy.

Similarly, a number of PharmD programs include opportunities for students to experience global health, through either elective courses or medical mission outreach. In their review of the curricula at US institutions, Bailey and DiPietro Mager (2016) found only eight PharmD programs that required global health competencies covering topics such as planning and implementation of medical missions, travel medicine, and global health research and policy development.

DUAL AND CONCURRENT DEGREES

The AACP lists 34 schools offering a combined PharmD and master of public health (MPH) degree in 2016–2017 (AACP, 2015). This represents an increase of 11 institutions over the 23 reported by the 2011–2012 AACP Public Health SIG survey (Gortney et al., 2013). At the time of the survey, one-third of these PharmD/MPH programs had been in existence for less than a year, indicating that there is indeed a growing interest in the United States. Combining a PharmD with a master of science in biomedical or health informatics is less common, with only four institutions listed in the AACP report (ACPE, 2015). In addition, many institutions have specialty certifications or areas of concentration in public health, informatics, medication therapy management, immunization, point-of-care testing, and substance abuse/tobacco cessation. This does not account for individuals who pursue an MPH or health informatics degrees outside of a formal PharmD program.

Dual degrees are available at some institutions combining the PharmD with global health. "Global health" is sometimes used interchangeably with "public health," but institutions offering this program emphasize the unique health issues that face pharmacists working in transnational or international environs. Global health tracks are more commonly available for students pursuing a concurrent MPH.

POSTGRADUATE TRAINING: RESIDENCIES

Licensing requirements for postgraduate continuing education provides avenues for pharmacists to increase their expertise in public health. Options range from continuing education classes to pursuing board certification in a specialty related to public health. Individuals interested in obtaining more formal certification or credentials for advanced practice in public health may do so by participating in advanced training programs in topics such as travel medicine, patient care, or immunization delivery.

PharmD graduates may choose to participate in one- to two-year residency or fellowship programs either as an end in themselves or with the goal of obtaining board certification. ASHP has developed an accreditation program for residencies that matches potential candidates with accredited residencies each year. Residency candidates select from a Postgraduate Year One (PGY1) program, a Postgraduate Year Two (PGY2) program, or a PGY1 and PYG2 combined program. For the residency year beginning in 2016, 1,708 accredited residency programs participated in ASHP's matching program and a total of 3,954 residents were placed into programs (ASHP, 2016a). PGY1 programs are geared toward generalist practice with programs focused on community pharmacy, managed care pharmacy, or pharmacy.

The PGY1 residency program has four required competency areas, but programs may elect to include the elective competency of Health, Wellness, and Emergency Preparedness, which requires residents to "design and delivery programs that contribute to public health efforts" and contribute to "organizational procedures for emergency preparedness" (Commission on Credentialing of the American Society of Health-System Pharmacists, 2014, p. 14). In addition, public health experience may be gained by completing the PGY1 residency at an institution that specializes in public health, such as a public health department or system, or with specific populations, such as in a prison or military hospital. In the second year of residency, programs emphasize specialty practices. Some ASHP-accredited PGY2 residencies include public health as a primary educational outcome, and these are discussed next.

Ambulatory care pharmacy prepares residency graduates to plan and manage the care needs of patients with chronic conditions, disease states, or illnesses that do not require hospitalization. The fourth educational outcome (ASHP, 2006a, p. 13) for the ambulatory care residency program establishes that pharmacists who specialize in ambulatory care will focus on establishing a long-term partnership with the patient to improve health and wellness and work together to prevent disease. Many ambulatory care pharmacy and infectious disease pharmacy residencies offer subspecializations in areas such as HIV/AIDS, chronic hepatitis C treatment, anticoagulation management, diabetes management, and addiction medicine.

As might be expected, public health is of primary importance for pharmacists who specialize in *infectious diseases pharmacy*. The first educational outcome (ASHP, 2006a, p. 3) lists prevention of infectious diseases along with promotion of health improvement and wellness. Specific objectives for this specialty are to "reduce the spread of antibiotic resistance and vaccine preventable disease" (ASHP & Society of Infectious Disease Pharmacists, 2007, p. 1).

Geriatric pharmacy and *pediatric pharmacy* include goals of improving health and wellness, as well as preventing medication-related problems that are unique or more prevalent, among specific age groups (ASHP, 2008; ASHP & Pediatric Pharmacy Advocacy Group, 2016). Four percent of the Pediatric Board exam is devoted to pediatric pharmacists' responsibilities to advocate for "age-appropriate formulations" of medications and participate in public education regarding issues that impact infants, children, and adolescents directly, such as poison prevention and vaccination (Board of Pharmacy Specialties, 2015c).

PGY2 residencies in *pharmacy informatics* do not specify public health outcomes per ASHP. The specialty does have many public health–related implications, such as improving the medication use system, identifying trends, and making interdisciplinary health care decisions possible (ASHP, 2006b; Shapiro, Mostashari, Hripcsak, Soulakis, & Kuperman, 2011).

In addition to the above targeted PGY2 residencies, other ASHP-accredited programs that may include public health training are cardiology, critical care, drug information, emergency medicine, health system pharmacy administration, internal medicine, medication use safety, nuclear medicine, nutrition support, oncology, pain management and palliative care, psychiatric pharmacy, and solid organ transplant (ASHP, 2016b).

POSTGRADUATE TRAINING: BOARD CERTIFICATION

The Board of Pharmacy Specialties offers eight board certifications to pharmacists, most of which involve a public health component. Specialties in ambulatory care or pharmacotherapy require more in-depth knowledge of population and public health topics such as patient education strategies, quality improvement programs, and emergency preparedness (Board of Pharmacy Specialties, 2015a, 2015d), while specialties in pediatric or oncology pharmacy have a smaller public health and advocacy component (Board of Pharmacy Specialties, 2015b, 2015c).

POSTGRADUATE TRAINING: CERTIFICATES AND CONTINUING EDUCATION

Certificate training programs are available for advanced professional training to pharmacists in specific practice areas of delivering medication therapy management services, pharmacy-based cardiovascular disease risk management, pharmacy-based immunization delivery, and patient-centered diabetes care (American Pharmacists Association [APhA], 2016a). Most state licensing boards require practicing pharmacists, as well as student licensees, to have current certification in cardiopulmonary resuscitation or basic cardiac life support prior to administering vaccinations to patients (APhA, 2016b). Basic Life Support for Healthcare Providers training may also be required, depending on state requirements.

Public health-related certificates not specific to pharmacy are available, such as certified diabetes educator or certified asthma educator. These are typically available from the national organization associated with the disease, such as the American Diabetes Association or the National Asthma Education Certification Board.

Career Options in Public Health Pharmacy

All pharmacists are public health pharmacists to some extent, particularly those in community or hospital settings who work directly with patients. However, there are jobs that specifically require public health pharmacists. Within the United States, many positions are part of government programs. Federal opportunities include working in the Veteran's Administration, as military pharmacists, in Indian Health Services, or in one of the health-related federal agencies, such as the Centers for Disease Control and Prevention, the Food and Drug Administration, or the U.S. Agency for International Development. Federally Qualified Health Centers (FQHCs) and departments of health at the state and local levels also have public health pharmacist positions. International agencies, such as the World Health Organization and Doctors without Borders (Médecins San Frontières), look for pharmacists with training and experience in global health pharmacies.

Even without a formal job description in public health, there are other examples of ways for pharmacists to participate in and affect public health. Many public health and community organizations welcome pharmacist representation in their councils, committees, and boards. Due to pharmacists' unique and trusted position in the community, they are often the first line in the surveillance of public health issues. Many pharmacists contribute to public health initiatives by promoting adherence, monitoring for adverse drug effects, and facilitating continuity of care.

The Need for Public Health Education and Training in Pharmacy

Growing opportunities for pharmacists in public health initiatives requires an understanding of the core competencies and public health functions. Facilitating cross-training for all health care providers has been highlighted through approaches such as the Interprofessional Education Collaborative (2016), which provides guidance for students and health care professionals on the development of collaborative approaches to care. Higher education is a pivotal area to develop and model the curricula for future health care providers, as well as utilizing those providers currently in practice to elicit the needed change to improve population health outcomes. The ability to enhance experiences within the health care system combined with health care initiatives available to at-risk communities will improve the judicious allocation of health care spending. Developing strong teams leads to effective programming and interventions that improve overall outcomes and fosters sustainable interventions that prevent disease and promote a culture of health.

The American Public Health Association (APHA), APhA, and ASHP all provide governance through policy statements that specifically address pharmacists' roles in public health. These statements describe the essential contributions of the pharmacist yet the ongoing deficiency is formal recognition as a profession in the public health workforce (APHA, 2014). The unique placement in the community for many pharmacists allows them to serve as the point of entry into the health care system. The growing body of patients needing medications for chronic diseases further requires the education and expertise of pharmacists within the community to provide education for prevention of complications and successful management of their health. In addition, the ability and accessibility of pharmacists to provide screenings facilitates early detection of disease or progression. Understanding the framework of public health programming can enhance the recognition of services needed in a given community or within a target population that integrates the pharmacist in the public health workforce.

Calls for workforce enhancement, relative to pharmacists' roles, are implicated through the practice shift from one of disease management to one that mirrors other health professions in disease prevention. Multiple opportunities exist outside of formal public health organizations, such as FQHCs and departments of health, for pharmacists to address population health issues and community health issues they see in everyday practice. Whether it is working in the capacity of health care planning and program development or through the implementation and surveillance of health care initiatives, pharmacists are uniquely qualified to strengthen the health care system at local, regional, and national levels through innovative and coordinated services (National Center for Chronic Disease Prevention and Health Promotion, 2012). By partnering pharmacists with other providers, as well as their patients, institutional impacts can be made to enhance care and services, improve safety, increase health literacy, and promote successful transitions of patients back into the community setting.

Health care cost containment with cross-trained providers is increasing at the state level in efforts to curb health care spending and optimize patient outcomes. Public health partnerships among clinicians and public health professionals strengthen the workforce and are essential in the wake of shortages of primary care providers. Enhanced education and training of pharmacists and those entering the pharmacy workforce increase the impact of pharmacists in medication management but, more importantly, increase the impact of pharmacists in the development and implementation of health care initiatives targeted for a specific community that foster self-efficacy. Public health initiatives for pharmacists include health optimization or comprehensive management beyond dispensing roles. These initiatives also speak to the evolving workplace and integration of preventive medicine services, which include immunization, chronic disease prevention, smoking cessation, adherence programs to reduce disease progression, and monitoring for adverse effects or unintended side effects of medications (Lai, Trac, & Lovett, 2013).

The development and integration of public health concepts in the pharmacy curricula across the country and increasing numbers of dual degree options through collaborations of pharmacy and public health programs further support the efforts of The APHA, APhA, and ASHP are taking action to prepare pharmacists for the public health workforce.

Leadership

For those pharmacists who wish to develop their leadership skills in public health, there are a number of strategies, including formal programs in pharmacy, leadership programs outside of pharmacy, informal personal development, and work within the APHA. Participating in a formal leadership program provided by one of the pharmacy organizations (e.g., ASHP, American College of Clinical Pharmacy [ACCP], AACP, or APhA) builds leadership skills, develops relationships with like-minded colleagues, and offers credentialing opportunities.

The ASHP provides leadership training through the ASHP Foundation, which is a nonprofit arm of the organization (www.ashpfoundation.org). The ASHP-Pharmacy Leadership Academy provides programming ranging from finance to technology in its leadership training. This organization focuses on acute and ambulatory health care settings and provides a foundation in leadership that could help an individual lead public health change.

The ACCP offers a Leadership and Management Certificate Program in conjunction with its national meetings. The training focuses on the knowledge, skills, and attitudes that will help an individual pursue leadership roles in clinical pharmacy, often in hospital and patient care settings. Much like the ASHP program, this certificate program includes a focus on pharmacy, but, unlike the ASHP, the ACCP provides a credential that helps individuals promote their leadership interests and their commitment to personal development of leadership skills.

The AACP offers the Academic Leadership Fellows Program, a yearlong commitment that develops leaders in pharmacy education (http://www.aacp.org). Fellows receive institutional support with an endorsement from the dean of their program. The focus of the fellowship training is for both general leadership skills and those of special interest to individuals in higher education. While not every individual becomes a college dean or university president, many of these individuals have leadership roles, including roles in public health.

The APhA has a program designed for pharmacy students who are chapter officers in the Academy of Student Pharmacists (APhA-ASP). The APhA-ASP Summer Leadership Institute develops leadership skills with a primary focus in advocacy for the profession. The APhA has additional programs and academies that would be of interest to pharmacists or pharmacy students who want to pursue leadership roles at the national level.

In addition to national professional organizations colleges and schools of pharmacy and private corporations have their own programs that develop leadership skills relevant to public health. Outside of the field of pharmacy, universities and other organizations offer leadership development programs as well, in areas such as health care systems management or not-for-profit organizational leadership. In this case, the individual should consider matching personal goals and interests with those of the program or degree.

Turning directly to public health and APHA, one of the most exciting leadership opportunities exists within the Special Primary Interest Group (SPIG) in Pharmacy. This group of pharmacy-oriented individuals (not all are pharmacists) has generated enough interest to develop a SPIG, with the intention of becoming a member section in the future within the APHA. Sections represent different interest groups within public health and are one of the key ways that the APHA organizes its members to promote public health issues (www.apha.org). Having an official pharmacy section raises awareness of pharmacy issues and promotes pharmacy as an integral part of the health care team. While pharmacists have been involved in other sections of the APHA for decades (the Medical Care section is one good example), now is an ideal time to develop leadership skills in areas directly linked to public health. The APHA also plays a major role in health care advocacy, taking a leadership and advocacy position in health promotion and disease prevention initiatives. The APHA also offers student internships (unpaid) for students interested in learning more about public health.

While there are more formal ways of building leadership skills, many pharmacists have taken the more "informal" way and simply started working in public health areas, trying to improve the health of their communities. At the 2016 APHA meeting, Project IMPACT Immunizations: IMProving America's Communities Together was presented, which was piloted in the state of Washington, supported by the APhA foundation and involving a community pharmacy owner, Kirk Heinz, who was able to improve the health of the members of rural areas by providing vaccinations and working in cooperation with area physicians/health care providers. Leading change does not always require a special degree if one has a will to succeed and help others.

As another example, one of the authors of this chapter (Dr. Garcia) has been able to work as a public health pharmacist without working in a department of health or a formal government entity. She is the Member-At-Large for her state's public health association and has sat as a member of the Board of Directors for three years. She supports collaborations with clinicians when discussing priority issues at the state level of this organization. She works to support education and training programs and to recruit other clinicians to join public health organization efforts despite the fact they do not hold an MPH or work in a formally recognized "public health capacity."

Implications for Public Health and Pharmacy Practice

The emerging importance of public health in pharmacy has many implications for pharmacists, both those already in practice and those who will enter practice in the future. The advances in education and training related to public health in pharmacy are indicative of the skills pharmacists will need to approach complex public health issues in changing practice environments. Shifts have occurred already through the integration of public health–focused programs, such as immunization training in pharmacy schools and immunization delivery in community pharmacies. Although many other roles of the pharmacist, particularly in the community pharmacy setting, remain tied to dispensing, that model is changing. Technology and automation are increasingly integrated into these traditional roles, allowing more time for pharmacists to focus on patient care and other clinical activities.

In a policy statement "The Role of the Pharmacist in Public Health," the APHA (2014) highlights knowledge and skills that pharmacists bring to public health. This document speaks specifically to roles pharmacists can play in essential public health services, public health preparedness, and prevention. National pharmacy organizations, like the APhA and ASHP, also have policy statements relating to the role of pharmacists in public health.

One issue specifically addressed in the APHA policy statement that also represents a major movement within the pharmacy profession is provider status. Currently, pharmacists are not recognized as patient care providers by portions of the Social Security Act and therefore are excluded from participating in Medicare Part B (APhA, 2013). This limits patient care services that pharmacists can provide and bill for reimbursement. Each state regulates pharmacy practice differently, and several states have recognized pharmacists as providers in various capacities (Gebhart, 2016). However, recognition of pharmacists as providers at the federal level is key to advancing the profession as a whole and to promoting further integration of pharmacists into the public health system. Although Congressional committees have proposed bills that would amend the Social Security Act to cover pharmacist services, particularly in medically underserved populations, no such amendments have yet been made (H.R. 592, 2015). Passage of a bill of this nature would recognize pharmacists as providers at the national level and would allow further integration of the profession into the public health workforce.

As the pharmacy profession continues to evolve, trends in this evolution point to an increased role and further opportunities for pharmacists in public health. Pharmacy education now includes specific public health topics and training, pharmacy practice is expanding in both patient care and public health activities, and new career and leadership opportunities for pharmacists in public health are now available. Pharmacists are poised to and should be prepared to become integral parts of the interdisciplinary public health team.

References

Accreditation Council for Pharmacy Education. (2015). *Accreditation standards and key elements for the professional program in pharmacy leading to the doctor of pharmacy degree.* Chicago: Author. Retrieved from https://www.acpe-accredit.org/pdf/Standards2016FINAL.pdf

American Association of Colleges of Pharmacy. (1998). *Center for Excellence in Pharmacy Education (CAPE) educational outcomes.* Alexandria, VA: Author. Retrieved from http://www.aacp.org/resources/education/cape/Documents/CAPE%20Outcomes%20Document%201998.pdf

American Association of Colleges of Pharmacy. (2004). *Center for Excellence in Pharmacy Education (CAPE) educational outcomes.* Alexandria, VA: Author. Retrieved from http://www.aacp.org/resources/education/Documents/CAPE2004.pdf

American Association of Colleges of Pharmacy. (2013). *Center for Excellence in Pharmacy Education (CAPE) educational outcomes.* Alexandria, VA: Author. Retrieved from

American Association of Colleges of Pharmacy. (2015). Table 4: Dual degrees. Alexandria, VA: Author. Retrieved from http://www.aacp.org/resources/student/pharmacyforyou/admissions/admissionrequirements/Documents/Table%204.pdf

American Pharmacists Association. (2013). *The pursuit of provider status: What pharmacists need to know.* Washington, DC: Author. Retrieved from http://www.pharmacist.com/sites/default/files/files/Provider%20Status%20FactSheet_Final.pdf

American Pharmacists Association. (2016a). APhA training programs. Retrieved from http://www.pharmacist.com/apha-training-programs

American Pharmacists Association. (2016b). Frequently asked questions about certificate training programs. Retrieved from http://www.pharmacist.com/frequently-asked-questions-about-certificate-training-programs

American Public Health Association. (2014). *The role of the pharmacist in public health.* Washington, DC: Author. Retrieved from http://www.apha.org/policies-and-advocacy/public-health-policy-statements/policy-database/2014/07/07/13/05/the-role-of-the-pharmacist-in-public-health

American Society of Health-System Pharmacists. (2006a). *Educational outcomes, goals, and objectives for postgraduate year two (PGY2) ambulatory care pharmacy residency programs.* Bethesda, MD: Author. Retrieved from http://www.ashp.org/DocLibrary/Residents/RTP-PGY2-AmCareProgram.pdf

American Society of Health-System Pharmacists. (2006b). *Educational outcomes, goals, and objectives for postgraduate year two (PGY2) pharmacy informatics pharmacy residency programs.* Bethesda, MD: Author. Retrieved from http://www.ashp.org/DocLibrary/Residents/RTP-Informatics.pdf

American Society of Health-System Pharmacists. (2008). *Educational outcomes, goals, and objectives for postgraduate year two (PGY2) pharmacy residencies in geriatrics.* Bethesda, MD: Author. Retrieved from http://www.ashp.org/DocLibrary/Residents/RTP-Geriatric.pdf

American Society of Health-System Pharmacists. (2015). *Model curriculum for pharmacy technician education and training programs.* Bethesda, MD: Author. Retrieved from http://www.ashp.org/DocLibrary/Technicians/Model-Curriculum.pdf

American Society of Health-System Pharmacists. (2016a). PGY2 competency areas, goals and objectives. Retrieved from http://www.ashp.org/menu/Residency/Residency-Program-Directors/PGY2-Competency-Areas-Goals-and-Objectives.aspx

American Society of Health-System Pharmacists. (2016b). Summary results of the match for positions beginning in 2016 combined phase I and phase II. Retrieved from https://www.natmatch.com/ashprmp/stats/2016progstats.html

American Society of Health-System Pharmacists, & Pediatric Pharmacy Advocacy Group. (2016). *Educational outcomes, goals, and objectives for postgraduate year two (PGY2) pediatric pharmacy residencies.* Bethesda, MD: Author. Retrieved from http://www.ashp.org/DocLibrary/Residents/Pediatric-Pharmacy-2016.pdf

American Society of Health-System Pharmacists, & Society of Infectious Disease Pharmacists. (2007). *Educational outcomes, goals, and objectives for postgraduate year two (PGY2) pharmacy residencies in infectious diseases.* Bethesda, MD: Author. Retrieved from http://www.ashp.org/DocLibrary/Residents/RTP-Infectious-Diseases.pdf

Anderson, D. C., Draime, J. A., & Anderson, T. S. (2016). Description and comparison of pharmacy technician training programs in the United States. *Journal of the American Pharmacists Association, 56*(3), 231–236. doi:10.1016/j.japh.2015.11.014

Babb, V. J., & Babb, J. (2003). Pharmacist involvement in Healthy People 2010. *Journal of the American Pharmaceutical Association, 43*(1), 56–60. doi:10.1331/10865800360467051

Bailey, L. C., & DiPietro Mager, N. A. (2016). Global health education in doctor of pharmacy programs. *American Journal of Pharmaceutical Education, 80*(4), Article 71. doi:10.5688/ajpe80471

Board of Pharmacy Specialties. (2015a). *Content outline for the ambulatory care pharmacy certification examination.* Washington, DC: Author. Retrieved from http://www.bpsweb.org/wp-content/uploads/2015/11/content_ambulatory.pdf

Board of Pharmacy Specialties. (2015b). *Content outline for the oncology care pharmacy certification examination.* Washington, DC: Author. Retrieved from http://www.bpsweb.org/wp-content/uploads/2015/11/content_oncology.pdf

Board of Pharmacy Specialties. (2015c). *Content outline for the pediatric pharmacy certification examination.* Washington, DC: Author. Retrieved from http://www.bpsweb.org/wp-content/uploads/2015/11/content_pediatrics.pdf

Board of Pharmacy Specialties. (2015d). *Pharmacy specialist certification content outline/classification system.* Washington, DC: Author. Retrieved from http://www.bpsweb.org/wp-content/uploads/bps-specialties/pharmacotherapy/pharma_fall.pdf

Bureau of Labor Statistics. (2015a). Pharmacist. In Bureau of Labor Statistics (Ed.), *Occupational outlook handbook* (2016–2017 ed.). Washington, DC: U.S. Department of Labor. Retrieved from http://www.bls.gov/ooh/healthcare/pharmacists.htm.

Bureau of Labor Statistics. (2015b). Pharmacy technicians. In Bureau of Labor Statistics (Ed.), *Occupational outlook handbook* (2016–2017 ed.). Washington, DC: U.S. Department of Labor. Retrieved from http://www.bls.gov/ooh/healthcare/pharmacy-technicians.htm.

Calis, K. A., Hutchison, L. C., Elliott, M. E., Ives, T. J., Zillich, A. J., Poirier, T., . . . Raebel, M. A. (2004). Healthy People 2010: Challenges, opportunities, and a call to action for America's pharmacists. *Pharmacotherapy, 24*(9), 1241–1294.

Commission on Credentialing of the American Society of Health-System Pharmacists. (2014). *Elective competency areas, goals, and objectives for postgraduate year one (PGY1) pharmacy residents.* Bethesda, MD: Author. Retrieved from http://www.ashp.org/DocLibrary/Residents/ASO-Elective-Competency-Areas-Goals-and-Objectives.pdf

Dennis, V. C., May, D. W., Kanmaz, T. J., Reidt, S. L., Serres, M. L., & Edwards, H. D. (2016). Pharmacy student learning during advanced pharmacy practice experiences in relation to the CAPE 2013 outcomes. *American Journal of Pharmaceutical Education, 80*(7), Article 127. doi:10.5688/ajpe807127

Gebhart, F. (2016). Provider status: Keep the pressure on lawmakers and push for payment. *Drug Topics, 160*(6). Retrieved from http://drugtopics.modernmedicine.com/drug-topics/news/provider-status

Gibson, M. R. (1972). Public-health education in colleges of pharmacy: I. The background and the problem. *American Journal of Pharmaceutical Education, 36*(2), 180–200.

Gortney, J. S., Seed, S., Borja-Hart, N., Young, V., Woodard, L. J., Nobles-Knight, D., . . . Nash, J. D. (2013). The prevalence and characteristics of dual PharmD/MPH programs offered at US colleges and schools of pharmacy. *American Journal of Pharmaceutical Education, 77*(6), 116. doi:10.5688/ajpe776116

Healthy People Curriculum Task Force. (2015). *Clinical prevention and population health curriculum framework.* Washington, DC: Association for Prevention Teaching and Research. Retrieved from http://c.ymcdn.com/sites/www.aptrweb.org/resource/resmgr/HPCTF_Docs/Revised_CPPH_Framework_2.201.pdf

H.R. 592, 114th Congress (2015). Retrieved from https://www.congress.gov/bill/114th-congress/house-bill/592/text

Interprofessional Education Collaborative. (2016). *Core competencies for interprofessional collaborative practice: 2016 update.* Washington, DC: Author. Retrieved from https://ipecollaborative.org/uploads/IPEC-2016-Updated-Core-Competencies-Report__final_release_.PDF

Lai, E., Trac, L., & Lovett, A. (2013). Expanding the pharmacist's role in public health. *Universal Journal of Public Health, 1*(3), 79–85. doi:10.13189/jph.2013.010306

Lenz, T. L., Monaghan, M. S., & Hetterman, E. A. (2007). Therapeutic lifestyle strategies taught in U.S. pharmacy schools. *Preventing Chronic Disease, 4*(4), A96.

National Association of Boards of Pharmacy. (2016a). *Content areas of the Pharmacy Curriculum Outcomes Assessment® (PCOA®).* Mount Prospect, IL: Author. Retrieved from https://nabp.pharmacy/wp-content/uploads/2016/07/PCOA-Content-Areas-9.6.16.pdf

National Association of Boards of Pharmacy. (2016b). *The 2015 United States schools and colleges of pharmacy curricular survey: Summary report.* Mount Prospect, IL: Author. Retrieved from https://nabp.pharmacy/wp-content/uploads/2016/09/2015-US-Pharmacy-Curricular-Survey-Summary-Report.pdf

National Center for Chronic Disease Prevention and Health Promotion. (2012). *A program guide for public health: Partnering with pharmacists in the prevention and control of chronic diseases.* Atlanta, GA: Centers for Disease Control and Prevention. Retrieved from http://www.cdc.gov/diabetes/pdfs/programs/stateandlocal/emerging_practices-work_with_pharmacists.pdf

Naughton, C. A., Friesner, D., Scott, D., Miller, D., & Albano, C. (2010). Designing a master of public health degree within a department of pharmacy practice. *American Journal of Pharmaceutical Education, 74*(10), Article 186. doi:10.5688/aj7410186

O'Neil, C., & Berdine, H. (2007). Experiential education at a university-based wellness center. *American Journal of Pharmaceutical Education, 71*(3), Article 49. doi:10.5688/aj710349

Patterson, B. Y. (2008). An advanced pharmacy practice experience in public health. *American Journal of Pharmaceutical Education, 72*(5), Article 125. doi:10.5688/aj7205125

Shapiro, J. S., Mostashari, F., Hripcsak, G., Soulakis, N., & Kuperman, G. (2011). Using health information exchange to improve public health. *American Journal of Public Health, 101*(4), 616–623. doi:10.2105/ajph.2008.158980

Whitley, H. P. (2012). Active-learning diabetes simulation in an advanced pharmacy practice experience to develop patient empathy. *American Journal of Pharmaceutical Education, 76*(10), Article 203. doi:10.5688/ajpe7610203

Woodard, L. J., McKennon, S., Danielson, J., Knuth, J., & Odegard, P. (2016). An elective course to train student pharmacists to deliver a community-based group diabetes prevention program. *American Journal of Pharmaceutical Education, 80*(6), Article 106. doi:10.5688/ajpe806106

Index